MATERNITY AND REPRODUCTIVE HEALTH *in Asian Societies*

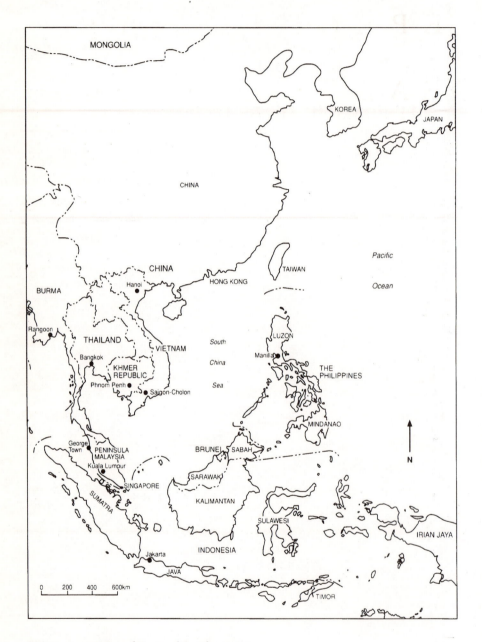

FRONTISPIECE: Map of East and Southeast Asia

MATERNITY AND

REPRODUCTIVE

HEALTH *in Asian Societies*

edited by

PRANEE LIAMPUTTONG RICE

*Centre for the Study of Mothers' and Children's Health
and School of Sociology and Anthropology
La Trobe University
Melbourne, Australia*

and

LENORE MANDERSON

*Australian Centre for International and Tropical
Health and Nutrition
University of Queensland
Brisbane, Australia*

hdap
harwood academic publishers
Australia Canada China France Germany India Japan Luxembourg Malaysia
The Netherlands Russia Singapore Switzerland Thailand United Kingdom

COPYRIGHT © 1996 by OPA (Overseas Publishers Association) Amsterdam B.V.
Published in the Netherlands by Harwood Academic Publishers GmbH.

Emmaplein 5
1075 AW Amsterdam
The Netherlands

British Library Cataloguing in Publication Data

Maternity and Reproductive Health in Asian Societies
    1.Motherhood – Asia, Southeastern 2.Human reproduction – Asia, Southeastern
    3.Obstetrics – Asia, Southeastern 4.Hygiene, Sexual – Asia, Southeastern
    I.Rice, Pranee Liamputtong II.Manderson, Lenore
    612.6'0095

    ISBN 90-5702-021-1

Cover: Village in Lombok
Photograph: Jocelyn Grace

Contents

v

List of Illustrations

List of Tables

Acknowledgments

Over the years, many people have provided us with inspiration and assistance in what has been, for us both, an enduring interest in women's bodies, women's health, and in birth, reproduction and sexuality.

The production of this book, however, has more immediate debts. Our thanks extend to the publisher for continued support and for bringing the project to life. We thank the Centre for the Study of Mothers' and Children's Health, La Trobe University, and the Australian Centre for International and Tropical Health and Nutrition, The University of Queensland, for institutional and practical support. We are very grateful to Tanya Mark for her thoroughness, enthusiasm and tenacity in checking bibliographic entries and locating source material, and to John Richter for his meticulous proof-reading and word processing assistance.

Pranee Rice adds the following: I wish to extend my deep gratitude to my mother, Yindee Liamputtong, and to my five sisters, whose life experiences are part of the personal context of this book. I also wish to extend my thanks to my two daughters, Zoe Sanipreeya Rice and Emma Inturatana Rice, whose births prompted me to study women's birthing experiences and reproductive health, who have always been patient with my busy schedule, and who have appreciated my work greatly.

Lenore adds: I want to thank my mother, Mardi Manderson, for inspiring me in many different ways, and for all that is implied in a book on motherhood. And I thank my children, Toby and Kerith, for the rich personal meanings they have given me of reproduction and of mothering.

Pranee Liamputtong Rice
Lenore Manderson

Introduction

Pranee Liamputtong Rice and Lenore Manderson

In the past decade or so, a number of publications have brought together ethnographic accounts of birth and reproduction. Brigitte Jordan's work (1978) is one of the first comprehensive comparative studies, written relatively recently, that draws attention to the diverse ways of managing birth and nurturing the new mother in different social and cultural settings — Yucatan, Sweden, the United States and the Netherlands. Subsequent anthologies by Kay (1982), MacCormack (1982) and Michaelson (1988), among others, highlight women's experiences of pregnancy, childbirth, the postpartum and the days of early mothering, and draw attention to the degree to which these events of reproduction are cultural and social as much as they are biological. They highlight too the extraordinary variability across cultures of the roles played by others — kinswomen, husbands, children, traditional birth attendants — in the management and care of the new mother and the unborn/newborn child.

Works such as these highlight the importance of reproduction to women with respect to their personal identity and social status, and in terms of the ways in which their lives have centred around events of biology. For women in pre-industrial societies, early marriage and lack of means of birth control has meant that the cycles of conception, pregnancy, birth, and lactation have dominated their adult lives. Women's work has therefore been structured around the home, their labour spent in activities which allowed them to combine infant and child care, food production, and income generation.

Everywhere, the accessibility and use of effective contraceptive technology has had major impact on women's lives, shifting women's roles away from those primarily associated with mothering, and enabling them to play a greater role as productive workers in a working environment separate from domestic life. Pregnancy and birth have been transformed from recurrent events that absorb much of women's adult lives, to rarer but no less important occasions. Significantly, the frequency of reproduction does not appear to correlate with its positive cultural evaluation, and birth remains a critical life event in the lives of women everywhere, regardless of social formation, family structure, or their other activities and roles.

Concern with ensuring the health (and survival) of the mother and child are evident in the various rituals that are observed throughout pregnancy and following delivery in all cultures. In nation states, this concern has parallel expression in the medicalisation of reproduction. Over the past century, women and children have been increasingly subject to health programs designed to reduce maternal and infant mortality, which emphasise ante-natal care, supervision of birth and the regulation of

1

midwifery, and the monitoring of early infant care and feeding (Davin, 1978; Lewis, 1980; Manderson, 1992, 1996). These programs focus on women's role as mother and the presumed links between different ways of mothering and the health of infants. The maternal and child health programs that exist today, including those described in this volume, share this long history: in former colonial states such as Indonesia, the Philippines and Malaya, colonial governments established antenatal clinics and home visiting to monitor indigenous women and to encourage the management of birth and infancy along the lines of contemporary medical views.

Pregnancy and birth are emphasised — culturally, in health programs, and in the scholarly literature — at the expense of other aspects of reproductive and sexual health, and by bringing them together we hope to widen our understanding of the workings of women's bodies. A relatively small literature exists on non-reproductive aspects of women's bodies and women's health. There are, for example, a few anthropology and history collections concerned with infant care and breastfeeding (e.g. Hull and Simpson, 1985; Fildes, Marks and Marland, 1992), and a number of articles on menstruation and menopause (Skultan, 1972; Flint, 1974; Snow and Johnson, 1977, 1978; Chu, 1980) which explore this particularity of women's experience. In Emily Martin's book (1992), menstruation, reproduction and menopause are treated together, as logical contrasting surfaces of the one phenomenon. Yet surprisingly, this approach is rare, and more commonly, menstruation, menopause, lactation, and particularly sexual health problems and functions, ordinary discharges, reproductive tract infections, and women's care of their own bodies, are unspoken. The silence which maintains discretion and privacy is one which also controls, and the dominance of medical understandings of women's bodies reinforces this control, creating an illusion of discharges as abnormal; sexual dysfunction as aberrant; blood and other exudations as dirty and polluting; fertility, infertility, and the end of fertility mysterious and frightening. In this process, women's health is jeopardised. Women resist from reporting and seeking care for sexual health problems, for example, out of embarrassment and for fear that any abnormality will be interpreted as social aberrance, physical symptoms of disease as evidence of breaches in propriety. Frequently, women themselves assume that changes in bleeding, discharge, and so on, are evidence of immorality, perversion or sin; negative constructions of women's bodies are always internalised. Lack of education about reproductive and sexual health maintains the silence and hence the discomforts that women experience. Concern with these silences, and the confinement of understandings and interest in women's bodies to reproduction, has lead Jacobsen (1991:5) to write of a "widespread and deepening — but largely neglected — crisis", and to draw attention to what continues to be the limited improvement of women's health globally, despite the focus on reproductive health issues within primary health care programs.

We have noted above that women's reproductive success determines their social status, the roles they play in a given society, and indirectly, the control they can exercise over their own lives and those of their children, and their continued well-being. Women's status — a broad term which we use here to include their economic standing and the power they are able to exert domestically and publically

— affects their access to property and resources, but also their access to health care, their access to information that influences treatment seeking behaviour in the event of illness, choices about whether and when to have a child or children, and their ability to control their own bodies.

Women's reproductive and sexual health is of particular interest in terms of preventive health, not just because of the cost to individual women of poor health, but because of its wider social costs. Women's health has an economic value, since ill health affects women's ability to work and so their productivity; although the nature of their work too may cause ill health. Similarly reproduction may both compromise and be compromised by women's health status: that is, women's ability to conceive and carry to term is impaired by ill health (e.g. anaemia), and conversely, women's lack of control of reproduction (e.g. frequent pregnancies) may result in ill health. Women's health is also important because of their position as custodians of family health. Women are carers and nurturers within the household, responsible for the everyday health and care of other members of the family, by producing food, cooking, and so on, and by ministering to the ill (see Koblinsky, Timyan and Gay, 1993; Leslie, 1992a; Rathgeber and Vlassoff, 1993).

The focus on reproductive health has reinforced a supposition that reproductive health and women's health are synonymous, and typically, "women's health" has been understood to refer to pregnancy, childbirth and contraception, leading to interventions such as safe motherhood and family planning programs. But as a consequence of this, there has been continued neglect of other aspects of women's health, including the way in which gender influences the risk of most if not all infections. All health problems are affected by gender, since morbidity and mortality rates reflect not so much sex differences in the biology of disease, but the mediation of disease through cultural and social circumstances. Being female or male affects the risk of infection, the social experience of illness, and care and outcome, resulting in what Ojanuga and Gilbert refer to as the "significant disparities" that exist between women and men (1992:613; see also MacCormack, 1988, 1992; Fitzpatrick and Manderson, 1989; Leslie, 1992b; Rathgeber and Vlassoff, 1993; Vlassoff and Bonilla, 1994).

The conflation of women's health and reproductive health restricts and ignores the complexity of gender. Still gender issues constellate around issues of reproduction and sexual health, as the papers in this volume illustrate. Hence the focus in this volume on the most conventional aspects of being female — aspects which, because of their cultural and personal significance, are also profoundly meaningful to women.

THE MANAGEMENT OF PREGNANCY AND BIRTH

Reproduction is not a solely biological affair, but rather "is socially constructed and formed by political and economic processes" (Browner and Sargent, 1990:228). Pregnancy and birth are culturally patterned, and women's knowledge, beliefs and behaviours are shaped in this context (Cosminsky, 1982). But pregnancy is also a "natural" state, normal rather than pathological, one which needs supervision but usually not medical care. This may explain why women are often reluctant to attend antenatal care and have a poor comprehension of its purposes, and why campaigns for regular prenatal attendance in order to reduce infant and maternal mortality have not been entirely successful (MacCormack, 1982; see also papers by Cabigon, Grace, and Hunter, this volume). As Jirojwong (this volume) demonstrates with respect to southern Thailand, women seek prenatal care primarily if they believe that their health and/or that of the foetus is compromised, although their decision to attend is further confounded by problems of access to care (transport, finances, childcare) and other circumstances. Further, even in industrialized countries where literacy is high and information concerning pregnancy and birth is readily available, women seek antenatal care for reassurance in the majority of cases, rather than medical care (e.g. in Britain, see Homans, 1982; in Australia see Crouch and Manderson, 1993a; Brown, Small, Lumley and Atsbury, 1994), and attendance at antenatal clinics has ritual rather than clinical significance for such women (Crouch and Manderson, 1993b).

Women are typically encouraged by family members to observe various rules to ensure their health and safety, successful conception and viability of the pregnancy, an easy delivery, and a healthy child. Local understandings of the nature of conception and the development of a child underpin these rules. In Japan, conception and birth were influenced in the past by belief in the cyclical nature of birth/death/rebirth, and belief in the arbitrariness of conception. This contrasts with modern beliefs in the intentionality of the individual, which emphasise the role of the individual in deciding to become pregnant, to carry to term, and to deliver successfully (see Nakayama, this volume). This latter belief system is clearly more in sympathy with practices of contraception, reproductive technology, and the medical management of pregnancy and birth. Jirojwong (this volume) also describes various traditional beliefs relating to pregnancy and delivery, in Thai communities influenced in part by Buddhist beliefs concerning the cyclic nature of birth/rebirth and the importance of *karma* in influencing birth outcome. To the extent that karma influences pregnancy outcome, medical intervention is considered to have little effect. Again, Symonds (this volume) argues that issues of birth, death, and the social system are inextricably linked to Hmong views of the cosmos, whereby the world is divided into that of the living and that of the spirits, with the "souls" of the dead re-entering the world of the living through appropriation of the body of a newborn infant.

Women traditionally have given birth at home where they have had control over their own bodies, and where childbirth and delivery have been an affair of women — the parturient woman, her female kin, and midwives. In her study of childbirth among peasant women in the Yucatan Peninsula of Mexico, for example, Jordan (1978) argues that home birth provides women with support in a time of crisis because of the extensive assistance of female relatives, neighbours and the traditional midwife. The process of home birth also fits with cultural understandings of female modesty, and minimises medical procedures which may often be regarded as unnecessary and frightening. Townsend and Rice, Symonds, Grace, Hunter, and others (this volume) describe contexts where home births are still usual. Home birth remains a preferred option for most women because of their dislike and fear of hospitals, the importance of the traditions that might only be followed in the home, and the continuity of care offered by a midwife (Jordan, 1978; Manderson, 1981; Kay, 1982; MacCormack, 1982; Rice, 1993, 1994a).

Birth has increasingly moved from a familial and social domain to that of hospital-based medicine, for many an alien institutional setting and knowledge base. Oakley (1975) for the UK, Shorter (1984) for the USA, and others, have documented the transition of the control of birth from midwife to doctor, and the increasing medicalisation of birth that has been part of this process in industrialised countries from the late 19th century. In most industrialised countries, pregnancy and childbirth are seen as a diseased state, a physical bodily disturbance (Cosminsky, 1982:225); the woman's body is the subject of control by medical professionals and technology (Davis-Floyd, 1987; Michaelson, 1988; Martin, 1992). A woman is required not only to give birth in hospital where she may have little or no control, but she is also given the message, as Davis-Floyd (1987:479) points out, about her powerlessness, "defectiveness", and her dependence on science and technology. This shift in understanding of birth, and the care of the pregnant and parturient woman, is arguably even more alien in non-Western states, where obstetric definitions of pregnancy and birth as "unnatural events of illness" are diametrically opposed to indigenous understandings of birth as natural and normal.

The appropriation of childbirth by medicine ignores women's own beliefs and the social and cultural meanings of childbirth, or rather, medicine declares such beliefs ill-informed, ignorant or irrelevant. Contemporary health systems emphasise instead the importance of machines and institutions over the woman's body, reflected within the labour ward where the midwife's hands are replaced by foetal monitors and forceps. However, government policy in many countries has supported traditional birthing to some degree, since hospital systems would be unable to meet the demand if all women were to seek hospital deliveries. Hence the emphasis in current policy on antenatal care as a mechanism of surveillance, by which to identify women at risk of complication and to encourage those women, primarily, to give birth in hospitals (Clark, Ketteritzsch and Mills, 1993; Begum, Seguerra and Hasan, 1994; Grace, Hunter, this volume). The various policies relating to antenatal care and monitoring suggest the ways in which this has been translated in contemporary Asian societies.

TRADITIONAL MIDWIVES

A report of the World Health Organization in 1978 (cited in Helman, 1990) indicated that worldwide, two-thirds of babies are delivered by traditional midwives, and as we already note, still the majority of woman give birth with the assistance of traditional birth attendants or other, non-specialist, older women and female kin. Serving as a medical and ritual specialist, the traditional midwife plays a vital role in managing the woman's body during childbirth, and in many cases, providing continued care from early pregnancy through the early months of the newborn's life. In Guatemalan society, as described by Cosminsky (1982), the midwife is responsible for ensuring conception, maintaining the pregnancy, caring for the pregnant woman and preparing her body for birth, and supervising labour and delivery. Postpartum, the midwife's role is even greater in ensuring the woman's recovery and future health. In India, the *dai*'s work in supervising childbirth involves not only the "polluting" work of cutting the umbilical cord, disposing of the placenta, and cleaning up the birth blood and clothes (McGilvray, 1982; McConville, 1988; Islam, 1989), but she also massages the woman, cooks for her family, cleans and washes the house, and takes part in "bathing" and "stepping out" ceremonies (Jeffery, Jeffery and Lyon, 1989). Laderman's (1983) description of Trengganu midwifery and Paton's (1988) work in Central Java provide further examples from Asia of the important role that older women play in providing health care and social support for the pregnant, parturient and newly delivered mother. These findings echo the representation of the traditional midwife's role as "an expanded role, part of a support system that includes social, ritual and psychological components" in the care of childbearing women (Cosminsky, 1982).

The midwife's status varies in different cultures, and is closely linked with general attitudes towards women, their bodies, and bodily functions. Where menstrual and childbirth blood are seen as polluting, the midwife's status may be rather low. In the Indian sub-continent, for example, the *dai* has low status — as the above reference to pollution suggests. In contrast, Malay *bidan* do not have particularly low status, but rather, are reverred as professionals who enjoy especial skills and knowledge. As Laderman (1983:150–1) describes, the *bidan* nurtures the woman throughout pregnancy and takes charge of various ritual and ceremonial activities, supervises labour and helps the mother to deliver; if labour is prolonged, she might intervene by offering "hot" medicine to drink, or massaging the abdomen, and will massage again to help expel the placenta. While the *bidan* is a key player, control remains with the labouring woman. Her role is neither predetermined nor usurped by the midwife even in the event of a difficult labour or a problematic delivery (Laderman, 1983:172). Balinese women healers also enjoy considerable status, although they are denied access to some of the more prestigious ritual roles (Connor, 1983); and in Cambodia, the *chmop* (traditional midwife) also has high status (Townsend and Rice, this volume).

The discussions of conception, pregnancy, birth and the postpartum in many of the chapters in this volume further illustrate the important roles played by the traditional birth attendant, and the very different functions — and relationships between individuals — of antenatal clinics, labour wards, and infant health centres. As some of the chapters illustrate (e.g. Jirojwong, Cabigon, and Townsend and Rice), women use government services primarily because of perceived practical advantages. Lack of fully trained staff and services mean, however, that the traditional birth attendant remains a key person in village births throughout much of Asia, and today as in the past many women receive antenatal care from them and deliver with their assistance in preference to government medical services. It is in recognition of this, as well as the lack of alternatives, that the World Health Organization has supported their further training and aimed to integrate them into health programs in developing countries. Townsend and Rice (this volume) describe the role of traditional midwives working at the Maternal and Child Health Centres in Site 2 Refugee Camp in Thailand, all of whom have basic training in modern obstetric care. Grace (this volume) also portrays the work of traditional midwives, provided with additional biomedical training by the Indonesian Government in recognition of their social and ritual importance as well as their established community role in the maintenance of women's health.

BODILY SUBSTANCES: MENSTRUATION AND MENOPAUSE

In many societies, parts of the woman's body, as well as bodily products, are regarded as "ritually polluting and unclean" (Ahern, 1975:193), and these body parts have the power to inflict harm. Women's sexual organs and their emissions are regarded as particularly powerful and dangerous. Hence the rules that pertain in various Asian countries regarding the separation of women's and men's garments, as well as the importance of the positioning of the bodies of women and of men, and women's ability to exploit these fears of pollution at times to their own advantage (e.g. Spiro, 1977).

Beliefs about menstrual blood provide a good example of this. Snow and Johnson (1977, 1978) point out that menstruation in some cultures is seen to function to cleanse the "impurities" of the body, in which context the retention or cessation of the flow of blood is a sign of pathology, leading, for example, to the blood rotting in the uterus and eventually turning into cancer. This belief in the cleansing function of menstruation is by no means confined culturally; Chu (1980) documents the same belief among Chinese women in Taiwan, as do Chirawatkul and Manderson (1994) for northeast Thailand. There are of course variations in these beliefs, and in the way in which menstruation is managed. Blood may be polluting, strength-giving, strength-depleting, sexually enhancing, purifying, health-giving or -taking. Chirawatkul (this volume), for example, argues that cultural beliefs of blood influence women's interpretation of health and illness, and also influence women's practices with regard to menstruation, childbirth, and menopause. In menstruation, the beliefs affect women's choice of self-care and ways to absorb and dispose of menstrual blood; in childbirth and menopause too, beliefs of blood influence women's practices to maintain "good health" (Chirawatkul and Manderson, 1994; see also Jennaway and Whittaker, this volume).

Blood from menstruation and childbirth is often regarded as immensely powerful (Douglas, 1966; Ahern, 1975). Due to the perceived potential of women to cause harm through pollution which might be effected by contact with blood, women may be banned from certain activities when they are in an "unclean" and "dangerous" state. A menstruating woman or a woman who has just given birth in Taiwan, for example, is not allowed to worship the gods (Ahern, 1975). While menstrual blood may be regarded as dirty and polluting, it is also commonly considered powerful because of its association with procreation: it "creates flesh and bones" of the foetus. Lochia (childbirth blood) is the "residue of the creation process", hence it is also powerful and endangers others. In this context, Kang-Wang (1980) recalls that when she was pregnant and a midwife in a birth station in Taiwan, older women rejected her not only as a midwife responsible for delivering the babies of their daughters-in-law, but were also displeased that she was present in the birthing room.

Attitudes towards menopause need to be understood in the context of understandings of reproduction. In most societies, procreation is a woman's greatest achievement and the means by which she gains some power; at times, it may be the only means by which she has any authority. The birth of a first child is critical since it alters a woman's status within the family, ensuring the continuity of the lineage. Women gain status when they bear children, or secure their personal status within their husband's lineage because of their success in producing a child from their own body (Kang-Wang, 1980; Rice, 1995; Jennaway, this volume).

Yet in precisely these societies where importance is placed on reproduction, so women gain authority and autonomy with ageing. Menopause is a universal event in the lives of all women. But Lock's (1982, 1986, 1991) research on menopause highlights the social meanings attached to this event. Menopause, like other reproductive health events, is also a social and cultural event, in which the physiological changes associated with the climacteric are only part of the experience and ascribed meaning. Woman's social status, sex roles, personal circumstances, life history and state of health influence their experiences of the menopause and their position in society post-menopausally.

Kaufert (1976) argues that these factors in turn affect the symptomatology of menopause. A number of studies indicate differences cross-culturally in the perception and reports of signs and symptoms of menopause. An example is hot flushes, which is very commonly regarded as a sign of menopause in western cultures. Yet in some cultures, there are no reports of hot flushes; elsewhere, hot flushes are reported but not as commonly as other physiological changes (Flint, 1974, 1975; Beyene, 1986; Lock, 1986; Chaiphibalsaridhi, 1990; Chirawatkul and Manderson, 1994). This difference may relate to biological differences among women, but may also relate to differences in the significance accorded to various bodily signs and symptoms.

Hence menopause is constituted both by biological changes and events, and by beliefs, attitudes and values that inform a woman's life cycle and her roles over its course. While factors such as diet, general health, and use of contraceptives may affect the production and equilibrium of hormones in a woman's body (Beyene, 1986), cultural factors such as status acquisition and the removal of taboos, or alternatively, loss of status and cultural devaluation, play an important role in how women perceive menopause (Flint, 1974, 1975; Brown, 1982, 1985). Cross-cultural data are limited but suggest that in general the experience of menopause is conditioned by the cultural context that shapes the pattern of a woman's role, and this in turn is subject to the effects of industrialisation and urbanisation. Menopause offers to many women a range of economic, political, social, and personal opportunities denied to them during their reproductive years, and is therefore a welcomed event. Rice's paper (this volume), for example, illustrates that for Hmong women, menopause is regarded unproblematically as part of growing old. Although having many children is highly valued, women do not see menopause negatively since they have already borne many children and ensured the continuity of their lineage. Chirawatkul, however, indicates that widespread changes in farming and patterns of everyday life have led villagers to perceive illness and diseases rather differently than in the past, and an increasing acceptance of health care, while resulting in clear improvements in maternal, infant and child health, has also had the effect of medicalising other health states. In this context, menopause is increasingly shifting from being regarded as a natural condition of older women, to one of a deficiency illness.

SEXUAL HEALTH

Increasing attention has been given to reproductive and sexual health in recent years (Jacobson, 1991; Gray and Underwood, 1991; Cook, 1993; Abernethy, 1994) as a consequence of a number of political, economic and public health concerns: high population growth and continued high fertility, women's continuing poor health — particularly maternal mortality despite several decades of maternal and child health programs, and increased concern about reproductive tract infections (RTIs), cancer of the reproductive system, and HIV infection. Reproductive tract infections (RTIs) and sexually-transmitted diseases are increasingly being recognised as a widespread health problem. These infections cause not only pain and discomfort, but may result in marital disruption, social stigma, and a range of serious and potentially fatal health consequences including infertility, ectopic pregnancy, miscarriage and stillbirth, increased risk of HIV infection, and cervical cancer. Despite their prevalence and consequences, they remain largely invisible due, Dixon-Mueller and Wasserheit (1991) argue, to taboos associated with such infections, and a belief among many that such symptoms are part of the price of being female. It is widely held that women should endure symptoms such as vaginal discharge, discomfort during intercourse and chronic abdominal pain, along with other reproductive health problems such as menstrual difficulties, side effects of contraception, miscarriages, and stillbirths (Dixon-Mueller and Wasserheit, 1991:11). The intense focus on AIDS has arguably obscured reproductive tract infections (Jacobson, 1991), and in Southeast and East Asia, as elsewhere, the development of approaches to the prevention, diagnosis and treatment of reproductive tract infections remains at an early stage. Traditional herbal remedies exist for these illnesses, attesting to their prevalence, but women often do not seek clinical treatment because of fear or embarrassment, and because such infections are often regarded as something women should bear as a natural part of "being a woman". Hence "a culture of silence" pertains in many parts of the world.

Our knowledge of the distribution of reproductive tract infections is limited because of women's reluctance to present for diagnosis or treatment health problems that include genital or urinary involvement. Women will often disguise symptoms such as swollen labia, swelling in the groin, and pain for fear that these are signs of sexually transmitted diseases, or because of fear of disapproval of others, including health workers as well as kin. Strong taboos also prevent many women from gaining familiarity with their bodies, to detect signs of disease and to differentiate the source of blood, and not all women notice minor bleeding. Further, many women suffering from reproductive and urinary health problems are reluctant to report possible infections to others — such as mothers-in-law — who hold both power and the economic resources that might enable treatment to occur. Studies including ones conducted in rural India (Bang, Bang, Baitule, Choudhary, Sarmukaddam, *et al.*, 1989) and Indonesia (Hull, Widyantoro and Fetters, this volume) draw attention to this. Poor care or lack of appropriate care, as documented by Whittaker (this volume), also influence women's decisions to seek help even where they perceive irregularity or signs of disease.

Improved understanding of ethnogynaecology and the cultural construction of sexual health will provide an important step in developing programs to encourage women to recognise and seek treatment. In her study of local understandings of common gynaecological conditions in a remote rural village community in northeastern Thailand, Whittaker (this volume) indicates that there is a rich indigenous understanding of women's health. Women's descriptions and narratives are invested with complex meanings concerning their fertility, and reveal the links between women's health and the changing socio-economic context of their lives. A number of gynaecological complaints are identified by the women. Vaginal discharges are of great concern and are viewed negatively as signs of lack of uterine cleanliness and ill-health. They are treated with both traditional humoral medicine and cosmopolitan medicine. Older women also commonly suffer from uterine prolapse, a health problem that has been virtually ignored outside of the gynecological literature.

A contemporary growing interest in reproductive tract infections and sexually transmitted diseases relates to the association between STD and risk of HIV infection. As of mid-1994, 2.5 million people in Asia were estimated to be infected with HIV, and proportionately more women and more poor people are among those with HIV infection and AIDS (Over and Piot, 1990). At the time of writing, the largest numbers of people known to be affected in Asia are in India, Burma and Thailand. Of these countries, knowledge of the epidemiology and social risk factors of infection, and experience of intervention programs, is best in Thailand. The government of Thailand estimates that by 2000, between two and four million Thais will be infected with HIV, and surveys in the early 1990s indicated that around 50–60 percent of commercial sex workers and injecting drug users were already infected (Weniger, Khanchit Limpakarnjanarate, Kumnuan Ungchusak *et al.*, 1991; Thailand, Ministry of Public Health, 1992). The rapid spread of HIV infection in Thailand has resulted, in the space of a few years, in dramatic changes, including the rise of indigenous NGOs to develop and deliver preventive health education and care interventions (Cohen, 1988).

Limited testing indicates that HIV already also has a foothold in the Lao People's Democratic Republic, an impoverished, land-locked country in the hub of Southeast Asia. Prevention programs are undermined by poverty and lack of infrastructure, and are compounded for Lao women by social and cultural factors which limit their capacity to protect themselves from infection. These are elaborated in Savage's chapter (this volume), which examines the risks of HIV infection to urban, ethnic Lao women in the Lao PDR, and the implications for planning and implementing AIDS prevention strategies. HIV transmission is linked with women and their culturally unacceptable, "uncharacteristic" or "immoral" behaviour. Obstacles to preventive behaviour are compounded by other factors, including financial considerations. Such factors pertain elsewhere in the region where there are similar changes effected through the opening of borders, expanding economic opportunities, improved transport, and the increased circular migration of people (e.g. in Northeast Thailand, see Lyttleton, 1994; in Burma, see Porter, forthcoming).

HEALTH SERVICES, CHOICES AND CONSTRAINTS

In many parts of the developing world, family planning programs were initiated to improve health and reduce population growth. However, these programs have failed to improve reproductive health. At one level, this is largely due to the fact that the programs have been too limited to meet women's varied needs. However, at a political level, it is, as Jacobson (1991:39) argues, due to "the limited mandate under which programs operate and the equally limited criteria by which they gauge success. In practice, deepening concerns about population growth and its potential to undermine development efforts result in a heavier emphasis on fertility control than health". In Bangladesh, for example, the government has only recently introduced "more secure" contraceptive methods to the women. These methods include mainly intra-uterine devices (IUDs) and tubal ligation (sterilisation) to reduce birth rates, with little regard for women's reproductive health or personal desires. It remains true that broader contraceptive choice, management of contraceptive side effects, and continuity and effectiveness of contraceptive practice have received little emphasis (Germain, 1987:20).

Despite government attempts, programs face a number of resource constraints. Many women have difficulties attending clinics due to the traditions of "seclusion" which limit their movement outside the home, or because of difficulties in taking time off from work, childcare and household responsibilities. At the national level, countries face limitations of "infrastructure, transport, logistical systems and personnel" (Germain, 1987:20).

A prime goal of government programs is to reduce the birth rate. State health policy in Indonesia identifies women as primary recipients of national health services only insofar as they have reproductive potential; and family planning and the concept of "family" are part of a state ideology in relation to population control rather than women's reproductive health. Hunter (this volume) describes the links between the state, women's voluntary organisations, and village practices, as these exist in an East Lombok rural mountain village. Here, services are provided through the *posyandu* (the integrated village health service post).

In North Bali, women's reproductive health is again closely monitored (Jennaway, this volume). Mass contraception, particularly the IUD, has been vigorously promoted through nationwide education campaigns conducted through the mass media as well as by community health clinics. Indigenous political structures have been enlisted to achieve initial contraceptive compliance and encourage birth spacing aimed at limiting ultimate family size. However, as Jennaway describes, individual women are not entirely compliant, and may use maternal health services instrumentally to achieve sexual and reproductive goals of their own.

Above, we have referred at a number of points to women's variable use of health services, whether for pregnancy care, the treatment of reproductive tract infections, or the provision of family planning advice. While the major problem in much of the developing world remains a lack of services, it is also apparent that where services for reproduction and sexual health are available, women are often reluctant to use them. What can account for this?

Grace (this volume) describes the use made by Indonesian women in many rural communities of both traditional and modern practitioners and treatment. However an examination of their preferences for contraception, pre-natal care and assistance during birthing indicate a relatively low level of acceptance of government (modern) health services. Grace argues that a kind of pluralism has evolved, which, rather than being planned, is the result of uneven access to government health services. The health department is in fact antagonistic toward traditional practitioners, and aims eventually to convert villagers from seeking their services to using only those offered by the government. But poverty, lack of formal education, and inadequate dissemination of information about health matters and the formal services available, and the value that women place on traditional midwifery practice, means that many women continue to seek treatment only from those practitioners they know, trust, can afford, and to whom they have easy access.

Antenatal care is not utilised if women do not see its relevance or if it is too far from home, as Jirojwong (this volume) found in Southern Thailand. Long distances to health services, sometimes made worse by poor roads, lack of public transport, and its costs, prevent women from receiving prenatal care.

Quality of care is another important factor for women's decision to or not to seek care. The lack of emotional support and privacy, and differences in languages, social class, and cultural expectations between women clients and health professionals, explain women's lack of use of services in many places (see Clark, Ketteritzsch and Mills, 1993; Begum, Seguerra and Hasan, 1994), and use of services would appear to be higher where there is little social or cultural difference between clients and providers. In Site 2 Refugee Camp, traditional birth attendants were the main care givers for Cambodian women in Maternal and Child Health (MCH) Centres (Townsend and Rice, this volume). These midwives share social and cultural norms with their clients and provide emotional and physical support throughout pregnancy and childbirth, resulting in their greater use by women. But in addition to women's appreciation of the value of antenatal care to ensure safe pregnancy and delivery, in this case the women also sought care to secure a "pass" to ensure that they would receive a food portion for the infant after she/he is born; without this legitimate "pass", they would not be able to get food for their child. Symonds provides a similar example of the pragmatic benefits of the use of health services in her chapter.

In addition, health services are used where they are perceived to be relevant to women's needs, although women's needs may not be consistent with medical understandings of birth and delivery. Further, traditional and modern practices of childbearing are not always in opposition to each other; rather, new technologies and approaches are incorporated into traditional understandings and practices. For example, Muecke (1976) illustrates the use of a heat lamp by women in Northern Thailand to replace traditional means of "roasting" and heating (Manderson, 1981), and Rice (1994b) similarly describes Hmong and Vietnamese women who have settled in Australia, who use electric heaters to regain heat lost in childbirth, as they are no longer be able to practice "mother-roasting" (see also Sargent, Marcucci and Elliston, 1983). Chu (this volume) points to the popular use of "sitting the month" centres among Taiwanese women. Due to rapid social changes in Taiwan, including the decrease of extended families and increase of nuclear households, the traditional "sitting the month" ritual, as described by Pillsbury (1978), has become difficult for women to observe. The emerging of "sitting the month" centres enables women to continue to do so. As McClain (1982:25) argues, women have attempted to "preserve valued traditional beliefs and practices even as they accept innovations in birth location and management" in response to social and cultural changes.

CONCLUSION

The chapters in this volume represent some of the research currently being conducted in the areas of reproduction and sexual health in East and Southeast Asia. The cover they offer is only partial, of course, but it reflects the interest in placing women's health in a social context, and in linking aspects of women's physical health with cultural understandings of gender, sexuality and the feminine body. We have argued that women's health has largely centred around pregnancy and birth, both in discussion and programmatically. This derives, at least in part, from the tremendous social and personal importance given to reproduction, as much as to any state interest in maternal or infant mortality. Beyond pregnancy and birth, with the exception of family planning programs, women's reproductive and sexual health has received little serious attention, and women's health consequently remains poor (Jacobson 1991:57).

In general, "women's health" has been conflated with issues of maternal and infant mortality, foetal outcome, and fertility control, and these associations are maintained in various government health programs. Other health problems which women experience are self-treated or ignored, since they are considered as minor irritants only, not sufficient to prevent them from undertaking their usual tasks. Health care provided at the primary level (at rural health posts, midwifery centres, and so on), which includes a means to elicit information about women's general health when providing treatment for specific reported problems, may help address difficulties relating to reluctance to report. But the ability of a health worker to undertake this task, as well as other duties, is problematic where the health worker is already inundated with a variety of clinical and administrative duties, and where improved services for women may require additional training and support. Means need to be found to streamline primary health worker duties to maximise their effectiveness without simply adding new tasks.

In most Asian countries, social and cultural changes have occurred rapidly. These changes have, in turn, affected women's reproduction and sexual health, and childbirth in most developing countries is increasingly under the control of western trained health professionals (McClain, 1982). The chapters in this volume explore the tensions that exist as states in Asia modernise and industrialise, in which context women's bodies are often situated between tradition and modern medicine, the midwife and the doctor, and home therapist and government health service.

This book is organised in the following manner. The first four chapters, grouped together as "Birth and its inflections", explore folk and medical understandings of reproduction, ideational and institutional settings of birth, and the changes that have occurred with the evolution of health care systems. Nakayama's paper focuses on the significance of a linguistic shift in speaking of conception and pregnancy — from *sazu-kara* (conception through the volition of the gods) to *tsuku-ru* (human acts of intentionality) — that has occurred with changes in economy and technology across Japanese society. Jennaway's paper explores understandings of fertility and reproductive health in a North Balinese village, and she provides a rich ethnographic description of reproduction and sexuality in Bali. Jirojwong (for southern Thailand) and Cabigon (for the Philippines) examine women's health beliefs and understandings of pregnancy and birth, and the way in which these influence their use of antenatal services set up to monitor reproduction and to improve pregnancy "outcome", in ways that are not always consistent with women's own needs and desires.

In Part II, "From her womb ...", we focus specifically on pregnancy and birth, and offer a number of different accounts of reproduction: Symonds on Hmong women, Townsend and Rice on Cambodian women in a refugee camp in Thailand, Grace on antenatal, birthing and postpartum care in rural East Lombok, Chu on provisions for the postpartum in contemporary Taiwan, and Hunter on maternal and child health in a Sasak village, also in Lombok, Indonesia. In Part III, we turn our attention to other aspects of women's reproductive and sexual health, and include chapters on ethnogynaecology in northeast Thailand (Whittaker), reproductive tract infections in Indonesia (Hull, Widyantoro and Fetters), menopause among Isan (northern Thai) and Hmong women (chapters by Chirawatkul and Rice), and finally and importantly, a paper addressing HIV and AIDS (Savage). This final chapter implicitly, we hope, underlines the value of the volume. We will not be able to develop or introduce interventions that will effectively prevent the transmission of HIV, or provide women with safe means of controlling their fertility, or address other health problems, until we are able to discuss reproductive and sexual health in ways that extend beyond pregnancy and birth and that appreciate the social and cultural significance of these events.

The chapters in this volume share several common themes. First, most chapters are based on ethnographic inquiries which utilise participant observation and interviews, and all authors describe societies in which we have lived for extended periods of time. As a result, the chapters offer insights into women's points of view, in ways that are not possible through the objective distancing of survey-based research. At the same time, all authors are women and we write our chapters from this particular subject status (Roberts, 1981). Many of us also write of our own cultures, and these are very much chapters from "insider" perspectives. They are not the only ways to speak of women's experiences. But they open a window into those experiences even so, inviting the reader to learn more about women in Asia, the role of reproduction in their lives, the rhythms of the life cycle, the rituals of pregnancy, birth and confinement, and the changes and disorders of the body.

REFERENCES

Abernethy, V. (1994) Population and women's health. *Healthcare Forum Journal*, January-February, 30–34.

Ahern, E.M. (1975) The power and pollution of Chinese women. In *Women in Chinese Society*, edited by M. Wolf and R. Witke, pp. 193–214. Stanford: Stanford University Press.

Bang, R.A., Bang, A.T., Baitule, M., Choudhary, Y., Sarmukaddam, S., *et al.* (1989) High prevalence of gynecological diseases in rural Indian women. *The Lancet*, 1, 85–87.

Begum, K., Seguerra, J., Hasan, I. (1994) *Birthing Choices: A Perspective from Southern Thailand*. Unpublished MTH report, Brisbane: Tropical Health Program, The University of Queensland.

Beyene, Y. (1986) Cultural significance and physiological manifestations of menopause: a biocultural analysis. *Culture, Medicine and Psychiatry*, 10, 47–71.

Brown, J.K. (1982) Cross-cultural perspectives on middle aged women. *Current Anthropology*, 23, 143–154.

Brown, J.K. (1985) Introduction. In *In Her Prime: A New View of Middle-Aged Women*, edited by J.K. Brown and V. Kerns, pp. 1–12. South Hadley, MA: Bergin & Harvey.

Brown, S., Small, R., Lumley, J., Atsbury, L. (1994) *Missing Voices: The Experience of Motherhood*. Melbourne: Oxford University Press.

Browner, C.H., Sargent, C.F. (1990) Anthropology and studies of human reproduction. In *Medical Anthropology, Theory and Practice*, edited by T.M. Johnson and C.F. Sargent, pp. 215–229. New York: Greenwood Press.

Chaiphibalsarisdi, P. (1990) *Self-care Responses of Rural Thai Perimenopausal Women*. Unpublished PhD thesis, Chicago: University of Illinois.

Chirawatkul, S., Manderson, L. (1994) Perceptions of menopause in Northeast Thailand: contested meaning and practice. *Social Science and Medicine*, 39(11), 1545–1554.

Chu, C.M.Y. (1980) Menstrual beliefs and practices of Chinese women. *Journal of American Folklore*, 100, 479–495.

Clark, L.A., Ketteritzsch, K., Mills, G. (1993) *Malay childbirth: Determinants of choice in Bachok, Kelantan*. Unpublished MTH report, Brisbane: Tropical Health Program, The University of Queensland.

Cohen, E. (1988) Tourism and AIDS in Thailand. *Annals of Tourism Research*, 15, 467–486.

Connor, L.H. (1983) Healing as women's work in Bali. In *Women's Work and Women's Roles: Economics and Everyday Life in Indonesia, Malaysia and Singapore*, edited by

L. Manderson, pp. 53–72. Southeast Asian Monograph Series No 32. Canberra: Development Studies Centre, Australian National University.

Cook, R.J. (1993) International human rights and women's reproductive health. *Studies in Family Planning*, **24**, 73–86.

Cosminsky, S. (1982) Childbirth and change: a Guatemalan study. In *Ethnography of fertility and birth*, edited by C.P. MacCormack, pp. 205–229. London: Academic Press.

Crouch, M., Manderson, L. (1993a) *New Motherhood: Personal and Cultural Transitions in the 1980s*. Chur: Harwood Academic Press.

Crouch, M., Manderson, L. (1993b) Parturition as social metaphor. *The Australia and New Zealand Journal of Sociology*, **29**, 1–18.

Davin, A. (1978) Imperialism and motherhood. *History Workshop*, **5**, 9–66.

Davis-Floyd, R.E. (1987) The technological model of birth. *Journal of American Folklore*, **100**, 479–495.

Dixon-Mueller, R., Wasserheit, J. (1991) *The Culture of Silence: Reproductive Tract Infections among Women in the Third World*. New York: International Women's Health Coalition.

Douglas, M. (1966) *Purity and Danger*. London: Routledge and Kegan Paul.

Fildes, V., Marks, L., Marland, H. (editors) (1992) *Women and Children First: International Maternal and Infant Welfare 1870–1950*. London: Routledge.

Fitzpatrick, J., Manderson, L. (1989) Women, health and development in Southeast Asia and the Pacific: an overview. In *Women's Health, Women's Development*, edited by J. Browett, pp. 7–28. Centre for Development Studies Conference Paper Series No 6. Bedford Park: Flinders University of South Australia.

Flint, M. (1974) *Menarche and Menopause of Rajput Women*. Unpublished PhD thesis. New York: Department of Anthropology, City University of New York.

Flint, M. (1975) The menopause: reward or punishment. *Psychosomatic*, **XVI**, 161–163.

Germain, A. (1987) *Reproductive Health and Dignity: Choices by Third World Women*. New York: The Population Council.

Gray, J., Underwood, Y. (1991) *Women in Danger: A Call for Action*. Washington, DC: National Council for International Health.

Helman, C.G. (1990) *Culture, Health and Illness: An Introduction for Health Professionals*, 2nd edn, Oxford: Butterworth Heinemann.

Homans, H. (1982) Pregnancy and birth as rites of passage for two groups of women in Britain. In *Ethnography of Fertility and Birth*, edited by C.P. MacCormack, pp. 231–268. London: Academic Press.

Hull, V., Simpson, M. (editors) (1985) *Breastfeeding, Child Health and Child Spacing: Cross-cultural Perspectives*. London: Croom Helm.

Islam, S. (1989) Rural women and childbirth in Bangladesh: the social cultural context. In *Gender and the Household Domain: Social and Cultural Dimensions*, edited by M. Krishnaraj and K. Chanana, pp. 233–254. New Delhi: Sage Publications.

Jacobson, J.L. (1991) *Women's Reproductive Health: The Silent Emergency*. Worldwatch Paper 102. Washington, DC: Worldwatch Institute.

Jeffery, P., Jeffery, R., Lyon, A. (1989) *Labour Pains and Labour Power: Women and Childbearing in India*. London: Zed Books.

Jordan, B. (1978) *Birth in Four Cultures*. Montreal: Eden Press.

Kang-Wang, J.F. (1980) The midwife in Taiwan: an alternative model for maternity care. *Human Organization*, **39**, 70–79.

Kaufert, P.A. (1982) Myth and the menopause. *Sociology of Health and Illness*, **4**, 141–166.

Kay, M.A. (1982) Writing an ethnography of birth. In *Anthropology of Human Birth*, edited by M.A. Kay, pp. 1–24. Philadelphia: F.A. Davis Company.

Kitzinger, S. (1982) The social context of birth: some comparisons between childbirth in Jamaica and Britain. In *Ethnography of Fertility and Birth*, edited by C.P. MacCormack, pp. 181–203. London: Academic Press.

Koblinsky, M., Timyan, J., Gay, J. (editors) (1993) *The Health of Women. A Global Perspective.* Boulder: Westview Press.

Laderman, C. (1983) *Wives and Midwives: Childbirth and Nutrition in Rural Malaysia.* Berkeley: The University of California Press.

Leslie, J. (1992a) Women's lives and women's health: using social science research to promote better health for women. *Journal of Women's Health*, **1**(4), 307–318.

Leslie, J. (1992b) Women's time and the use of health services. *IDS Bulletin*, **23**, 1, 4–7.

Lewis, J. (1980) *The Politics of Motherhood: Child and Maternal Welfare in England, 1900–1939.* London: Croom Helm.

Lock, M. (1982) Models and practice in medicine: menopause as a syndrome or life transition? *Culture, Medicine and Psychiatry*, **6**, 261–280.

Lock, M. (1986) Ambiguities of aging: Japanese experience and perceptions of menopause. *Culture, Medicine and Psychiatry*, **10**, 23–46.

Lock, M. (1991) Contested meanings of the menopause. *The Lancet*, **337**, 1270–1272.

Lyttleton, C. (1994) Knowledge and meaning: the AIDS education campaign in rural northeast Thailand. *Social Science and Medicine*, **38**, 135–146.

McClain, C. (1982) Toward a comparative framework for the study of childbirth: a review of the literature. In *Anthropology of Human Birth*, edited by M.A. Kay, pp. 25–59. Philadelphia: F.A. Davis Company.

McConville, F. (1988) The birth attendant in Bangladesh. In *The Midwife Challenge*, edited by S. Kitzinger, pp. 134–153. London: Pandora.

MacCormack, C.P. (1982) Biological, cultural and social adaptation in human fertility and birth: a synthesis. In *Ethnography of Fertility and Birth*, edited by C.P. MacCormack, pp. 1–23. London: Academic Press.

MacCormack, C. (1988) Health and the social power of women. *Social Science and Medicine*, **26**, 677–684.

MacCormack, C. (1992) Planning and evaluating women's participation in primary health care. *Social Science and Medicine*, **35**(6), 831–837.

McGilvray, D.B. (1982) Sexual power and fertility in Sri Lanka: Batticaloa Tamils and Moors. In *Ethnography of Fertility and Birth*, edited by C.P. MacCormack, pp. 25–74. London: Academic Press.

Manderson, L. (1981) Roasting, smoking and dieting in response to birth: Malay confinement in cross-cultural perspective. *Social Science and Medicine*, **15B**, 509–520.

Manderson, L. (1992) Maternal and child health in colonial Malaya. In *Women and Children First: International Maternal and Infant Welfare 1870–1950*, edited by V. Fildes, L. Marks and H. Marland, pp. 164–177. London: Routledge.

Manderson, L. (1996) *Sickness and the State. Health and Illness in Colonial Malaya, 1870–1940.* Cambridge and Melbourne: Cambridge University Press.

Martin, E. (1992) *The Woman in the Body.* Boston: Beacon Press.

Michaelson, K. (editor) (1988) *Birth in America: Anthropological Perspectives.* South Hadley, Mass.: Bergin and Garvey.

Muecke, M. (1976) Health care system as socializing agent: childbearing the North Thai and Western way. *Social Science and Medicine*, **10**, 377–383.

Oakley, A. (1975) Wisewoman and medicine man: changes in the management of childbirth. In *The Rights and Wrongs of Women*, edited by J. Mitchell and A. Oakley, pp. 17–58. Harmondsworth: Penguin Books.

Ojanuga, D.N., Gilbert, C. (1992) Women's access to health care in developing countries. *Social Science and Medicine*, **35**(4), 613–617.

Over, M., Piot, P. (1990) HIV infection and other sexually transmitted diseases. *International Planned Parenthood Federation Medical Bulletin*, **24**, 6.

Paton, V.A. (1988) *Mbah Cipta's Gift. Healing in a Central Javanese Village*. Unpublished PhD thesis, Nedlands: Department of Anthropology, University of Western Australia.

Pillsbury, B. (1982) Doing the month: confinement and convalescence of Chinese women after childbirth. In *Anthropology of Human Birth*, edited by M. Kay, pp. 119–146. Philadelphia: F.A. Davis Company.

Porter, D. (Forthcoming) A plague on the borders: HIV, development, and travelling identities in the Golden Triangle. In *Sites of Desires/Economies of Pleasure. Sexualities in Asia and the Pacific*, edited by L. Manderson and M. Jolly. Chicago: University of Chicago Press.

Rathgeber, E.M., Vlassoff, C. (1993) Gender and tropical diseases: new research focus. *Social Science and Medicine*, **37**(4), 513–520.

Rice, P.L. (1993) *My Forty Days*. Melbourne: The Vietnamese Antenatal/Postnatal Support Project.

Rice, P.L. (1994a) Childbirth and health: cultural beliefs and practices among Cambodian women. In *Asian Mothers, Australian Birth*, edited by P.L. Rice, pp. 47–60. Melbourne: Ausmed Publications.

Rice, P.L. (1994b) When I had my baby here! In *Asian Mothers, Australian Birth*, edited by P.L. Rice, pp. 117–134. Melbourne: Ausmed Publications.

Rice, P.L. (1995) *Cultural Reaction to Motherhood: Fertility and Infertility in Hmong Women*. Unpublished paper presented at the Workshop on Southeast Asian Women, Monash University, Melbourne, 14 July.

Roberts, H. (editor) (1981) *Doing Feminist Research*. London: Routledge and Kegan Paul.

Sargent, C., Marcucci, J., Elliston, E. (1983) Tiger bones, fire and wine: Maternity care in a Kampuchean refugee community. *Medical Anthropology*, 7, 67–79.

Shorter, E. (1984) *A History of Women's Bodies*. Harmondsworth: Penguin Books.

Snow, L.F., Johnson, S.M. (1977) Modern day menstrual folklore; some clinical implications. *JAMA*, **237**, 2736–2739.

Snow, L.F., Johnson, S.M. (1978) Myths about menstruation: victims of our own folklore. *International Journal of Women's Studies*, **1**, 64–72.

Spiro, M. (1977) *Kinship and Marriage in Burma. A Cultural and Psychodynamic Analysis*. Berkeley: University of California Press.

Thailand, Ministry of Public Health (1992) *Summary of the Survey on HIV Infection in Dec 1991*. Unpublished mimeograph. Bangkok: Ministry of Public Health.

Vlassoff, C., Bonilla, E. (1994) Gender-related differences in the impact of tropical diseases on women: what do we know? *Journal of Biosocial Sciences*, **26**, 37–53.

Weniger, B.G., Khanchit Limpakarnjanarate, Kumnuan Ungchusak, *et al.* (1991) The epidemiology of HIV infection and AIDS in Thailand. *AIDS*, **5**(Supp. 2), S71–S85.

PART I:

BIRTH AND ITS INFLECTIONS

CHAPTER 1

Japanese Women's Views on Having Children: The Concepts of *Sazu-Karu* and *Tsuku-Ru*

Makiko Nakayama

On 26 July 1978, the evening editions of Japan's major newspapers reported on the front page that a British medical team had succeeded in delivering the world's first test-tube baby, named Louise Brown, through *in vitro* fertilisation. In response to the successful implementation of this reproductive technology, the editorial of the *Asahi Shimbun* commented on the following day that the long-held belief that babies are gifts from gods, or *sazu-kari-mono* in Japanese, was shattered; babies are now something we can do away with or "make" at will — *tsuku-ru* in Japanese.

In reporting news on reproductive technology, the mass media always raises the question of whether babies are something given or made. The opinion at the time of birth of the first "test-tube baby" was that the idea of *sazu-karu* (to be given children by a supernatural being) had been replaced so that children had now become "something that we are free to make or destroy as we please" (leader from *Asahi Shimbun*, 27 July 1978). Similarly, when the medical team at Tohoku University succeeded in delivering the first Japanese *in vitro* baby in 1983, and again in 1986 when experimental research by Keio University showed that a child's sex could be engineered to a very high rate of success using the Parcole method,[1] the question "Are we entitled to make children?" was invariably raised as counter to the belief that "by nature children are bestowed from above [by a supernatural being]". At such times, the concepts of *tsuku-ru* and *sazu-karu* are positioned antithetically, symbolising respectively "activity" and "passivity" of the actions and perceptions involved in having children. This is reflected in articles about parents who have had "their own child" after successful fertilisation, who joyfully assert that the child was *sazu-kari-mono* (given from the supernatural being). A diachronic analysis of these key terms will be given below.

With this background, what does having children mean to the Japanese, especially in terms of the birth of a new life? How do they conceptualise it? How are the two crucial expressions, *sazu-karu* and *tsuku-ru*, to be related to the views of the Japanese? Have the opinions of the Japanese public on having children changed as a result of the recent rapid advances in reproductive technology? This chapter addresses these hitherto unexplored questions.

In the first section of this paper, I summarise the views Japanese people held in the past on life and childbirth, based on a database compiled by Japanese folklorists in

21

the 1930s. In the second section, I present how Japanese women who bore babies in the 1980s conceptualised their first pregnancies, focusing on the two words, *sazu-karu* and *tsuku-ru*; I use a series of interviews I conducted to illustrate my point. In the last section, I discuss the historical changes in cognition of Japanese women and men, triggered by advances in reproductive technologies and the pervasive clinical application of those technologies; I compare the trends before and after the 1980s when the views about getting pregnant, giving birth and having babies, presented by Japanese folkloric literature, had begun to fade (Nakayama, 1995).

FINDINGS OF JAPANESE FOLKLORISTS IN THE 1930s

Japanese Views on Life-cycle in Terms of "Rites of Passage"

The views on life cycle held by ordinary Japanese who lived between the mid-19th century and the 1930s are best shown in the studies by Japanese folklorists pioneered by Kunio Yanagita (1875–1962).[2] In the 1930s, a nationwide survey was conducted which collected lexicons used to express various customs and folk beliefs of the Japanese, mainly of rice paddy farmers who composed the majority of the population at that time. Local informants were interviewed to elicit what their grandparents and parents used to say and what they themselves used to do in their childhood (Imperial Gift Foundation of Boshi-Aiiku-Kai, 1975).[3]

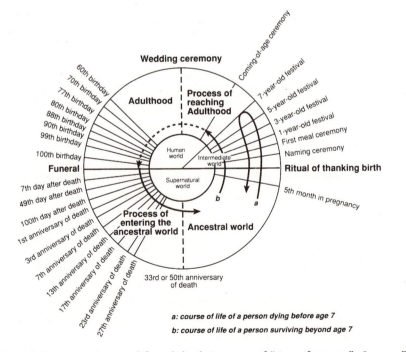

FIGURE 1.1 Japanese views on life and death in terms of "rites of passage". Source: Tsuboi (1984).

One of Yanagita's disciples, Hirofumi Tsuboi (1984:173), represented the life cycle of the Japanese in this period schematically, as set out in Figure 1.1. I have modified Tsuboi's original diagram where appropriate. There are two possible courses of life as indicated by the two arrows 'a' and 'b'. People believed that a baby was born from the ancestral world, and reaches adulthood after passing through various rites of passage. The baby is regarded as *sazu-kari-mono* (gift) from the gods or supernatural beings, and would temporarily stay in the human world as a godlike being until the age of seven, which marked a watershed in the life cycle of the Japanese. The soul of a baby or child who died before it reached the age of seven was returned to the ancestral world by the hands of its family members, in the hope that the baby would be reborn as another child (arrow 'a').

A child surviving beyond age seven would experience the coming-of-age ceremony, a wedding ceremony, and several special birthdays in old age. After death, a person's soul was believed to begin a journey in the supernatural world to the ancestral world, and eventual rebirth, while the descendants observed rituals to promote a smooth journey after death (arrow 'b').

In summary, the human soul travels cyclically between the supernatural world and the human world, directed by gods and the supernatural beings but not by human beings.

Having Children: Expressions and Folk Techniques

I analysed expressions describing people's experiences of having children from the database on customs and folk beliefs concerning childbirth and childcare (Imperial Gift Foundation of Boshi-Aiiku-Kai, 1975). Among 16 verbs, *ninshin-suru* (to get pregnant) was most widely and most frequently used; *sazu-karu* (be given by the superior) ranked second, followed by *deki-ru* (to conceive). No example of *tsuku-ru* ("make" as human conduct) was found.

I wish to examine more closely three words, *sazu-keru*, *sazu-karu*, and *sazu-kari-mono*. *Sazu-keru* originally meant that the superior, in this case gods or supernatural beings, gives something to the inferior, in this case human beings, while *sazu-karu* means to be given something by the superior being. The noun, *sazu-kari-mono*, meant a gift given as a result of *sazu-karu* (see Phase A in Figure 1.3). To illustrate this, in a comical essay, *Ukiyo-buro* (conversations of people at public baths in Edo) by Shikitei Sanba, published between 1812 and 1823, an old woman wishing to have a grandchild laments of her helplessness that she just has to wait since "a child is *sazu-kari-mono*" (Shikitei, 1989:96).

The concepts of *sazu-keru*, *-karu*, *-kari-mono* existed in the early 19th century (Hara and Wagatsuma, 1974), and were functioning in the minds of the Japanese in the 1970s and 1980s when the mass media like *Asahi Shimbun* was commenting on new reproductive technology (see Phase B in Figure 1.3). The messages in the 1970s and 1980s were generally positive toward *sazu-keru*, *-karu*, *-kari-mono*, while negative toward *tsuku-ru*. In this context, it was generally held that women should accept the arrival of babies and the subsequent "duties" of childbearing.

Two means of conceiving and carrying a child existed, magical and folk health techniques:

(1) praying to gods or some greater power (e.g. going to Shinto altars, praying to a *jizo* stone, Buddha [guardian deity of children], to deities that enshrine cedar trees, to the male phallus, small ball-shaped stones, etc.)

(2) adopting a child in order to conceive a child oneself

(3) stepping over a placenta or sitting on the place where a placenta has been buried

(4) sharing the luck of puerperal women (wearing a pregnant woman's girdle, sleeping in the bed of a woman who has given birth, eating food left over by a woman who has given birth, eating with her cutlery, etc.)

(5) other forms of charm or magic (sleeping with a doll or Buddhist statue, or husband and wife eating rice-cakes, eggs, plums, etc. together)

(6) attention to the woman's body, mainly methods of warming the body or keeping it from getting cold, such as healing treatment at spa baths, burning moxa on the skin, etc.

As can be seen, what is common to all but the last contrivances is that they are methods that rely on magical or spiritual forces. Such contrivances are extensive on Honshu, Kyushu and Shikoku (see Figure 1.2). In contrast, health techniques are less often described, and no description is found in regard to the act of intercourse, other sexual conduct, or the manipulation of concrete reproductive technology.

WOMEN TALKING ABOUT CHILDBIRTH IN THE 1980s

Now let us move to the present. The Japanese economy has passed through a period of high-level growth since the Pacific War, and by the 1970s/80s had arrived at a period of stable growth. The employment and economic structure of Japanese society has changed dramatically, and various aspects of our lives (e.g. work, education, family) have gone through some astonishing changes. There has been a dramatic decline in infant mortality and maternal mortality rates, a shift from home births to hospital births, improvements in medical care for childbirth, alternative birthing movements, and many other transformations. In terms of the number of children born, there is, following the peak of the post-war baby boom, now a pronounced trend towards fewer births and fewer children. According to a survey by the Japanese Ministry of Health and Welfare, the total fertility rate in Japan was 1.75 in 1980 and 1.53 in 1990.

Under these dramatic changes, do the concepts of circulation and regeneration, as well as the beliefs in the supernatural world, continue to exist in the minds of Japanese?

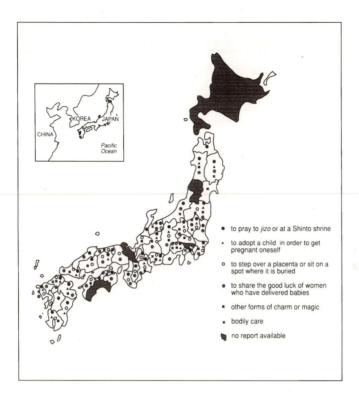

FIGURE 1.2   Techniques for having a child in Japan, c. 1930.

Women's Views on their Pregnancies

From 1987 to 1990, I conducted semi-formal interviews with 15 Japanese women who gave birth to their first baby in the 1980s, whose attributes are given in Table 1.1. From this data, I have analysed how informants expressed their feelings when they were first informed of their pregnancy, and how they conceptualised their experiences of pregnancy (Nakayama 1991, 1992). Below I cite several examples along with my interpretations.

Yoko (informant no. 11) works as an architect. She espouses a simple lif and her main diet consists of wild rice and fresh produce. Just before turning 30, she made her final decision to have a child of her own. She said:

> I deliberately *tsuku-tta* [past tense of *tsuku-ru*] it [a child]. It's within my control. It's not that I was *sazu-katta* [past tense of *sazu-karu*] by others. A baby is sort of durable goods. It's something we enjoy for leisure... I feared I might change my mind when it is too late to have one. It's all for myself. I desperately wanted to have fun raising a child. It's like, sort of buying something really expensive, like purchasing my own house. You are the one to make a choice. It's perfectly all right not to have children.

Yoko commits herself to the concept of *tsuku-ru* and uses the term to claim that she was the one to select the course of life. Thus she chose to *tsuku-ru* a baby.

Satoko (informant no. 10) was told by her doctor, immediately after her retirement from work before marriage, that she would have difficulty with conception. However she got pregnant seven months after her marriage. She said:

> It's true that I *tsuku-tta* my first baby, but it's something beyond that. I must admit the feeling of *sazu-karu* co-existed within myself. I might say in between: partly *sazu-karu*, partly *tsuku-ru*. Even though the feeling of *tsuku-ru* predominates in myself, I cannot use the word *tsuku-ru* because it sounds unethical. You know, it has to do with sex and the feeling of *tsuku-ru* appears to devalue precious human life.

Satoko states that although the word *tsuku-ru* more precisely expresses her inner feelings and her actions involving pregnancy, she hesitates to use the term in discussing ethical issues. To explain her feelings, she uses another term instead — *sazu-karu* — which in her opinion is free from sacrilegious connotations.

Keiko (informant no. 15) and her husband both wanted a child, and although they made plans and took steps to conceive, they were worried that they might not be able to.

> We both thought that if we couldn't have our own child, we would be happy with someone else's [by adoption]. We both felt that our own child would be a gift *sazu-kari-mono*, you see.

Both say that they were worried that they were infertile and might not be able to have children. In such a context, a child born to them is perceived as being a gift, a *sazu-kari-mono*. Yuko (informant no. 4) did not want to get pregnant for the first year of marriage:

> When I got pregnant [against my wish], everybody was telling me *sazu-kari-mono* [it was a godsend]. They'd say I should see it *sazu-katta* [past tense of *sazu-karu*]. And I'd think, "What? *Sazu-karu*? Where's the blessing in that? How dare they say such a thing to me!" When I look back on it now, that word makes me feel uncomfortable more than anything. At the time it sounded repulsive. But, well, now I can be honest with myself and I view a child as *sazu-katta*.

In this case, the word *sazu-karu* serves to give comfort, encouragement, and ease to a woman disappointed at the fact of her unwanted pregnancy, while others make the woman conceptualise her pregnancy as *sazu-karu* or the woman herself conceptualises it thus.

Sakiko (informant no. 13) took steps for three years after getting married, to improve her health and physical strength before planning her pregnancy.

> Well yes, *tsuku-ru*, it was like we were making the child. It shows you are actively involved, you know. Active involvement. The idea of *sazu-karu* [a child as a godsend], in contrast, is somehow passive. The word sounds passive, doesn't it? It seems to mean that you somehow are irresponsible for your own doings. It is you who *tsuku-ru*.

TABLE 1.1 Individual attributes of informants.

Informant	Year of birth	Age of Husband[1]	Year of Marriage	Year of birth of first child	Place of delivery	Educational record*		Occupation*		Domicile[2],*
						Informant	Husband	Informant	Husband	
1	1962	0	1987	1989	Private obstetric clinic	University	University (incomplete)	None	Company employee	RAN(Ur)
2	1962	+2	1987	1988	General hospital	University	University	Private school teacher	Private school teacher	RAN(To)
3	1962	+5	1984	1988	Private obstetric clinic	Senior high school	University	Food market employee	Company employee	RPN(Ma)
4	1961	0	1989	1990	General hospital	University	University	None	Company employee	RAN(Ka)
5	1960	+3	1987	1990	General hospital[†]	University	University	Uni. office staff[#]	Company employee	CAN(To)
6	1958	0	1984	1987	General hospital	M.A. (incomplete)	University	None	Company employee	OAN(Ta)
7	1958	–1	1985	1988	General hospital[3],[†]	M.A.	University	University teacher[#]	Company	CAN(To)
8	1957	+1	1984	1987	Christian obstetric clinic[4]	Senior high school	University	None	Company employee	RAN(To)

TABLE 1.1 Continued.

Informant	Year of birth	Age of Husband[1]	Year of Marriage	Year of birth of first child	Place of delivery	Educational record*		Occupation*		Domicile[2,*]
						Informant	Husband	Informant	Husband	
9	1956	+1	1986	1988	Christian obstetric clinic[4]	University	University	None	Company employee	OAN(To)
10	1956	+3	1982	1984	University hospital	University	M.A.	None	Company employee	OAN(To)
11	1956	0	1983	1987	General hospital[4,†]	Junior college	University	Architect	Architect	RIN(To)
12	1956	+10	1983	1984	University hospital	University	University	None	Company employee	RAN(Ni)
13	1956	+10	1979	1982	Private hospital[5]	M.A.	University	University research	Company employee	OIG(Ur)
14	1953	0	1982	1983	General hospital	Junior college	University	None	Civil servant	OAN(To)
15	1949	+2	1987	1988	Private obstetric hospital[6]	M.A.	M.A.	None	University lecturer	RAN(To)

[1] Compared to informants.
[2] R = Rent; C = Company accommodation; O = Own house; A = Apartment; P = Public housing; I = Individual house with garden; N = Nuclear family; G = Three generation stem family; (Ur) = Urawa; (To) = Tokyo; (Ma) = Matsudo; (Ka) = Kashiwa; (Ta) = Takatsuki; (Ni) = Nishinomiya.
[3] Japan Red Cross affiliated.
[4] Japan Obstetrics Association late first childbirth (over the age of 30).
[5] Obstetrics and psychiatry department. [6] World Health Organization late first childbirth (over the age of 35).
* At start of research; † Previous miscarriage; # Part time.

Women like Sakiko, who interpret the word *sazu-karu* as defined in dictionaries, tend to dislike the passive meaning attributed to *sazu-karu*, and thus emphasise that their pregnancy is the result of their *tsuku-ru* action.

Analysis of Two Key Words

Below, I summarise my analysis of conversations with those women who spoke of their experiences of conception and birth (see Phase C, Figure 1.3).

Firstly, women who conceived and gave birth in the 1980s frequently used the expression of *tsuku-ru* when they spoke to me. Here the expression of *tsuku-ru* had the sense of "paying attention to the whole sequence of events [such as the intention, planning, performance, and action] leading to pregnancy, and perceptions based on a factual awareness of these events". In this respect, these women's notions of agency are not dissimilar to those of women in other industrialised countries, where all aspects of conception, pregnancy and labor are represented as controllable (see e.g. Michaelson 1988; Crouch and Manderson, 1993a, 1993b).

Secondly, it was extremely rare for these women to use expressions such as *sazu-karu* in their everyday speech. But they occasionally used this expression as "a means of expressing their innermost feelings" when they found out that they were pregnant. This expression was not used in the sense that appears to have operated in the past — to suggest that conception was beyond human control, something over which humans have no power. Rather, in the minds of these women, the meaning of the word *sazu-karu* is determined by the context in which the individual woman had been placed, and accordingly the word might have various meanings. For example, a woman may be trying to conceive a child of her own volition, and had proved unable to conceive as planned, so that she worried that she or her partner might be infertile, or felt that she had been waiting "too long" for pregnancy, or had heard stories about people who had difficulty in conceiving and thought of this as applying to herself. When such a woman discovered that she was finally pregnant, she used the expression *sazu-karu* to express her joy and relief. Meanwhile, women who had intended and planned not to conceive (for the time being), and discovered that they were pregnant, also used the expression of *sazu-karu* to reflect their dismay or surprise, but also to become reconciled to being pregnant.

Thirdly, some women used the expression *sazu-karu* to express passivity towards conceiving a child, something "for which we rely on, seek, or borrow the luck of gods or some greater power...not something that we ourselves can have any power over". In other words, *sazu-karu* is a passive act of having children, although even these women tended to stress that their pregnancy was the result of their own volition.

Fourth, in some cases the two concepts of *sazu-karu* and *tsuku-ru* may co-exist in the minds of individual women, who were unable to decide on either meaning, as, for example, in cases of women who said that conception and childbirth were "partly *sazu-karu*, and partly *tsuku-ru*", or that "pregnancy is something planned, but a baby is *sazu-kari-mono*".

Overall, although these two key words, *sazu-karu* and *tsuku-ru*, have been considered as mutually exclusive (Kudomi and Sato, 1985), analysis of the interviews demonstrates that the two words differ in perspective and connotation, and should be considered to refer to two different phases of women's cognition. These two phases can co-exist and overlap; in fact, in the cognition of one of my informants, the two did not conflict with each other but were in harmony. These two independent phases are structurally dynamic: for some women, they have a complex structure, for some they co-exist, for others they are in conflict.

Women's Views on Reproductive Technologies

Let us turn to informants' views on today's new reproductive technology, citing relevant statements from two informants (lower half of Phase C, Figure 1.3).

Akemi (informant no. 9) had practiced contraception by mutual consent with her husband for a year and a half after marriage. Then, longing for a baby, she stopped using contraceptives and became pregnant, during which time the new technology of sex selection began to be hotly debated. She said: "I think you should not apply the technology to your first child. Because babies have an aura of *sazu-kari-mono*. It sounds manipulative, I feel it's against human nature".

Naoko (informant no. 12) retired from paid work when she married to enjoy life as a housewife. She practiced contraception during the first six months of her married life. Immediately after she and her husband decided to have a baby and she stopped using contraceptives, she became pregnant. She explains: "In my opinion, those people for whom the *in vitro* fertilisation is the only viable method, should not try to have a baby. If I may be allowed to ignore the feelings of would-be mothers suffering from infertility, and set aside their desire to have a baby, then generally speaking, I think you should not challenge the rules of nature. This applies as much to childbearing as to other things".

Women like Akemi and Naoko, who planned their pregnancies to fit in with their life plans and successfully conceived, contended that they saw conception by the use of reproductive technology as a product of *tsuku-ru*, whereas natural conception was the result of *sazu-karu*. However, *sazu-karu* has undergone major semantic changes over time to cover various concepts associated with pregnancy, and women who gave birth to babies in the 1980s did not necessarily use the term as defined in dictionaries, but rather modified its meaning in light of their personal experiences. In addition, with the increased possibilities of pregnancy using reproductive technology, the idea of *tsuku-ru* in its original sense has lost its meaning. This is due to the appearance of much more powerful manipulative technology for *tsuku-ru* and has to be seen in the context of contrasting forces, viz. the difference of manipulative technology and the degree of human intervention between the former and the latter eras. Thus the meaning of *tsuku-ru* is weakening. The expression *sazu-karu*, in contrast with this, relates to loss of passivity of the person involved and the "miracle" of conception and pregnancy that involves a lack of self-determination. In contrast to *tsuku-ru* reflecting manipulative technology, *sazu-karu* has taken on a new and

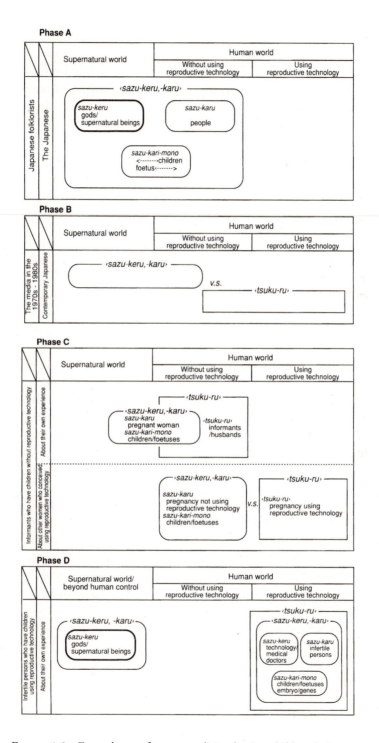

FIGURE 1.3   Four phases of conceptualising having children in Japan.

different meaning, and its use is now dependent on the context of individual life stories being told, and the extent of intentionality in these contexts. In other words, the expressions *sazu-karu* and *tsuku-ru*, that are used in connection with having children, today are a means of expressing an awareness. In doing so, the individuals who use them change the meanings of the expressions to suit their own biographies.

WILL REPRODUCTIVE TECHNOLOGY CHANGE JAPANESE PERCEPTIONS OF LIFE? — FOUR PHASES OF VIEWS

Let us now review the changing views of having children, which can be categorised into four phases (see Figure 1.3). First it is worth mentioning the tacit understanding concerning mother and child which has existed up to the present. A child is an invaluable treasure. Therefore, many women have been and are under considerable pressure to bear babies, and a woman without childbearing and childrearing experience is still deemed immature.

Now we will examine each phase in turn. As proposed by the Japanese folklorists, Phase A represents views on having children held by the Japanese who lived between the mid-19th century and the 1930s. Here gods or supernatural beings *sazu-keru* a child to people in the human world, as shown in the block on the upper left. In other words, people *sazu-karu* a child as a *sazu-kari-mono* from the gods and the supernatural beings, as the block on the upper right shows. The lower block illustrates the *sazu-kari-mono* in the form of a foetus, moving from the supernatural world to the human world, and remaining in the intermediate world as a godlike being until it reaches age seven.

Phase B shows the discourse seen in the mass media in the 1970s and 1980s in reaction to the advances in reproductive technology, particularly *in vitro* fertilisation. The mass media in this period started their argument with the following premise of phase A: A baby or a child is a *sazu-kari-mono*; therefore, women who bear babies should passively accept their role as mothers and raise their children in harmony with both the supernatural world and the human world. The media were concerned that women might begin to associate childbirth — as a result of reproductive technology — with *tsuku-ru*, like the production of a material object at their disposal.

Phase C represents the view of my informants, all of whom had conceived. First, the notion of regeneration is completely absent; instead they vaguely perceive the existence of something beyond human control. Second, they attach different senses to the two key terms, *sazu-karu* and *tsuku-ru*, when talking about their own childbearing experiences and when talking about others who had conceived by reproductive technology. In the first case, the meanings of *sazu-karu* and *tsuku-ru* overlap or cross-cut.

Furthermore, the two words are used flexibly to express various feelings depending on the context. In the second case, however, the meanings of the two words are strictly determined regardless of the context: pregnancy using reproductive technology is conceptualised as *tsuku-ru*; pregnancy without using reproductive technology is *sazu-karu*. As in Phase B, they are opposed to the idea of *tsuku-ru* and favor the word *sazu-karu*.

Phase D represents the view of women and men who succeeded in having a baby using reproductive technology. The left block shows that they regard their child as a *sazu-kari-mono* from the supernatural world, outside of human control. Their view is that reproductive technology and their medical doctors *sazu-keru* the baby (Ohinata, 1992:110; Ohtsuki, 1990:210). Moreover, *sazu-kari-mono* is interpreted to have a wider connotation, and includes babies, foetuses, embryos, and even genes.

In conclusion, the connotation and denotation of the words *sazu-keru*, *sazu-karu*, and *sazu-kari-mono* are changing. It should be noted that these four phases are chronologically ordered but they all exist in contemporary Japan.

DISCUSSION

The historical changes in Japan with regard to life circumstances including those related to having and rearing children indicate the gradual diminishing of our perception of the existence of a supernatural world when we think about having children. We are gradually coming to perceive life within the limitations of the time in which we are physically living in the human world, i.e. the conceptual time scale for life, including having children, appears to be much narrower than it used to be. As a result, it is possible that our ways of perceiving birth and having children will become concentrated within the human world, and the perception of children as being reborn and journeying between the supernatural world and the human world will be lost.

The views of women who had children without using reproductive technology in the 1980s cannot be illustrated by the circular conceptual diagram posited by Tsuboi (1984). This is because, in order to form the circle, we need to have a perception that life continues beyond the single lives of individuals, and we also need to perceive repeated transmigration between the supernatural and human worlds.

Tsuboi (1984:503) states that "the Japanese since the Second World War have progressively compartmentalised '*Ie*'[4] and the 'ancestors', and have a fixed conception of human life as starting at birth and ending at death, thus the idea of a cyclical structure has become extremely weak"; as a result, "the cognition that our own individual world starts at birth and is completed at death is becoming universally imposed". Tsuboi's assertions have been reinforced by others (Nakamura and Hirose, 1987; Tamaru, 1989).

Nakamura and Hirose (1987:158) point out that the Japanese "feel quite uncomfortable with the debate in search of the 'moment' of the birth of new life, namely the question 'when does life start' in western culture with its emphasis on the relationship between god and the individual". They argue too that this is because "in traditional Japanese society, the birth of life was regarded as a process, and this process has been incorporated in its entirety in social relationships such as parents, families, and communities".

While there is still room for the former "cyclical perception", the tendency today is to perceive of life linearly. This "linear perception" of life leads to an attitude that clarifies the progress of a being from creation to demise. The fact that the life of an individual is thus clarified means that the limitations (whereby the individual's life starts at birth and ends at death) and "discontinuity" of life (whereby all individual lives are limited within themselves) will also be clarified.

The following comments were spoken by a Japanese woman once she knew that she was infertile.

> I feel as if I've been cut off from human society and the natural world. Human beings receive life from their parents, and pass it on to their children, their children in turn to their own children, forming a chain of life. This process can span hundreds of years. And while the people around me have all become parents and have become part of the chain in this way, I get a feeling of alienation that I alone have been cut off from all of that. Trees and plants all send out new buds when spring comes. Because I can't have children, I feel as if I can't even put myself on the same level as those plants (Ohinata, 1992:174).

These comments reveal that individuals who realise the discontinuity of their own lives seek continuity in life. There is a sense of loneliness which results from an individual seeking continuity in the existence of "one's own child". However, since this cannot be materialised, life must be spent as an individual and nothing more. I think this idea demonstrates how strongly people seek continuity (limitlessness) when they realize the discontinuity (limitation) of their own life, at the same time, the form in which non-continuous individuals try to seek continuity in life.

Japanese people are gradually changing their understandings of having children that they are thought to have had in the past, i.e. the philosophy that human existence is continuous and cyclical, transcending individual lives. In this context, as reproductive technology and its clinical application advances, cognition of the "non-continuous individual" will become clearer, while greater importance will be placed on "certifying continuity" such as proving the true parenthood of specific individuals.

ACKNOWLEDGMENTS

This chapter is based on my paper *Kodomo wo motsukoto to wa* [What it means to have children in Japan], in *Tsuku-rareru Seisyoku Shinwa* [The Myth of Reproduction] (Asai and Tsuge, 1995). I would like to express my special thanks to Professor Hiroko Hara and Professor Miwako Shimazu for giving me useful comments and reviewing my English drafts.

ENDNOTES

1. The Parcole method is a method developed by Dr Rihachi Iizuka of Keio University in which a Parcole solution is applied to sperms to separate the xx genes from the xy genes before centrifuging them.

2. Kunio Yanagita (also pronounced Yanagida) is the founder of Japanese Folklore Studies (*minzokugaku*), an avid traveler and prolific writer (over 100 books and 1000 articles). He contributed many articles to journals over the period 1868–1912. A unifying theme to his work is the search for the elements of tradition that explain Japan's distinctive national character (see Yanagita, 1970).
3. This material is the only edited compilation of nationwide survey material on pregnancy, childbirth, and upbringing in Japanese folklore from around mid-19th century to the 1930s. There is, to date, still no survey material on a nationwide scale that supersedes this book. However, the disadvantage of the book is that it is not easy to detect whether the testimony of the people who supplied the material has been recorded without modification.
4. Traditional primary unit of social organisation in Japan. *Ie* is often translated as "family", but the term "household" comes close to conveying the Japanese concept of *Ie*. Once established, *Ie* is expected to exist through generations.

REFERENCES

Crouch, M., Manderson, L. (1993a) *New Motherhood: Cultural and Personal Transitions in the 1980s*. Chur: Harwood Academic Press.
Crouch, M., Manderson, L. (1993b) Parturition as social metaphor. *The Australia and New Zealand Journal of Sociology*, **29**(1), 1–18.
Hara, H., Wagatsuma, H. (1974) *Shitsuke* [Child Discipline]. Tokyo: Kobundo.
Imperial Gift Foundation of Boshi-Aiiku-Kai (1975) *Nihon Saniku Shyuzoku Shiryo Shyusei* [Collected Material on Folk Customs on Childbirth and Children's Upbringing in Japan]. Tokyo: Dai-ichi Hoki Shuppan.
Kudomi, Y., Sato, G. (1985) Saniku ni kansura chosa [Research on childbirth education]. In *Kashiwa City Education Basic Research Report on Education to Effect the Kashiwa City Educational Plan*, edited by Y. Hisatomi, G. Sato. Chiba: Research Committee.
Michaelson, K. (editor) (1988) *Birth in America: Anthropological Perspectives*. South Hadley, Mass.: Bergin and Garvey.
Nakamura, K., Hirose, Y. (1987) Seimei no hajimari ni tsuite [The beginnings of life]. *Karada No Kagaku* [Body Science], **138**, 154–158.
Nakayama, M. (1991) Seikatsu-shi kara mita koumi [The first pregnancy of women's life history]. *Meijro Gakuen Joshi Tanki-daigaku Kiyo* [Memoirs of Mejiro Gakuen Junior Women's College], **28**, 199–223.
Nakayama, M. (1992) Ninshin taiken-sha no kodomowo motsu ishiki [The cognitions of pregnant women; the concepts of "sazu-karu" and "tsuku-ru"]. *Hattatsu Shinrigaku Kenkyu* [The Japanese Journal of Developmental Psychology], **3**(2), 51–64.
Nakayama, M. (1995). Kodomo Wo Motsukoto To Wa (What it means to have children in Japan). In *Tsuku-rareru Seishoku Sinwa* (The Myth of Reproduction), edited by M. Asai, A. Tsuge, pp. 16–53, Tokyo: Dojin-sha.
Ohinata, M. (1992) *Bosei Wa Onna No Kunsho Desuka* [Is Motherhood a Badge for Women]? Tokyo: Sankei Shimbun-sha.
Ohtsuki, H. (1990) *Taigai-jusei Nikki* [Diary of "*in vitro* Fertilization"]. Tokyo: Shufu to Seikatsu-sha.
Shikitei, S. (1989) *Ukiyo-buro* [Chit-chats of the people at public baths], edited by K. Jinboo. Tokyo: Iwanami Shoten.

Tamaru, N. (1989) Seimei-kan no mondai [Problems of views on life]. In *Atarashii Seimei-rinri Wo Motomete* [Quest for New Bioethics], pp.61–86. Tokyo: Hokuju Shuppan.

Tsuboi, H. (1984) Mura shakai to tsuuka-girei [Village community and rites of passage]. In *Mura To Murabito: Nihon Minzokugaku Taikei* [Villages and Villagers: A Collection of Works in Japanese Folklore] **8**. Tokyo: Shogakkan.

Yanagita, K. (1970) Chiisaki-mono no koe [The voices of little people]. *Teihon Yanagita Kunio Shu* [Selected Works of Kunio Yanagita]. Tokyo: Chikuma Shobo.

CHAPTER 2

Of Blood and Foetuses: Female Fertility and Women's Reproductive Health in a North Balinese Village

Megan Jennaway

Male cultural constructions of female fertility in North Bali relate to the womb and its products: uterine blood is invested with negative significance, foetuses are positive. The relatively recent introduction of cosmopolitan medicine may modify this view. Biomedical constructions of maternity are more equivocal about the value of foetuses, and indifferent to the meaning of uterine blood. However, biomedical ideologies centering around women's reproductive health have, in the Indonesian context, assumed the right to intrude upon women's reproductive autonomy and may compound local prejudices against women's blood.

While they may not actively contest these ideological constructions, women are not acquiescent when they impinge upon their daily lives. In North Bali, women's perceptions of their own fertility are to some extent permeated by male ideologies of female sexuality and procreation. However, male cultural perspectives do not adequately account for women's own experiences of fertility and the alternative discourses they construct. Grounded in the body, these discourses are primarily concerned with female health and subjective well-being. Women's views of blood and foetuses differ from those of men and relate to the way the loss of uterine blood and the nourishing of a foetus within the womb impose burdens on their bodies. Both circumstances produce symptoms of tiredness and fatigue, and deplete a woman's life-force. In a structural sense, therefore, far from constituting an inverse relation, these apparently contrary elements — blood and foetuses — are for women more or less equivalent.

Moreover, women's perspectives again contrast with dominant biomedical constructions of female fertility. Specifically, women are not always prepared to tolerate the intrusions of biomedicine in the form of birth control; by invoking culturally-sanctioned notions of harmony and compatibility, women are able to deploy a defensive discourse which justifies contraceptive non-compliance.

In this paper, I seek to demonstrate these assertions by examining some key phases of female fertility — those of menstruation, conception, contraception/abortion and pregnancy — as viewed by North Balinese women. My account is based on data collected during twelve months of ethnographic fieldwork conducted in 1992 in a rural village in Buleleng, North Bali. Techniques for the elicitation of information included participant observation and unstructured interviews with women on maternal and general health.

THE SETTING: *DESA PUNYAN WANGI*

Desa Punyan Wangi (pseudonym) is a rural village about 12 kilometres west of Singaraja, the capital of the *kabupaten* (region) of Buleleng in North Bali. In 1992 it had a population of 3622 (1142 males, 1244 females) and a mixed agricultural economy based mainly upon cash-crop clove and coffee production. Most (78%) of the population are farmers involved in agricultural production. Despite only being 2–5 kms from Lovina, a major tourist centre situated along the coastline to the north, as yet Punyan Wangi has not prospered by this proximity to any significant degree, with few tourist dollars being injected into the relatively depressed local economy. Most villagers under the age of 45 are bilingual in both Indonesian and Balinese, alternating between the two according to context.

INDIGENOUS CONSTRUCTIONS OF FEMALE FERTILITY

In Desa Punyan Wangi, indigenous constructions of female sexuality and fertility define an inverse relation between uterine blood and foetuses. The wombs of women are ambiguously conceived of as presenting a potential risk to men, depending on whichever of these two elements occupies the womb space at the time. Sexual activity is culturally proscribed whenever a woman is menstruating, expelling lochia, or during mid-cycle bleeding. By contrast, sex is actively condoned in relation to a foetus, whether potential or actual. Not only is sex deemed necessary to conception, it is also thought essential for the healthy development of the foetus and for the reinforcement of paternal identity. At a conceptual level, the potential for or realisation of a foetus implies the absence of blood from the womb, rendering it "safe" for sex. Blood is culturally constructed as an impure, defiling substance and poses a threat to male sexual and social integrity. Foetuses, on the other hand, proclaim a man's procreative powers and enhance his sexual and social prestige.

In relation to fertility, sex can be seen as providing an index of female purity. Moreover, it operates as the vector which determines the inverse relation between the two opposed elements of blood and foetuses in social space. But whereas sex is negatively correlated with blood, it is positively correlated with foetuses.

To some extent, women acquiesce in these male constructions of their fertility, affirming their ascribed impurity during menstruation and cooperating in the limited forms of sequestration required of them at such times. But these notions of pollution pervade women's consciousness at a deeper level to (dis)colour womens' subjective perceptions of themselves and their own bodies: they see themselves as literally "dirty" when they are menstruating. Yet women are not inordinately preoccupied with this negative self-image; rather they are concerned with bodily health and vitality, in particular, with the condition of their *bayu* or "life-force".[1]

Whenever their womb undergoes biological transformation, women experience a corresponding loss of energy, both physical and spiritual. They become tired and fatigued (*lemet, kenyel, kiap*) and their vitality (*bayu*) is dissipated (*oon*). This occurs when they lose blood from the womb and also when their wombs are burdened with a foetus. The greater the quantity of blood lost, or the larger the foetus becomes, the more depleted their *bayu*. For the women of Desa Punyan Wangi, preserving their personal vitality and maintaining a sense of bodily well-being is of far greater concern than any imputed state of pollution.

These points will be made clearer below in my discussion of the specific phases in the female fertility cycle. However, women's overriding concern with bodily health is also well illustrated by their responses to the specific biomedical constructions of maternal health which have emerged within the cultural context of postcolonial Indonesia.

BIOMEDICAL CONSTRUCTIONS OF WOMEN'S REPRODUCTIVE HEALTH

The notion that "womens' reproductive health" constitutes a genuine biomedical category has been subject to some criticism. Several critics see this as a means to medical intervention in the management of aspects of maternity (e.g. Zola, 1972; Stephens, 1986; Martin, 1987). Zola, for instance, suggests that pregnancy, in particular, provides the "most illuminating illustration" of the way in which modern medicine has laid claim to:

> a whole host of related processes; not only to birth but to prenatal, postnatal and paediatric care; not only to conception, but to infertility; not only to the processes of reproduction but to the processes and problems of sexual activity itself; not only when life begins (in the issue of abortion) but whether it should be allowed to begin at all (e.g. in genetic counselling) (Zola, 1972:496).

Martin (1987) affirms this view in her critique of biomedical models of female reproduction which denigrate various aspects of women's bodies and their functions, especially menstruation and menopause. Moreover, the impact of these models upon Western obstetric practice has served to disinherit women of control over their bodies, thereby alienating them from the birth process (Martin, 1987:51,63; cf. Zola, 1972; Stephens, 1986:70; Jordan, 1988). In one view, the body in labour is viewed mechanically, as an analogue to an amorphous collection of workers on a factory floor, bereft of supervision.[2] In this metaphor, only biomedicine can provide the managerial skills essential to successful reproduction. In justification of its appropriation of the reproductive capacities of the female body, Western biomedicine has successfully constructed maternity as an illness, a "sick" condition which can be "treated" by modern medicine (Oakley, 1979; Crouch and Manderson, 1993). To the extent that the women of Punyan Wangi are preoccupied with the health effects of maternity, Western biomedicine's focus on maternity is in sympathy with their concerns. Although women experience the effects of menstruation, pregnancy and the related phenomena of fertility upon their bodies as debilitating, they disavow all claims to sickness. Fatigue and depleted energy levels do not constitute illnesses for village women, but merely reasons to rest and take care of themselves.

On the other hand, village women find certain practical biomedical intrusions upon their lived bodies — such as contraception — rather less sympathetic. While they may acknowledge the benefits of contraception in relieving them of the burden of frequent childbearing, which, as noted, they perceive to exact a toll upon their bodies, women are aware that such relief comes at a price. To the extent that the costs of contraception upon their bodily health and personal subjectivity are too high, women tend to resist contraception in the form offered to them under the national maternal health system.

MENSTRUATION

Blood — particularly menstrual blood — is construed as a highly polluting substance in Hindu-Balinese cosmology (Covarrubias, 1989:133; Lovric, 1987:255). Menstruating women are deemed ritually impure (*sebel*)[3] for the duration of menstruation and must endure a degree of sequestration. This extends only to the ritual domain; in most other respects they may go about their activities as normal. *Sebel* women are debarred from participating in temple activities and in the past were forbidden to prepare food. However in Desa Punyan Wangi this second restriction no longer appears to be enforced.[4]

A woman views menstruation (*nyebelin raga*) in two quite distinct ways: first, she feels her vitality to be diminished and her body feels fatigued, and second, she feels dirty and impure. This would seem to imply an overflow of association from ritual impurity to a general sense of uncleanliness: some women speak of feeling extremely dirty. Moreover, women not only *feel* dirty but *think of themselves* this way whenever they are menstruating. These connotations of defilement pervade women's self-image; rather than their *bayu* becoming soiled, they themselves become dirty and impure.

Yet women were not overly concerned with their ascribed "dirtiness"; this was simply acknowledged. In general, women were far more preoccupied with their felt physical condition during menstruation than with any notional state of impurity. Invariably, they described experiencing feelings of tiredness and lassitude associated with their low energy levels. Menstruation thus impacts dually upon a woman's body, first by diminishing her life-force (*bayu*) and second and consequently, in causing her to feel tired, lethargic and even sleepy.

There is an overt taboo upon sexual relations during menstruation. All my informants affirmed that it is forbidden for a couple to engage in sex while the woman is menstruating because it is not appropriate (*sing pantes*) and feels dirty (*komel asane*). To breach this taboo can incur serious punishment: whoever defaults may be cursed or may become sick. The reason women gave for the prohibition was that it was forbidden to have sex with one's husband if you were still "dirty", i.e. menstruating. The recurrent ambiguity between ritual and bodily uncleanliness here would appear to reflect a consistent blurring of this distinction in women's minds. One woman indignantly responded that she was not a disgusting sort of person, implying that only such a person would wish to engage in sex at such a time.

Fear of menstrual contamination through sexual contact is reported elsewhere in the ethnographic literature on Bali (Covarrubias, 1989:156; Duff-Cooper, 1985a; Weck, nd.:182). Previously the menstruating wife was commonly ejected from the conjugal bed; women of affluent households slept on beds in a different balé (pavilion); poor women often slept on a mat on the floor beside their husband's bed. Covarrubias (ibid.) attributes this to men's fear of ensorcelment in that the woman might anoint his head with menstrual blood during the night, thereby cursing him with the worst of impurities.[5] In Punyan Wangi, separate sleeping was less common, although one of my informants always slept apart from her husband if she was menstruating.

Menstrual blood is therefore culturally constructed in Desa Punyan Wangi as highly defiling to a man, and contact with it jeopardises his sexual and spiritual integrity. For menstruating women, the stigma of defilement is not so acute, for their personal sexuality is not at stake. However, women's identification as impure colours their subjective reality at such times, such that they actually feel dirty. Overriding any ascribed quality of uncleanliness is their own bodily experience of menstruation, as enervating and a drain on their bayu, although women tend to use this time to advantage, by resting, catching up with light household chores, and enjoying the exemption from religious duties. Although menstruation has clear drawbacks, it also has sufficient advantages in terms of workload alleviation for women not to mind it overly much. Clearly, menstrual blood does not for women constitute the object of abhorrence that it does for men.[6]

CONCEPTION AND THE VALUE OF CHILDREN

While sex during menstruation is abhorrent to most villagers, sex at any other time is endorsed precisely because it might lead to conception. As seen above, in terms of preserving male sexual purity, sex in the absence of menstrual blood is construed as entailing no danger to the man. Further, in relation to the purity/impurity dichotomy, sex during the non-menstrual phase of a woman's fertility cycle is a neutral act: it only becomes charged with positive significance in relation to a foetus, i.e. if conception is at least the goal, if not also the outcome, of coitus.

Procreation in North Bali establishes a man's virility and perpetuates the lineage, thereby fulfilling a fundamental cultural imperative, and ideally, providing progeny for social and economic support in old age.[7] Neither women nor men achieve full adult status until they have reproduced. In their article on Balinese naming patterns, Geertz and Geertz (1964) recount that in the past, upon the birth of a couple's first child, the names of its parents were changed to reflect their new status. Childless adults were therefore easily identifiable by the retention of their childhood appellative. Their claim that in Bali considerable sociological importance attaches to children is based upon this status linkage. In Desa Punyan Wangi, as in other parts of Bali, the practice of teknonymy is now declining, but children are no less highly valued (e.g. Bateson and Mead, 1942:29; Streatfield, 1986:34; Covarrubias, 1989:132). Notwithstanding, Hull (1978:4–5) argues against this, by evoking a contrast between nuclear family systems of domestic organisation with the extended Balinese family, and then attempts to explain the apparent contradiction between the alleged value of children and the Balinese receptivity to birth control (see below). The two propositions are not inconsistent however: love of children does not have to translate to a desire for huge quantities of them. In Punyan Wangi at least, irrespective of the degree of individual families' commitment to birth control guidelines, the point remains that for most couples, it is essential to have at least one child. Banjar membership, for instance, is dependent upon such an outcome and at a cultural level, the contention by Geertz and Geertz (1964) that social identification as an adult begins with the birth of the first child holds true.

Symbolically, foetuses are invested with strong positive associations which contrast with those for menstrual blood. Foetuses enhance male social identity, menstrual blood endangers it. The antithesis between the two is revealed in relation to the permissibility of sexual intercourse: while sex is *proscribed* whenever the womb is voiding itself of blood, it is *prescribed* whenever the womb is devoid of a foetus. Men are encouraged to fill vacant wombs with foetuses, but must avoid all contact with female genitalia when those same wombs are full of blood.

In Punyan Wangi villagers believe that the foetus is the product of the father's sperm (*semara*) and maternal fluid (*yeh memene*). Specifically, it is constituted of a maternal contribution of fluids: blood (*getih*) and water (*yeh*); and a paternal one of solid elements, such as bones (*lung*), flesh (*be*), skin (*kulit*) and muscles or tendons (*otot, uwat*). Covarrubias' (1989:123) report serves to supplement this outline of indigenous understandings of the birth process. The confluence of sexual substances described above was believed to turn into blood in the womb, forming a ball which was further nourished by the mother's blood (a view which he finds remarkably close to the Western biological understanding of procreation) (cf. Streatfield, 1986:23; Weck, n.d.:186ff).

Despite some broad similarities, Covarrubias does not entirely accord with the conception beliefs expressed by villagers in modern-day Punyan Wangi. Punyan Wangi folk do not see the process of conception as merely a mechanical union between two complementary contributions from oppositely sexed bodies. For villagers, there is one significant element which permits conception to occur: the fact that the male's contribution of semen (*yeh muani, yeh bapane*), is already imbued with the divine life-force of the God of Love, Batara Semara. Similarly, the maternal fluid (*yeh luh, yeh memene*) contains the essence of Dewi Ratih, the female Goddess of Love and consort of Batara Semara.

Jane Belo (1970:102; cf. Streatfield, 1986:23) reports a widespread notion that inside every woman's womb is a *manik*, which means "gem" in both Indonesian

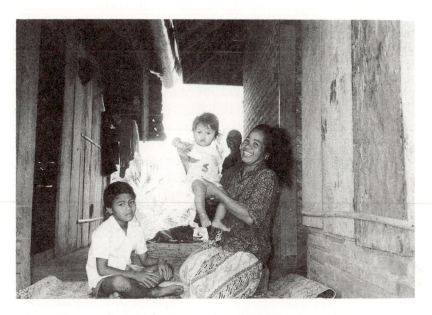

FIGURE 2.1 Women who are infertile may adopt children to protect their position within the family. Luh Wani was unable to conceive, and finally, at the age of 45, adopted a son. (Photo: M. Jennaway).

and Balinese. However, in Balinese it also conveys the alternative meaning of "ovary" (Dinas Pendidikan, 1990; Echols and Shadily, 1990). Upon being repeatedly "hit" during sexual intercourse, the *manik* grows to form a foetus.[8] Once the baby has been delivered, a new *manik* develops to replace the old one. In Desa Punyan Wangi the word *manik* is occasionally used to convey a meaning synonymous with both the Balinese word *belingan* and the Indonesian *janur* (both of which mean "foetus"), a use which is not inconsistent with its meaning of "ovum", if not precisely "ovary".

CONTRACEPTION AND ABORTION

The high fertility ratio witnessed for Bali in the past (Hull, 1978:5) implies that prior to the advent of the national family planning program, Balinese women did little to limit their fertility. This contrasts with the picture presented by Alexander and Alexander (1979) for Javanese women, who in the nineteenth century exercised considerable control over their fertility through prolonged lactation and post-partum sexual abstinence.

Presumably these contraceptive options were also available to Balinese women, but given the lack of data (Hull, 1978:2), it is difficult to establish whether they were consciously utilised in this way. Prolonged lactation, still prevalent today, may well have helped depress the fertility of Balinese women. However, the average period of post-partum sexual abstinence customary in Desa Punyan Wangi is much shorter than that for Java last century and the demographic impact of this questionable. The standard period of post-partum celibacy quoted to me by village women was one Balinese month, or 42 days (*abulan pitung dina*), and the setting of this mandatory minimum period seems to relate more to indigenous notions of ritual impurity than efforts to limit fertility. The passage of one Balinese month is to remove the stain (*ngilangang noda*) of childbirth, and sexual intercourse may be resumed subsequently without penalty to the male partner. The emphasis of post-partum sexual abstinence, therefore, seems to have been on preserving a man's spiritual purity rather than on its contraceptive value.

Indonesia has a long tradition of indigenous pharmacological knowledge which in Java is manifest in herbal remedies known as *jamu* (Hetler, 1986; Rahardjo, 1990). Contraceptive *jamu*, as well as natural abortifacients, are available from some indigenous midwives, although around Punyan Wangi only Javanese midwives (distinguished as *dukun bayiorang Islam*) were believed to possess these skills. Since abortion is considered a sin (*dosa*) by both Muslim-Javanese and Hindu-Balinese, neither contraceptive nor abortifacient *jamu* are available from the many commercial *jamu* outlets in Singaraja, the closest large town. Women seeking pharmacological remedies to suppress fertility in the past had to resort to the services of a Javanese midwife from among the many Muslim enclaves situated in and around Singaraja. The absence of such a resort from the reproductive histories of my women informants may imply that this option was seldom used. Alternatively, the stigma attached to taking such a measure (particularly abortion) might discourage women from admitting to ever having done so. In any case, the majority of my informants had the benefit of cosmopolitan contraception, as available through the state maternal health services, for most of their reproductive years, as they were quick to point out when questioned on this issue.

Hence formerly, village women had a high fertility rate and gave birth to a succession of children. This view finds preliminary support in my observations of older generation village women: those over the age of about 45 tended to have had large families, with heavy rates of infant loss. Within my own household for instance, my adoptive mother, Meme, had borne ten children of whom only seven had survived. In the past, women's wombs apparently bore a heavy reproductive load, with all the attendant impacts upon bodily health and vitality that this implies.

Cosmopolitan modes of contraception were introduced into the village through the Indonesian family planning campaign (KB: *Keluarga Berencana*) in 1970.[9] The campaign is managed by a semi-autonomous body, the National Family Planning Coordinating Board (BKKBN: *Badan Koordinasi Keluarga Berencana Nasional*), run under the auspices of the Department of Health (Hull, 1991). Family planning has constituted a major strategy of the New Order government's objective of population control (Hull, 1978; Hurdle, 1981; Hunter, this volume) and has achieved remarkable successes in a relatively short period of time (Hull, 1978, 1991; Hurdle, 1981; Poffenberger, 1983; Streatfield, 1986; Warren, 1986; Parker, 1993). Hull (1991:4) points out that the astounding transformation in Indonesia's contraceptive coverage from 18% in 1976 to 70% in 1989 is doubtless what earned President Suharto the 1989 UN Population Award.

In Bali especially, the KB program has been hailed as a spectacular success (Hull, 1978:1; Streatfield, 1986:1; cf. Poffenberger, 1983:43,59), although Hull (1978:5) notes that the dramatic decline in Balinese fertility achieved by the program began from a starting-point of very high fertility. Many factors may account for Bali's success, including the excellent design of the KB program itself (Hull, 1978:7; Streatfield, 1986:11),[10] community involvement through the agency of the *banjar* (indigenous local council) (Warren, 1986:216–217; Parker, 1993:18–19; cf. Streatfield, 1986:9–10, 153)[11] and exploiting the "single-strike" technology of the IUD (Parker, 1993:18) combined with the strong positive incentive of providing IUDs to women at no cost (Hull, 1978:1). While Hull (1978:6) applauds the effectiveness of the education initiative which accompanied the family planning campaign, Parker (1993:18) characterises the way the state provided information to local people as a "totalitarian method of disseminating information about contraception" to virtually preclude effective consideration of the alternatives (cf. Patten, 1992).

The heavy reliance of the KB program in Bali upon *banjar* cooperation is apparent in the scrupulous records maintained by the several *banjar* of Desa Punyan Wangi regarding contraceptive prevalence among members. Comprehensive lists are kept of all fertile couples (PUS: *pasangan usia subur*)[12] within the *banjar* and their contraceptive status. Several sources (e.g. Warren, 1986; Streatfield, 1986:9–10) suggest that in the establishment phase of the program, eligible couples identified by the banjar as resisting contraception were pursued with vigilance by local family planning officials to effect their compliance.[13] My Punyan Wangi informants claimed that when KB was just starting to be introduced into the village, recalcitrants were not only hounded by *petugas KB* (family planning officials) but also publicly reprimanded by the *banjar*, and in several cases fines were levied. Public humiliation therefore seems to have been effectively deployed by the *banjar* to achieve impressive levels of conformity to family planning objectives.

FAMILY PLANNING IN PUNYAN WANGI

In 1992, nulliparous married women in Punyan Wangi who did not wish to fall pregnant were generally placed on the pill, although alternatives such as condoms, diaphragms, contraceptive injections (Depoprovera) and implants (Norplant) were available. In conformity with the KB program's orientation towards IUDs, however, primiparous and multiparous women were still encouraged to use the IUD (Lippes Loop) on the assurance that it could be removed should they wish to become pregnant again.

Nationally the KB program urged women to limit family size to two children. My investigations of women using contraception in Desa Punyan Wangi indicate that it was used for birth spacing and to prevent further reproduction. There was

TABLE 2.1   Choice of contraception.

Contraception	Bali %	Buleleng %	Punyan Wangi %
IUD	71.5	63.6	81.3
The Pill	7.8	15.0	13.1
Condoms	2.1	2.9	1.8
Injection (Depoprovera)	9.2	11.3	2.8
Hormonal Implant (e.g. Norplant)	0.7	1.6	0.0
Other	8.7	5.6	1.0

Source: Bali, BKKBN, 1991: Table 6; Bali, Bappeda Tingkat II Buleleng, 1990:100.

widespread acceptance among both women and men of the view that families should limit their size to just two offspring: villagers cited economic scarcity as the main motivation. But the role of the local family planning official, Pak Santika, in ebulliently promoting this ideal, should not be overlooked: I witnessed him reducing to tears a woman who dared to contemplate having a fourth baby. He was equally energetic in securing compliance with the objective of birth spacing: often I observed him at *posyandu* or *pos penimbangan* sessions exhorting women, who were discussing the option of falling pregnant again, to wait until their first child had entered school.

IUDs continue to be the most prevalent form of contraception in Bali. In the two decades from 1971 to 1991, out of a total population of 352,828 contraceptive users, 252,469 (71.5%) used IUDs (Bali, BKKBN, 1991; see also Table 2.1). The free insertion of IUDs, combined with the prospect that they would require no further financial outlay, clearly persuaded many women to opt for it, and IUDs were inserted into married women's wombs with great zeal.

But the impressive levels of contraceptive coverage achieved by the family planning initiative may obscure certain problems in its implementation. Anecdotal evidence gives cause for concern as to the ways in which these results were achieved. For instance, one female doctor who worked with the BKKBN for many years, supervising and monitoring the program, told me a number of paramedics were content to implant the devices even without routine screening beforehand. It was a matter of constant anguish to this doctor that she was unable to get BKKBN support for a policy of pre-testing IUD recipients for prior infections. She was told that the suggestion was completely unfeasible, given the expense and the risk of losing a client in failure to follow-up.

No attempt was made to advise women of the need for regular checkups despite the comparisons provided by Western countries. Women who agreed to have an IUD inserted were not counselled either to have post-insertive checkups, or to change their IUDs regularly. Supporting this claim was the explanation I received from a KB official at the *kecamatan* (district) level: when he was asked, 22 years after the inception of the program, what recommendations had been made to women regarding the frequency of post-insertive IUD check-ups, he assured me that the IUDs used in the KB program had not yet reached the end of their lifespan. Hence many women had not had their IUD checked since the day of its insertion. One woman I met had had the same IUD inside her womb for eighteen years, another woman for twenty-one years, and periods of fifteen years were reasonably common.

In Kabupaten Buleleng the rate of participation in family planning is the second lowest in Bali (82.2%).[14] Among contraceptive users, the proportion using IUDs in Buleleng is also less than average (63.6% compared with 71.5%). Conversely, the proportion of couples using alternatives such as Depoprovera, condoms and the pill is higher than the average for Bali. For Depoprovera, Buleleng's use rate is 11.3% compared with the provincial average of just 9.2%; for the pill it is 15.0% compared with 7.8%; and 2.9% of Buleleng contraceptive users use condoms as compared with 2.1% throughout Bali (see Table 2.1).

Between April 1991 and January 1992, contraceptive coverage in Desa Punyan Wangi rose, placing it on a comparable footing with levels achieved for other parts of Bali (86.8%). It was also the highest level of KB participation among all villages within the district in which Punyan Wangi lies, that of Sukasada I. Unfortunately, such information as was available for this period was not disaggregated by contraceptive type. I have therefore had to rely on 1990 figures from an alternative source to provide an outline of the predominant trends in contraceptive preferences among villagers.

In 1990, 81.3% of contraceptive users were using the IUD, compared with 13.1% using the pill, while 2.8% opted for Depoprovera, and just 1.8% (9 individuals) claimed to be using condoms (see Table 2.1). The contraceptive picture for Desa Punyan Wangi was thus very different from that for Buleleng as a whole: the low relative reliance on IUDs for Buleleng was not replicated in Punyan Wangi, where IUDs represented the form of contraception used by more than four out of every five fertile couples. On the other hand, the prevalence of the pill (13.1%) was only slightly less than that for the whole region (15%), and likewise for condoms, viz. 1.8% in Punyan Wangi compared with 2.8% for Buleleng. But aside from IUDs, the only other striking discrepancy is in the number of people preferring to using contraception in the form of an injection; whereas in Buleleng overall 11.3% preferred Depoprovera, in Punyan Wangi — where this alternative is only available outside the village — only 2.8% of contraceptive users had opted for this method. It should not be assumed from this however that Depoprovera is an unpopular method of birth control among Punyan Wangi women: the ethnographic data I provide below indicates that more women would probably opt for Depoprovera were it more accessible.

WOMEN'S RESPONSES TO THE IUD

Given that 81.3% of the women on contraception in Punyan Wangi are using the IUD, much of the following discussion is concentrated upon women's responses to this particular contraceptive method. The pressure for women to start using an

IUD begins to be applied soon after the birth of their first child. The majority of my thirty-seven women informants had IUDs, which is consistent with the official picture of IUD prevalence in Punyan Wangi (see Table 2.1 above). Women speak of going on contraception as "having family planning" (*maKaBé: ma-KB*) but this is often shorthand to say they are going to get an IUD inserted. Alternatively they may specify that they are having a Lippes Loop put in (*maKaBé masang Loop*). But underlining the extent to which family planning is identified with IUDs in the minds of village women is the most common expression of all — *masang KaBé* — lit. "to have family planning inserted".

Many Punyan Wangi women reported difficulties with their IUD. IUDs worldwide are associated with higher rates of reproductive tract infections (RTIs) often leading to secondary sterility (Hull and Tukiran, 1976). While Streatfield (1986:122) did not find this to be the case in his 1982 survey, the local bidan in Punyan Wangi suspected a link between RTI manifestations, i.e. white or cloudy vaginal discharges symptomatic of vaginal infection and the increased use of IUDs. Vaginal infection (*keputihan*) was one of the problems with which women IUD users most frequently presented (see also Hull, Widyantoro and Fetters, this volume).[15]

Streatfield's (1986:122) survey detected many other problems among the 470 IUD-users in his sample of women, including prolonged and/or heavier menstruation, stomach cramps, fatigue, breakthrough bleeding and weight loss. Other problems he reports include discharge, dizziness, odour, fever, and disturbed vision. Punyan Wangi women who were experiencing problems voiced the opinion that for them, the IUD was inappropriate. None of them intended to use it for long and factors which caused them to vacillate between changing to an alternative or staying with the IUD included (a) expense i.e. alternatives must be paid for and (b) unreliability e.g. in the case of Depoprovera, women appreciate that there is a significant risk of pregnancy as its effects wear off.

For many women Depoprovera still represents the most attractive alternative because its few side-effects are positively evaluated in Balinese culture: blood flow is lessened (some women become amenorrheaic), and there may be weight gain (roundness, *moleh*, is considered attractive in a female). This positive cultural evaluation of a filled-out (but not fat) rounded form is underscored by a strong aversion to thinness (*berag*) in a woman. Women who gained weight on Depoprovera declared that it was *cocok* (suitable) for them because they believed it enhanced their appearance.

No women made such positive claims about the compatibility of the IUD. On the contrary, those who referred to the question of personal compatibility invariably denounced it as quite unsuitable (*sing cocok*). The majority of those who suffered weight loss caused by the IUD experienced this as a disturbing, even alarming, side-effect. Moreover, IUDs often fail to prevent pregnancy. For quite a few of my informants, the device simply fell out (cf. Streatfield, 1986:122).[16] Some of them realised this had occurred, for others the subsequent pregnancy was the first indication that it was no longer in place. In other cases, the device remained in the womb but an ectopic pregnancy ensued. Below I list some examples from my fieldnotes:

Ni Nengah Karti fell pregnant with her fourth child even with her IUD still in place; she had it removed and proceeded with the pregnancy. Ni Kadek Murni's IUD was inserted after her first birth. It fell out and she had it replaced. The second one then fell out as well and she found she was pregnant again before she had even got around to replacing it. After fifteen years on an IUD, Ni Made Restiki fell pregnant again with her device still in place. She went to hospital and had it removed before both having an abortion and getting a tubectomy : she already had two teenage boys. Ni Wayan Wiriani's IUD fell out three years ago but so far she hasn't fallen pregnant. Ni Ketut Murtining decided to limit her family to two because of poverty, but then her IUD fell out without her knowledge and she found herself pregnant again.

Besides the IUD, few other methods of contraception are practised in the village (see Table 2.1). The pill is too expensive and condoms are unpopular, considered to be a hassle (*repot sekali*). Diaphragms are not readily available. Hormonal implants (*susuk jarum*) are almost unheard of: I knew of only one woman who was using it as her preferred mode of contraception, having obtained it from the general hospital in Singaraja.[17] At present, the ease and popularity of contraceptive injections (*KB suntikan*) seems to make Depoprovera the most viable and likely alternative to IUDs, although again expense is a factor. Women must pay anew for each three monthly injection. The obvious drawback with Depoprovera is that it is not officially recommended for continuous use. Family planning guidelines recommend one shot six weeks after birth, and another three months later, giving post-natal coverage of just over seven months. After two consecutive injections, women are advised to try something else. Hence the Depoprovera option is not a perfect solution in that it needs to be combined with an alternative contraceptive.

The single greatest deterrent to using an IUD among the women was that it extended the length of time for which they were bleeding. Many women also suffered stomach cramps and complained of abnormally heavy blood loss, including mid-month bleeding. One woman was having cycles of only twenty days or so, with heavy menstrual flows each time. Another suffered extended menstrual periods that often lasted up to sixteen days in a month. Associated with this she was often tired and giddy, and after her third visit to the *bidan* the latter pronounced her to be suffering from anaemia and put her on the pill, having removed the IUD.

Women who experienced increased bleeding from the IUD must endure feeling dirty (*daki, reged*) for an extended length of time. This amplifies their sense of personal dirtiness and reinforces their negative self-image. Women experiencing increased bleeding had no doubt that the IUD was the cause. One woman explained: "Since going on the IUD my dirtiness has become excessive".

Women's way of dealing with their feelings of shame at their perceived unclean state and their abhorrence of excessive bleeding was to joke about it.

> Ny Kartiki had suffered from severe cramps and excessive bleeding ever since her IUD had been put in. Once a neighbour came to visit and as she squatted on the floor, chatting sociably prior to getting up and preparing coffee, she felt an enormous bloodrush descend to her groin, soaking her entire rear. She

remained immobile for two more hours, in great discomfort, talking to their guest. Finally her husband, knowing her problems with the IUD, guessed what must have happened. He apologised to his visitor that his wife was "too sick" to make coffee that day.

(His regret, however, did not extend to making it himself nor even to finding a ruse to lure his guest outside while she made a discreet exit.)

For the majority of fertile women of Desa Punyan Wangi, cooperating with the family planning program virtually translates to acceptance of an IUD. For most, other forms of contraception are an expensive and somewhat notional alternative. However, IUDs are increasingly being viewed with suspicion and in some cases, even repugnance. The increased blood flow associated with the Lippes Loop, experienced by many women, is viewed as an encumbrance and a nuisance. It extends the period of time for which their bodily well-being is compromised by fatigue and lassitude. But at a more profound level, it prolongs the disquieting sensation in women that their bayu, their life-force, is being eroded.

Many Punyan Wangi women are choosing to resist the imposition of IUDs upon their bodily well-being by the strategic deployment of a counter-ideology centring around the notion of compatibility (cocok). The theme of matching or personal compatibility is central to indigenous constructions of illness and healing in Bali (Ruddick, 1980:48; Macauley, 1984:151); it is also implicit in many other aspects of social life, such as in describing the relation between teachers and pupils (Connor, 1982), between members of the same patriline (Hobart, 1980:150–151), and so forth. The belief that compatibility is an essential prerequisite to social harmony is underpinned by a more general cosmological system which identifies harmony or order as the fundamental condition of the universe. Again harmony on a cosmic scale implies a balance between macrocosmic and microcosmic elements, a celestial matching which mirrors the element of matching or cocok in human relationships (Connor, 1982: 192–4; Gunawan, 1982; Muninjaya, 1982; Macauley, 1984:1–3,179).

By claiming that the IUD is not suitable for her body, a village woman is relieved of the obligation to use it and may legitimately have it removed. I did not hear of a single case in which a woman who had given up her IUD on these grounds attracted community censure. Having suffered with their IUD, however, many of these women do not seek alternative contraception, thereby in a passive way resisting family planning and undermining its population control objective.

PREGNANCY: *MASA BELING*

Indigenous models of the female body during pregnancy construe it as an organic entity expressing fecundity and fullness, as an ever-ripening seed. Villagers say that a pregnant woman is like *padi meling* (lit. "pregnant rice", a ripe stalk of rice). The abdominal swelling associated with pregnancy is not considered ugly or unattractive, given the cultural preference for a rounded, filled-out look in women. Yet, directed toward promoting the value of motherhood and children, it does not particularly reflect women's experience. Village women on the whole are less than delighted to be barefoot and pregnant, they experience the distension of their bellies as uncomfortable (*keweh*) and heavy (*baat*), and their bodily-energy (*bayu*) is depleted (*oon*). They look forward to birth as signalling the time when they can once again feel beautiful (*jegeg*), slender-waisted (*bangkiang lengkiang*) and light (*ingan*).

Covarrubias' (1989:123) comment that pregnant women were "free of any taboos" does not apply to the women of Punyan Wangi, if anywhere in Bali. In Punyan Wangi, many foods are proscribed or taboo, while there is a positive prescription or requirement to engage in regular sex. Most of the food taboos relating to pregnancy derive from the humoral notions of the body prevalent throughout Southeast Asia (Manderson, 1987). Foods which are excessively hot or cold are proscribed for pregnant women, lest they should harm the foetus. These notions even pervade the cosmopolitan medical system.

Pregnant women may only eat small amounts of watery fruits such as oranges, pawpaw, rambutan and mango. Even coconut milk — considered excellent for building up a mother's milk supply — must be consumed only sparingly during pregnancy. All these foods are classified as cool, verging on cold, and may be deleterious to the baby's health. On the other hand, "hot" foods, particularly red meat such as goat, buffalo, dog, and pig, are completely proscribed, with the exception of the purified pig meat that it is eaten on ceremonial occasions. Chicken is a neutral food, but spicy foods — particularly anything containing chilli — are dangerously hot. Alcohol distilled from palm sugar is forbidden (although women rarely consume this). Eggs have an ambivalent classification, some women avoiding them altogether, others asserting that Balinese eggs — a very small fine-shelled variety of egg which is 90% yolk — are beneficial if eaten raw and mixed with a small amount of honey. There was less consensus about fish, although most women concluded it was an appropriate food if taken in moderation.

Sexual Prescriptions: Night Work (*Magae Peteng*)

In Punyan Wangi, terms for sex are euphemistic. Often the expression *ngajak kurnane* (to "get together with" your spouse) is used, but equally women refer to sex as *magae peteng* (to labour at night/night labour). The most obvious explanation for this expression would seem to lie in the notion of the labour of making a baby. However, in Punyan Wangi it has an additional meaning.

As noted earlier, indigenous beliefs regarding procreation construe the foetus as being partially composed of maternal blood, and also as being nourished by it. Weck (nd:189) records a sophisticated view of conception among literate traditional healers (*balian usada*) as a process involving the enclosing of the "mixture" of the male seed and the female "within the chorionic membrane". He goes on to add that "this *locks up the blood* so that a pregnant woman has no more menstruation" (ibid.; my emphasis). This conceptualisation of maternal blood as being "absorbed" by the foetus renders the womb sufficiently pure to permit sexual intercourse during pregnancy, in contrast to the many other societies which proscribe it (cf. Spencer, 1977:292).

Punyan Wangi villagers not only affirm the admissibility of sex during pregnancy, they consider it mandatory. This stems from a belief that maternal blood alone is insufficient to nourish the foetus: the husband's sperm is also vital for foetal growth. One woman explained:

> It's appropriate to have sex with your husband while you're pregnant so that
> the baby in your belly will be strong.

Another explanation suggested that sex ensured against the baby's becoming weak and pale. One forty-seven year old woman warned that:

> If you don't have sex with your husband during pregnancy the baby in your
> belly won't thrive. People say it's because the foetus will not hear its [paternal]
> grandfather calling. [Hence] it's still better [for the foetus] to have sex with
> your husband.

Hence the imperative to maintain sexual intercourse during pregnancy seems to be connected with notions of paternal-patrilineal claims on the child, as though the single act of conception is not quite enough irrefutably to establish paternity. The sperm's continual "hitting" of the woman's *manik* may therefore be interpreted as meaning that the foetus must continually be reminded of its paternity during gestation by means of these recurrent coital "strikes", which symbolically represent the call of the offspring's patrilineal ancestors. According to the husband of one of my informants, such reminders are necessary in order that the foetus is able to recognise its father after birth. Hence the idea that sex is a form of labour carried out at night may stem from this injunction to have regular sex throughout pregnancy. By engaging in sex, men are working both to ensure the health of the foetus and to reinforce its patrilineal identity.

Notwithstanding these requirements to "work at night" for the benefit of the patriline, Punyan Wangi women emphasised that prenatal sex must still be approached with caution since an excess of it may harm the foetus. Sex during pregnancy should not be too frequent, although individual perceptions of what constituted the right level of frequency varied widely. Most women suggested that intercourse should occur at most twice a month, although one woman seemed to think that her average of fifteen times a month was not excessive. For this woman, however, the frequency with which she and her husband had sexual intercourse was always determined by the state of her *bayu*.

A number of women admitted that sex during pregnancy, especially in the late stages, is not particularly appealing to them. Even when their husbands pestered them for sex, they preferred to refrain. Only one woman claimed to find sex enjoyable during pregnancy, but even she found it a bit difficult as time went on.

The belief that sex is not only the precondition for conception but also necessary for continued foetal growth underlines the positive association between sex and foetuses in male ideologies of procreation. In mediating the oppositional relation between blood and foetuses, sex therefore enables men to appropriate female reproductive capacities and to assume progenitive powers far beyond the realm of mere biology.

Pregnant Bodies

While the gross body undergoes the physiological changes associated with each phase of fertility, women subjectively experience these changes through their *bayu* (vitality, life-force). Just as a woman's *bayu* is affected by menstruation, their *bayu* is likewise affected by pregnancy. Thus the terms in which women described the effect of sex upon their *bayu*, as depleting (*oon*) or weakening (*lemet*) it, are reminiscent of their depiction of menstruation, as seen above.

Most women preferred not to be pregnant because they felt uncomfortable and heavy. One woman however, said that she found the feeling of being naked and pregnant enjoyable; another claimed that she felt quite normal throughout pregnancy. But her view of "normal" encompassed a rather depressed level of well-being: her *bayu* was depleted and low, her stomach felt heavy and her body felt constricted (*robed*).

Nonetheless, although only one woman claimed actually to enjoy the physiological condition of pregnancy, Punyan Wangi women continue to fall pregnant, even now when they have the option to avoid it. A veteran of four pregnancies, two of them abortive, explained it in these terms: "It's not that I like being pregnant, but I'm scared not to have children".

Hence where necessary women will override both their personal disinclination for pregnancy, and the social pressures to adopt family planning, in order to reproduce. The possibility of polygynous marriage in some cases compels women not only to have children, but furthermore to produce a male heir in order to achieve long term social security (Jennaway, 1995). While a woman's subjective experiences of blood and foetuses as bodily tolls render these two substances in some ways equivalent, under certain circumstances the positive social benefits attaching to a foetus render it a preferable condition for a woman to be in. But once a woman has established her credentials as a successful childbearer — i.e. by giving birth to a son — the symbolic balance tends to shift back towards a preference for blood (in the sense that menstrual blood implies an absence of foetuses). Ideally, however, women prefer to be neither menstruating nor pregnant, so that they can escape the enervating effects of both menstrual blood and foetuses upon their embodied selves.

CONCLUSION

In this paper I have argued that in North Bali, blood and foetuses are structurally opposed elements within male cultural discourse, the one threatening to male sexuality by its associations of defilement, the other enhancing it by attributing inflated progenitive powers to men: sex is construed as essential for the baby in a woman's belly.

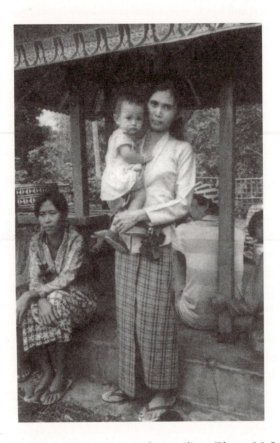

FIGURE 2.2   Sons are important to the patriline. (Photo: M. Jennaway).

Moreover, male social status is augmented by this notional demonstration of paternity, for children are essential in order to perpetuate the patriline. Hence from a male perspective, association with a foetus through the sexual act — not only for conception and subsequent growth but also to remind it of its paternity — is overwhelmingly positive. But association with blood, which represents the negation of all these (male) status affirming associations, is deplored.

Women's attitudes to blood and foetuses are not in accordance with such a cultural construction of these two elements as antagonistic. Inevitably, women's subjective consciousness is imbued by these negative cultural constructions of uterine blood as impure, such that women tend to view their own bodies as not only ritually but also physically unclean whenever blood flows from their wombs. But in some ways, acknowledgment of their impure state can be read as an indifferent concession to the dominant male view: women themselves appear to be more concerned with how they *feel* at such times. What matters to them in relation to fertility is the condition of their "life-force" — their *bayu* — which suffers equally from the imposition of either menstruation or pregnancy. Women's subjective perceptions of the effects of uterine bleeding — amplified by an unsuitable IUD — are virtually the same as that of gestation. Blood and foetuses place a similar tax upon women's wombs: their life-force is compromised, making them tired, listless and sleepy.

In the case of menstruation and pregnancy, women are prepared to accept these felt, bodily effects of fertility as an inevitable part of a woman's lot. However, they are less reconciled to them in the case of IUDs, alternatives to which increasingly are becoming available. Women of Desa Punyan Wangi are beginning to invoke cultural ideologies of harmony and compatibility (*cocok*) in their construction of a counter-discourse in which the IUD is branded as inappropriate or unsuitable (*sing cocok*) for their bodies. In so doing, they obtain exemption from the obligation to use the device, thereby regaining a measure of control over both their reproductive health and their inner vitality.

ACKNOWLEDGMENTS

This paper is based on field research conducted for a Ph.D (Medical Anthropology). I gratefully acknowledge funding provided by an AIDS Postgraduate Research Award (APRA) of the then Department of Health and Community Services and an Australian Award for Research in Asia (Australian Vice-Chancellors' Committee), and from the Tropical Health Program, The University of Queensland. I wish to thank my supervisors Professor Lenore Manderson and Dr Linda Connor for their encouraging comments. Thanks are also due to Dr David Dammery for permission to quote from his unpublished translation of the work of Wolfgang Weck, and my field assistant Ni Ketut Sumenadi for her help and insights.

ENDNOTES

1. The word *bayu* can be translated as "energy", "vitality" (e.g. Wikan, 1989), but it also connotes the "inner self" or "life-force" in the form of usage somewhat equivalent to "soul". However, in the more formal sense of referring to that which is believed to survive a human being after death, soul is better translated as *atma*.
2. This view also underlies biomedicine's approach to the treatment of women's reproductive bodies: seen as an agglomerate of divisible components the female body is therefore dismemberable (Shorter 1984; Manderson 1986:90–101). Bodies, like cars, can be tinkered with, by focussing upon the intimate workings of each separate part, such as the womb, in isolation from the rest.
3. See Lovric (1987:254–6) for a critique of the conventional interpretation of *sebel* as implying simply pollution. Lovric (ibid.) argues that the term *sebel* connotes a fundamental ambiguity: the ascription of *sebel* status to women signifies a recognition of both female power and female danger.
4. Post-partum women are similarly deemed impure; lochial blood is if anything construed as even more defiling than menstrual blood. Several of my female informants, for instance, denounced the lochia as the most impure substance of all.

5. See Connor (1990:353) and Bateson and Mead (1942:7) regarding the symbolic status of the head and the degrees of purity indicated by relative height: Balinese models of the body indicate its tripartite division into head, upper torso and lower body along a gradient of purity.

6. Compare with Duff-Cooper's (1985b) discussion of "disgust" in relation to the twin bodily functions of eating and defecation, wherein he somewhat pedantically argues eating is not considered "disgusting" in Bali. But even by Duff-Cooper's Oxford Dictionary definition, menstrual blood is culturally construed as disgusting.

7. Even in Punyan Wangi, this is beginning to weaken as local youth increasingly are assailed by the pressures of modernisation towards wage-labour, individualism and the progressive loosening of family ties.

8. I could not clearly establish whether it is the number of "strikes" per act of intercourse which counts, or the frequency of coitus.

9. In her history of Indonesia's family planning program (KB: *Keluarga Berencana*), Hurdle (1981:24) distinguishes three main phases: a pronatalist era under President Sukarno (1949-1965); a phase of "tacit approval" (1966–1969) in the early Suharto years; and the period of "total government commitment" to family planning objectives (post-1970). In this latter period the Indonesian government actively sought to redress the population explosion incurred by Sukarno's negative approach to fertility control.

10. To the inventory of factors contributing to the success of family planning in Bali given by Hull (1978), Streatfield (1986) adds the significant fact that the KB program had a higher per capita budget than did any other province. The other factors he cites, such as a higher ratio of clinics and fieldworkers per head of population, and the efficient dissemination of information, through the *banjar* system, would logically flow from this financial amenity. He also attempts to argue that the introduction of the KB program occurred at an "optimal moment" in Balinese history, when the Balinese were reeling with shock in the wake of the 1965 massacre of members of the communist party (PKI: *Partai Komunist Indonesia*). However his presumption that the collective insecurity engendered by these massacres in Bali encouraged the Balinese people willingly to embrace family planning is somewhat dubious.

11. Streatfield (1986:9–10, 153) however prefers not to place too much emphasis on the *banjar* system alone as being the crucial factor in Bali's achieving its outstanding family planning successes because similarly impressive fertility reductions were achieved — without *banjars* — in some parts of Java, particularly in the Yogyakarta region. Yet elsewhere Streatfield concedes that the Balinese *banjars* were "probably the single most important factor" in the program's success after all (1986:153).

12. PUS, lit. meaning "couples of fertile age", is something of a misnomer since it only refers to married couples in which the female partner is aged between 19 and 49 years. Obviously such a definition excludes a large group of fertile adolescent women; women whose fertile phase of life extends into their fifties; and unmarried women of any age. The term PUS has replaced the original English acronym "ELCO" — "eligible couple" — which may have permitted more latitude in its interpretation.

13. Warren (1990:197) provides a counter-example to this alleged collusion between state officialdom and the *banjar* in which a *banjar* head evoked nationalist (*Pancasila*) rhetoric to defend a non-compliant couple.

14. Only Karangasem is lower, with 77% of all fertile couples participating in the program (Bali, BKKBN, 1991).

15. There is no way of testing whether this result is a modern aberration or comparable with past RTI prevalence among Balinese women. The empirical data does not exist for such comparisons. But if this is in fact an increase on the past, it is tempting to attribute it to the manner in which mass IUD insertions were performed throughout Bali without adequate regard to women's prior gynaecological health. Evidence from elsewhere in Bali indicates that the rate of both RTIs and STDs among women is rising (Susanti 1990).

16. Of the 338 women found by Streatfield (1986:122) to have discontinued contraceptive use, 16% had done so because their IUDs had fallen out.

17. More surprising is the fact that this woman is of relatively low socioeconomic status: she was married to a *penyakap* (tenant farmer), had three children, had only had primary school education and lived high up in the hills towards the village's southern boundary. I was unable to ask her what factors had led her to choose Norplant.

REFERENCES

Alexander, J., Alexander, P. (1979) Labour demands and the "involution" of Javanese agriculture. *Social Analysis*, **3**, 22–44.

Bali, Bappeda Tingkat II Buleleng (1990) *Kompilasi Data Pembangunan Desa/Kabupaten di Semua Kecamatan. Kecamatan: Sukasada, Kabupaten: Dati II, Buleleng.* Buleleng, Bali: Bappeda Tingkat II Buleleng.

Bali, Badan Koordinasi Keluarga Berencana Nasional (BKKBN) (1991) *Laporan Hasil Pelaksanaan dan Pencapaian Gerakan Keluarga Berencana Nasional, Propinsi Bali, Bulan Oktober.* Denpasar, Bali: Badan Koordinasi Keluarga Berencana Nasional (BKKBN).

Bateson, G., Mead, M. (1942) *Balinese Character: A Photographic Analysis.* New York: New York Academy of Sciences.

Belo, J. (1970) A study of customs pertaining to twins in Bali [1936]. In *Traditional Balinese Culture*, edited by J. Belo, pp. 3–56. New York: Columbia University Press.

Connor, L. (1982) *In Darkness and in Light: A Study of Peasant Intellectuals in Bali.* Unpublished PhD thesis. Sydney: University of Sydney.

Connor, L. (1990) Seances and spirits of the dead: context and idiom in symbolic healing. *Oceania*, **60**, 345–359.

Covarrubias, M. (1989) *The Island of Bali* [1937]. Singapore: OUP.

Duff-Cooper, A. (1985a) Notes on some Balinese ideas and practices connected with sex from Western Lombok. *Anthropos*, **80**(4–6), 403–419.

Duff-Cooper, A. (1985b) Ethnographic notes on two operations of the body among a community of Balinese on Lombok. *Journal of Anthropological Society of Oxford*, **16**(2), 121–142.

Echols, J., Shadily, H. (1990) *Kamus Indonesia-Inggris* 3rd edn. Jakarta: Penerbit Pt Gramedia.

Geertz, C. and Geertz, H. (1964) Teknonymy in Bali: parenthood, age-grading and geneological amnesia. *Journal of Royal Anthropological Institute*, **94**, 94–106.

Hetler, C.B. (1986) *Female-Headed Households in a Circular Migration Village in Central Java, Indonesia.* Unpublished PhD thesis. Canberra: Australian National University.

Hobart, M. (1980) *Ideas of Identity: The Interpretation of Kinship in Bali.* Denpasar: Udayana University.

Hull, T. (1978) *Where Credit is Due: Policy Implications of the Recent Rapid Fertility Decline in Bali.* Working Paper No. 18. Yogyakarta, Indonesia: Population Institute, Gajah Mada University.

Hull, T. (1991) *Government and Society in Southeast Asian Family Planning Programs: The Cases of Indonesia, Vietnam and the Philippines.* Paper presented at the 1991 Annual Meeting of the Population Association of America. Canberra: Dept. Political and Social Change, Australian National University.

Hull, T., Tukiran (1976) Regional variations in the prevalence of childlessness in Indonesia. *Ethnos,* **6**(32), 1–25.

Hurdle, L. (1981) *The Indonesian Family Planning Programme (1949–1979): A Historical Study.* Unpublished MA thesis. Armidale: University of New England.

Jennaway, M. (1995) *Bitter Honey: Female Polygynous Destinies in North Bali.* Paper presented at the Third Indisciplinary Forum on Indonesian Women's Studies (WIVS) Workshop, Leiden, 25–29 September. The Netherlands: Leiden University.

Jordan, B. (1988) *Birth in Four Cultures: A Cross-cultural Investigation of Childbirth in Yucatan, Holland, Sweden and the United States.* Montreal: Eden Press.

Lovric, B. (1987) *Rhetoric and Reality: The Hidden Nightmare. Myth and Magic as Reverberations and Representations of Morbid Realities.* Unpublished PhD thesis. Sydney: Sydney University.

Macauley, A.P. (1984) *The Cultural Construction of Illness in Bali.* Unpublished PhD thesis. Berkeley: University of California.

Manderson, L. (1986) Edward Shorter and the disembodiment of women's history. *Canberra Anthropology,* **9**(1), 90–101.

Manderson, L. (1987) Hot-cold food and medical theories: overview and introduction. *Social Science and Medicine,* Special Issue, 4(9), 329–330.

Martin, E. (1987) *The Woman in the Body: A Cultural Analysis of Reproduction.* Boston: Beacon Press.

Parker, L. (1993) *Witches, Bees and IUDS: Sexuality and Fertility Control in Bali.* Unpublished paper presented at the State, Sexuality and Reproduction in Asia and the Pacific Conference, Canberra, July 16–18. Canberra: Australian National University.

Patten, J. (1992) *Informed Choice and Reproductive Health: An Investigation of the Extent of Understanding about Contraceptives and the Availability of Information Services among the Residents of Munduk Pakel.* Independent Study Project undertaken under supervision of Dr. Inne Susanti (UNUD, BKKBN), Denpasar, Bali.

Poffenberger, M. (1983) Towards a new understanding of population change in Bali. *Population Studies,* **37**(2), 43–59.

Rahardjo, Y. (1990) *Jamu Peluntur: Traditional Medicine for Menstrual Regulation and Abortion in Indonesia.* Paper presented to the Third International Congress in Traditional Asian Medical Systems, Bombay, January 4–7.

Ruddick, A. (1980) *Charmed Lives: Illness, Healing, Power and Gender in a Balinese Village.* Unpublished PhD thesis. Providence, Rhode Island: Brown University.

Shorter, E. (1984) *A History of Women's Bodies.* London: Pelican.

Spencer, R. (1977) Embryology and obstetrics in pre-industrial society. In *Culture, Disease and Healing: Studies in Medical Anthropology,* edited by D. Landy, pp. 289–299. New York: MacMillan.

Stephens, M. (1986) The childbirth industry: a woman's view. In *Visibility and Power: Essays on Women in Society and Development*, edited by L. Dube, E. Leacock, S. Ardener, pp. 70–84. Delhi: Oxford University Press.

Streatfield, K. (1986) *Fertility Decline in a Traditional Society: The Case of Bali*. Canberra: Department of Demography, Australian National University.

Susanti, I. (1990) *Indonesian Reproductive Tract Infections (RM) Study*. Denpasar, Bali: Proyek Keluarga Berencana Indonesia.

Warren, C. (1986) Indonesian development policy and community organisation in Bali. *Journal of Contemporary South East Asia* **8**, 213–230.

Weck, W. (n.d) *The Folk Medicine and Ethnography of Bali* (translated by D. Dammer). Unpublished manuscript.

Wikan, U. (1989) Illness from fright or soul loss: a North Balinese culture-bound syndrome. *Culture Medicine and Psychiatry*, **13**, 25–50.

Zola, I. (1972) Medicine as an institution of social control. *Sociological Review*, **20**(4), 487–504.

CHAPTER 3

Health Beliefs and the Use of Antenatal Care Among Pregnant Women in Southern Thailand

Sansnee Jirojwong

The goal of the Thai Government today is to increase the use of Maternal and Child Health (MCH) services to reduce perinatal and maternal mortality, and MCH services have been included in a series of National Economic and Social Development Plans. A minimum schedule of antenatal care (ANC) has been defined, according to which a woman should make no less than four visits to an ANC clinic. In addition, she is required to make the first visit by the sixth month of pregnancy. The three subsequent visits should be made on a monthly basis, from the seventh to the ninth month of pregnancy (Thailand, Ministry of Public Health, Family Health Division, 1987; Khamparnya, 1990). By the end of 1990, the government aimed to provide antenatal care to at least 75% of pregnant women. However only 54.5% of pregnant women used ANC services at that time (Niyomwan, 1991), falling considerably short of the national target, confirming an under-utilisation of ANC services, and women who have complications such as high blood pressure or anaemia may not gain benefits from screening procedures. In this chapter I will describe the health beliefs of pregnant women from Southern Thailand and discuss their use of antenatal care, including perceived benefits of ANC and barriers to ANC attendance.[1]

TRADITIONS OF BIRTH

Hmor Tamyae: Traditional Birth Attendant

Thai women hold particular beliefs and follow specific practices relating to pregnancy, birth and the puerperium (Rajadhon, 1961; Hanks, 1963; Muecke, 1976; Noonsuk, 1980; Rice, 1994). These beliefs and practices have been passed on from generation to generation. Women are encouraged by their close family members and other relatives to observe several rules to ensure their health and safety, and that of their infant, throughout pregnancy and delivery.

Traditional Thai medicine is derived from and known locally as Ayurvedic medicine, although it has been influenced by Chinese medicine as well as Sanskrit traditions (Thailand, Ministry of Public Health, 1972; Riley, 1977; Mulholland,

61

1979; Nukoonkit, 1986). The basic principle is that the body is comprised of four basic elements: earth, water, wind and fire; and an imbalance of hot and cold can cause illnesses. The use of herbal medicine, massage, and spiritual ceremony are the primary forms of treatment (Thompson, 1967; Kaetsingha, 1978; Golomb, 1985; Archananuparp, 1988a, 1988b; Whittaker, this volume).

Traditional Thai medicine was dominant until this century. Although, there were contacts between Thailand and western countries such as France, Holland, Spain, England, and Portugal from the 1650s, very little knowledge of biomedicine reached the country until the nineteenth century. The first government hospital, Siriraj Hospital, was opened to the public in April 1887; thereafter, biomedical facilities expanded rapidly. By 1986 three categories of government health care centres were operating under the Ministry of Public Health. These were regional and provincial hospitals, district and community hospitals, and community health centres (Health Association of Thailand, 1987). Obstetrics was the last branch of biomedicine to be adopted by the Thais.

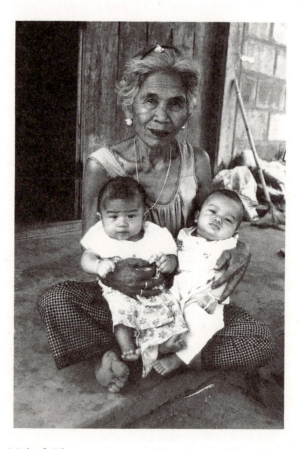

FIGURE 3.1   Midwife Thong nurses two infants she has delivered. (Photo: A. Whittaker).

Prior to the introduction of obstetrics care, *hmor tamyae* (traditional birth attendants — TBAs) played a major role in providing care during the perinatal period. Most TBAs are women who have children and are generally well known within the community. Their role in assisting deliveries has steadily decreased over the years. In 1971 it was estimated that about 64–79% of deliveries were assisted by TBAs; by 1991, this had decreased to 19% (Royston and Ferguson, 1985; Khanjanasthiti, 1986; Niyomwan, 1991).

In many communities, particularly in the South and Central Regions, a woman needs to visit the TBA throughout pregnancy; elsewhere TBAs may be involved only in delivery (Hanks, 1963; Muecke, 1976). When care is sought, the woman visits the TBA during the odd months of pregnancy (i.e. 3, 5, 7) to request her assistance during delivery. Generally a first-time pregnant woman will visit the TBA during the 5th month or the 7th month of pregnancy; a multigravid woman will visit the TBA during the 7th or the 9th month of pregnancy. The timing is crucial since the even number (*khuu*) (e.g. 6th or 8th months of pregnancy) is regarded as a synonym with twins (*khuu* or *faet*). Therefore, visiting a TBA during the even months of pregnancy may result in a twin pregnancy (Noonsuk, 1980).

During the initial visit, the woman is required to make some offerings to the TBA. These vary widely. The minimum items are areca nuts, betel pepper leaves, flowers and 9.00 Baht (US$0.36). Additional items may include palm sugar, cotton, dry grain rice and a coconut. The items are used to pay respect to the TBA and her teacher (*khong hwai khruu*). Before birth takes place, the TBA visits the pregnant woman at her home. If required, she will massage, lift or manipulate the abdomen. Coconut oil is made, blessed by traditional healers or monks, and is applied to the women's abdomen by the TBA or the woman herself during late pregnancy, to ensure an easy birth. The abdominal massage by TBAs may relieve discomfort, detect the baby's position, reposition it if necessary (e.g. if the foetus is transverse or breech), and check the movement of the baby (Fraser, 1966; Noonsuk, 1980). Again, fees for the service vary, from 20.00 Baht (US$0.80) to 100.00 Baht (US$4.00) depending on the TBA's reputation within the community.

A *hmor nuat* or a masseur is also called in to massage the pregnant woman. Her care is needed to relieve muscular discomfort during late pregnancy, but not to assist with deliveries. Malay traditional healers (*bomoh*) may be called by the TBA when spirit-caused illnesses cannot be handled by her (Fraser, 1966).

When birth is expected, the woman's husband or a female relative will call the TBA. She will assess whether the woman is in labour or not. Once labour is established, various ritual ceremonies are conducted by the TBA and the women's husband and relatives to ensure safe birth. The woman will offer a set of goods (*khong hwai khruu*) to pay respect to the TBA. Subsequently the TBA will pray and offer the goods, consisting of betel, pepper leaves, areca nuts and flowers to her teacher. The woman will drink blessed water made by the TBA. The TBA will apply coconut oil on the women's abdomen. All windows and doors are opened to ensure an easy delivery (Hanks, 1963). During labour, the TBA will pray, massage and reassure the woman. Female relatives or the woman's husband provide additional help, such as giving emotional support and encouragement, and provide practical help by offering the woman damp face washers or drinking water (Muecke, 1976).

After birth, the TBA will make an offering (*tang raad*) to her teacher to ensure that the woman and her newborn child will be healthy. The minimum required items are similar to *khong hwai khruu* in addition to dry grain rice and the fee. If a male child is born, a book and a pencil will be added. If a female child is born, a needle and a thread of cotton will be added.

As elsewhere in Thailand and in neighbouring Malaysia, the TBA will assist the mother to lie by the fire (*yuu fai*) (see also chapters by Whittaker, and Chirawatkul, this volume; cf. *ang pleung*, Townsend and Rice, this volume). This will help the blood and wind of the woman to return to their pre-pregnancy state, and to reduce muscle pain or weakness during and after middle age. Stones will be put on a fire; a heated stone will be wrapped with thick clothes and placed on the woman's abdomen; once cool, it will be replaced with a new hot stone. Three stones may be used to ensure a continual supply of heat. The application of hot stones on the woman's abodomen is aimed at ensuring that the woman's womb will descend into her pelvis. This is believed to take around nine days for a first time mother or a mother who has given birth to twins; a multigravid mother will require only five or seven days by the fire. Once the *yuu fai* is completed, a short ceremony is performed (*sabaad raad*). The TBA will visit the woman every day. She will mix herbs such as tamarind leaves with warm water and assist the woman to have a warm shower with this mixture. The TBA will bathe a newborn baby for three days or more and, if necessary, she will cook and look after older children. She will visit the child again when the umbilical cord is detached; the cord will be burnt and its ash will be mixed with water. Later, the child will drink it to ensure its future health.

Ritual and ceremonial behaviours of Malay Thais are slightly different. Neither the woman's husband nor other men are allowed in the house. Birth is handled by a traditional birth attendant (*bidan*), but a male traditional healer (*bomoh*) may be called to resolve births made difficult by supernatural agencies or spirits (Fraser, 1966; Manderson, 1981a; Laderman, 1987).

Beliefs and Practices during Pregnancy

More than 95% of Thais are Buddhists, who believe that life does not begin with birth and end with death, but is linked in a chain, each event conditioned by volitional acts (*kam* or *karma*) committed in a previous existence (Hanks, 1963; Noonsuk, 1980; Mahamakut Rajvitayalai, 1982). The success of conception is a consequence of the parents' acts. Both parents need to be aware of the consequences of daily life so that their good actions will result in healthy and safe births.

Giving birth is seen as a critical time for women. The chance of dying during birth is deemed to be equally as high as that for men going to war. This perception has undoubtedly influenced pregnant women's behaviour to ensure that they and their unborn child survive. It is very important for pregnant women to act cautiously and there are numerous suggestions of what is permissible and what is not. Some behaviour is prescribed to ensure easy birth. For example, a woman should not stop working, but should remain active in daily household activities; she should not eat too much and gain too much weight. In addition, she should not kill animals lest the baby be deformed; she should not take showers after dark lest she have too much amniotic fluid or water (*faet nam*); and she should not jump, fall, or walk briskly to avoid injury or miscarriage (Noonsuk, 1980).

A number of foods are prescribed during pregnancy to ensure a good looking baby. Coconut juice and papaya will help a baby have fair complexion. Palm sugar will make beautiful eyes. Food with names similar to "easy", "slippery", "flowing" are recommended, such as sweet potato (*hua man* or oily bulb), fresh water eel (*pla hlai* or flowing fish), and sago (*saa khuu*, which has slippery consistency). Twin fruits such as bananas are prohibited since they may cause a twin pregnancy. A few women also believe that durian can produce heat and may cause a miscarriage; hence it is also avoided (cf. Manderson, 1981b).

The Use of Preventive Health Measures and Illness Behaviours

As noted, use of antenatal services in Southern Thailand falls below the national target, despite the fact that such care may detect abnormalities early, provide treatment and prevent complications. If properly provided, ANC can improve maternal and child health outcomes (Caldwell, 1981; Mosley and Chen, 1984), and screening procedures, particularly among high risk pregnant women, are likely to reduce maternal and child deaths. The Thai Government has devised MCH policies to increase the coverage of ANC services (Thailand, Ministry of Public Health, Family Health Division, 1987; Khamparnya, 1990).

During pregnancy, women seek care from both biomedical and traditional care givers. For example, one study conducted in two major hospitals showed that about 60% of women received care from biomedical caregivers; 32% to 35% sought care from both biomedical caregivers and TBAs (Jirojwong and Skolnik, 1990). Most births are at hospitals; in Ratapoom, in Southern Thailand, 13% were at home and 87% were in hospitals in 1994. The majority of home births are likely to be attended by TBAs (Jirojwong and Skolnik, 1991; Begum, Seguerra and Hasan, 1994).

The Health Belief Model is a useful paradigm for investigating factors which influence the use of ANC clinics, although its main application has been to explain the use of preventive health measures such as the testing or prevention of tuberculosis, cervical cancer, dental disease, rheumatic fever, polio, and influenza (Rosenstock, 1974; Rosenblum, Stone and Skipper, 1981). Rosenstock's model (1974:330) proposed that for an individual to take action to avoid a disease, she or he needed to believe (1) that she/he was personally susceptible to it, (2) that the occurrence of the disease would have at least moderate severity on some component of her or his life, and (3) that taking a particular action would be beneficial by reducing susceptibility to the condition. If the disease occurred, the action would need to be regarded as beneficial in reducing its severity, and would not involve major barriers such as cost, convenience, pain or embarrassment. With respect to taking a test for early detection of a disease, the same factors were deemed necessary. But in addition, compliance involved the individual believing that she or he could have the disease even in the absence of symptoms.[2]

One issue to be considered when applying this model to antenatal care is the degree to which pregnancy is regarded as a healthy state rather than a risk for illness. Two general arguments are used to construct pregnancy: the first formalises reproduction, since most pregnancies and deliveries are normal; the second is that a small proportion of women have complications in pregnancy or delivery and these women constitute an "at risk" group. The concept of risk has lead to the introduction of several diagnostic techniques, algorithms and technologies to prevent morbidity and mortality of both mothers and infants. Pregnancy in this context is considered to be an illness, as if and treated as such.

The first approach uses a social-medical paradigm to argue that pregnant women did not act out sick roles in normal pregnancy (McKinlay, 1972), while Hern (1975) used the biomedical model to explain pregnancy as an illness, based on a small proportion of women who have a complicated pregnancy or delivery. Both these approaches begin from the biomedical model, however, in contrast to ethnographic accounts of pregnancy and birth (e.g. Kay, 1982; MacCormack, 1982) which insist on the cultural and personal perceptions of pregnancy, in which notions of "pregnancy-as-illness" are largely absent.

McKinlay (1972) has used his understanding of sick roles to insist on the "normalness" of pregnancy. He argues that pregnancy is different from illnesses in western society, based on behaviour exhibited when people get sick or are in a sick role, since pregnant women do not follow the four expectations of a sick role. These are: the sick person is exempt from the performance of normal social role obligations and responsibility for his/her own state; they must be motivated to get well as soon as possible; they should seek technically competent help; and they should cooperate with medical experts. McKinlay has been criticised because he did not include abnormal pregnancies or deliveries in this description; Hern (1975), in contrast, argued strongly that pregnancy was an illness, and that pregnant women required medical supervision. He defined pregnancy as an "episodic" and "moderately extended chronic condition" with definable mortality risk, changes and complications. The biomedical model was used in order to describe the illness parameters of pregnancy in relation to its etiology, pathogenesis, pathophysiology, clinical manifestations, laboratory findings, complications, differential diagnosis, treatment, prognosis, epidemiology, and behavioural aspects, including issues of induced abortions and preventability of pregnancy.

Thai women's perceptions differ markedly from these biomedical understandings (Rajadhon, 1961; Hanks, 1963; Muecke, 1976; Fraser, 1966; Noonsuk, 1980). Pregnant women maintain certain behavioural patterns in order to avoid "risks" to their health or their babies' health, as described above, but the prescriptions and proscriptions of pregnancy and birth treat these as extraordinary life events rather than illness. In consequence, women's perceptions of risk during pregnancy are not concordant with those of obstetricians, or of staff of antenatal services. This may explain at least some of women's disinterest in presenting for antenatal care.

THE STUDY

Study Design

A prospective study was conducted in Hatyai in Southern Thailand, 1990–1991. Pregnant women who made an initial ANC visit at three hospitals were approached and invited to participate in the study, and subsequently, interviews were conducted in homes by the author. Women's responses to questions were recorded on a designed interview schedule, which included both open-ended and closed-ended questions. The studies of Boonyanurak (1985) and Zweig, LeFevre and Kruse (1988) were used as guides in designing the questions. Five symptoms were selected in order to assess women's perceptions regarding their susceptibility to complications of pregnancy and birth, their ability to recognise signs of complications, the signs and symptoms of abnormal, and the benefits of ANC to prevent or cure the complications. The symptoms selected those which are as routinely and widely recognised as symptoms of normal pregnancy, such as nausea and vomiting, and swollen feet not higher than the ankles, and three symptoms which might require monitoring: vaginal bleeding, no intrauterine movement of an infant for two days, and abdominal pain before the ninth month of pregnancy. The symptoms were chosen to provide a wide range of symptoms from less to more harmful symptoms to mother or the baby's health, and distinguish between "normal" signs in the Thai context, and "abnormal" symptoms following biomedical approaches to pregnancy. Examples of questions are given in Appendix 3.1.

The three hospitals, Hatyai Hospital, Songkla Nagarind Hospital and Moon Nithi Mitraparp-samarkki Hospital, were selected for the recruitment of women into the study; at least 65.5% of pregnant women living in Hatyai sought care from these hospitals (Jirojwong and Skolnik, 1991). Two hundred and forty-eight pregnant women who made their first ANC visit at the hospitals were approached and invited to participate in the study. The first in-depth interview concerning health beliefs was conducted within seven days of the initial meeting. Two hundred and three women were interviewed. Data regarding the use of ANC clinics and TBAs were collected during the second interview, which was conducted within 6 weeks of giving birth. Only 177 women were able to participate; the major reason for non-participation being that the women had moved to other places.

PROFILE OF RESPONDENTS

Demographic and obstetric characteristics of the women and their spouses are presented in Table 3.1. The majority of women (62.1%) were 20-29 years of age,

TABLE 3.1   Personal characteristics of the women and their spouses.

Characteristics	Number	%
Maternal age (years) (average = 24.5 years)		
≤19	43	21.2
20–24	67	33.0
25–29	59	29.1
30–34	23	11.3
≥35	11	5.4
Number of pregnancy		
First time	82	40.4
Second time	65	32.0
Third time	39	19.2
Fourth time	12	5.9
Fifth time or more	5	2.5
Mothers' occupations		
Government officer	9	4.4
Trader	16	7.9
Employee	42	20.7
Home maker	29	14.3
Agriculture, land owner	21	10.3
Agriculture, labourer	86	42.4
Mothers' levels of education		
Primary level or lower	73	36.0
Secondary level	71	35.5
Grade 10	25	12.3
High school or equivalent	21	10.3
College graduate or equivalent	13	6.4
Husbands' age (years) (average = 28.4 years)		
≤19	11	5.6
20–24	56	27.6
25–29	68	33.5
30–34	39	19.2
≥35	29	14.3
Husbands' occupations		
Government officer	24	11.8
Trader	20	9.9
Employee	115	56.7
Agriculture, land owner	25	12.3
Agriculture, labourer	13	6.4
Unemployed and others	6	3.0
Husbands' levels of education		
Primary level or lower	53	26.1
Secondary level	49	24.1
Grade 10	45	22.1
High school or equivalent	39	19.2
College graduate or equivalent	11	5.4
Did not know	6	3.0

Total percentage is not equal to 100 due to rounding.

and only 5% were older than 34 years. The average age of women was 24.5 years. Forty percent of women were pregnant for the first time; only 2.5% were pregnant for the fifth or more time.

Consistence with the greater number of Muslims in southern Thailand compared with elsewhere in the country, 11% of the study sample were Muslims, while 88% were Buddhist and the remainder Christian or Hindu. About 53% of women were living in rural areas, defined as outside the municipality and development areas (*sukhaa-phibaan*). All women had received at least one year of formal education; 36% had completed the primary level of education or lower. About half the women (52.7%) were employed in the agricultural sector as land owners, labourers, or peasants; only 4.4% were government officers.

Eighty percent of spouses were aged 20–34 years. The majority (56.7%) were employees and engaged in the construction sector, were shop attendants, or were working in factories. Only 18.7% of spouses were engaged in agriculture as land owners or labourers. All spouses had at least one year of formal education. An average monthly family income was 4,623 Baht (approx. US$185).

Compared to national data and data from the Southern Region as a whole (Boonyanurak, 1985; Suwanwela and Sookthomya, 1988; Pimchaipong, Theepswang and Krisevatana, 1988; Pongnikorn, 1989), the women studied were more highly educated and a higher percentage were pregnant for the first time, but they had a similar monthly family income to other Thai families. It should be noted that there was a lower percentage of Muslims among the women studied compared to the province as a whole.

CAUSES OF THE SYMPTOMS: WOMEN'S PERCEPTIONS

Women perceived the causes of symptoms differently. A wide range of causes could be categorised into five major groups: those caused by the state of pregnancy, by the infant, by the woman's own actions, by heredity, and from other causes.

A number of symptoms are considered to be normal to pregnancy. Most of the women perceived that nausea and vomiting were usual, announcing to other people that a women is pregnant. This is quite important for the first time pregnant woman: "How could others know that you are pregnant if you don't vomit? It is a part of pregnancy". Swollen feet not higher than the ankles was also considered normal and having swollen feet three times during late pregnancy indicated that a woman was approaching delivery. Some women also perceived that vaginal bleeding, cessation of foetal movement for two days, and abdominal pain before the ninth month of pregnancy were normal. Vaginal bleeding indicated that maternal blood was washing the infant's face, after which the blood would pass through the vagina, or it might be considered as an indication that the woman would have a difficult, prolonged and painful labour. In contrast, amniotic fluid loss before delivery was understood to indicate an easy delivery.

The second cause of symptoms is the infant itself. Women referred this condition as *pheetdehk* or *aa-pheetdehk*. *Pheetdehk* is closely linked with nausea and vomiting and swollen feet not higher than the ankle. One woman explained that:

> It is because of *pheetdehk*. Different pregnancies will produce different symptoms. It's because of the baby. Last one I did not have any nausea, but with this one I did. If it is simply because of pregnancy, I should have the same symptoms during every pregnancy. When the pregnancy is more than three months, it [nausea] will be over by itself.

The third cause is related to maternal attributes or activities. Maternal activities of an extreme or unusual scale, such as eating too much, not having enough to eat or having an accident, can cause the infant to stop moving. This symptom is seen as normal since an infant may be tired and want to rest. The woman would then wait and see. The period of waiting may last a few days or even weeks.

> When you eat too much or are too full, the baby also will be full. Then he [the baby] will sleep and not move.
>
> If you are hungry or working too much. Like me, I collect rice on the farm all day, never stop, until late [in the day]. Baby will be very tired and stop moving.
>
> I fell off the bike when I was nine months pregnant. The baby did not move for a few days. My mother and neighbours said that the baby was frightened so she did not move.

Women's activities such as working too hard, being unhealthy, not being careful in daily activities, or lifting heavy things, can also cause vaginal bleeding. Women who stay in one position for too long, are not physically fit, or are too fat, may suffer from swollen feet, and women believe that city women are likely to have swollen feet since they have a comfortable life, do not work hard, and tend to stay in one position for "too long".

A woman's previous behaviour, such as trying to induce an abortion in a previous pregnancy, can cause a spontaneous abortion in the current pregnancy and loss of the child. It is seen as *kam* or a punishment because of their previous actions. In addition, either parent may be regarded as being *phii súa* or a demon, because of the date and time of their own birth, and this can cause vaginal bleeding and subsequent abortion. *Phii súa* is a spirit that takes its own children. Magic healers (*hmor weetmon* or *bomoh*) can perform a spiritual ceremony to ward off the demon, as a result of which the woman will have a successful pregnancy.

A woman who may have experienced a preterm birth in the past may have the same symptoms during a subsequent pregnancy. Similarly, swollen feet and vaginal bleeding may recur in subsequent pregnancies. Symptoms may also be caused by heredity. If a woman's mother, sister or close relatives experienced abdominal pain before the ninth month of pregnancy or vaginal bleeding, or if the baby had ceased moving for two days, it is also likely that the woman herself will develop these symptoms during pregnancy. Women also believe that if their spouses are promiscuous, they may develop vaginal bleeding during their pregnancy.

SUSCEPTIBILITY TO AND SEVERITY OF SYMPTOMS

The chances of women developing a symptom depends on the perceived causes and the evaluation of their conditions. When symptoms such as nausea, vomiting and swollen feet are perceived as "normal" or as a part of being pregnant, a higher percentage of women say that they have a chance of developing the symptoms. When the symptoms are caused by abnormal circumstances such as hard work or heredity, women rate their chances of having symptoms as low — from not having them at all, to probably having them.

Women mentioned strategies they used to ensure that they would have a normal pregnancy. These include being careful when conducting activities, seeking help from a traditional healer or attending ANC clinics.

> I don't think that anything will happen to me. I am very careful....very careful. Even when I defecate (woman, aged 32, 2nd pregnancy).
>
> When I first knew that I was pregnant, my elder son told me to go to a [ANC] clinic. He said I might have a mentally retarded child. He is in high school now. He knows a lot. I was scared so I went to the hospital very early [in my pregnancy]. How would I have problems again? I intend to go (to the hospital) as requested [by nurses or doctors] (woman, aged 40, 4th pregnancy).

Table 3.2 summarises the percentage of women who perceive that they are likely to develop the five symptoms. They range from 38.2% for nausea and vomiting to 13.8% for baby not moving for two days.

Although some symptoms were perceived as natural by some women, most of them expressed concerns when they had vaginal bleeding or when their unborn baby stopped moving for two days. They mentioned fear, anxiety and frustration since the symptoms could lead to the death of the babies or themselves. Vaginal bleeding could be severe and cause abortion or early delivery. Babies ceasing to move would cause concern if the symptom was prolonged. Table 3.3 shows the percentage of women who expressed their concern if they developed any of the five symptoms.

Concern does not necessarily lead to a woman seeking help from health professionals, and there is a wide range of responses if symptoms develop. Women may do nothing, treat themselves, rest, seek help from traditional caregivers, or seek advice from relatives or friends. Some women will simply "wait and see".

Seeking help from the biomedical system does not necessarily mean that treatment is being sought. Women may only need reassurance. They may go to the ANC clinic for an appointment and let doctors or nurses detect abnormalities. As one woman put it: "I will go to the clinic for the appointment. They [doctors or nurses] would see if I have swollen feet. If they don't say anything, it means I am all right" (woman, aged 23, 3rd pregnancy). Some women seek help from doctors whenever they experienced abnormal symptoms: "I will go there [hospital]. Whatever happens [to me], I will go there. I have had ANC already. I am scared. Tell them [doctors]. If they say it is all right, then I will be happy" (woman,

TABLE 3.2   Symptoms anticipated during pregnancy.

Symptoms	Perceived chance (%)
Nausea and vomiting	38.2
Swollen feet not higher than the ankles	22.1
Vaginal bleeding	18.3
Baby stopped moving for two days	13.8
Abdominal pain before ninth month of pregnancy	19.7

TABLE 3.3   Concern about symptoms compared to willingness to seek biomedical help.

Symptoms	Women who would be worried (%)	Women who would seek help from biomedical care givers (%)
Nausea and vomiting	34.5	16.4
Swollen feet not higher than the ankles	33.5	30.5
Vaginal bleeding	85.2	68.5
Baby stops moving for two days	79.8	61.6
Abdominal pain before ninth month of pregnancy	72.9	64.0

TABLE 3.4   Perceptions of doctors' and nurses' ability to prevent or cure symptoms.

Symptoms	Preventable (%)	Curable (%)
Nausea and vomiting	9.1	52.7
Swollen feet not higher than the ankles	3.0	24.6
Vaginal bleeding	36.9	72.4
Baby stops moving for two days	31.5	64.5
Abdominal pain before ninth month of pregnancy	25.6	53.3

aged 19, 1st pregnancy). Some women use herbal medicine such as tiger balm, or blessed holy water from Buddhist temples. Combinations of treatments were also used.

One woman said that she would respond to the baby ceasing to move for two days:

> I would wait for a week. See whether it [the baby] will move or not. My aunt said sometimes baby is tired and rest. If it does not move [after one week] I will see a grandmother [TBA] to let her touch my tummy. She will know whether there is anything wrong with the baby or not. If she says go to see doctors, I will go to the hospital.

Some women believe that the symptoms cannot be treated, particularly abdominal pain before the ninth month of pregnancy, and would take no action. They would regard the symptom as a sign of being in labour, and believed that nothing could be done to stop delivery, and that doctors or nurses could only provide treatments or assistance after the delivery. Percentages of women who would seek help from biomedical personnel when they experienced the symptoms are included in Table 3.4.

USE OF ANTENATAL SERVICES

Less than half of the women studied (47%) conformed to the ANC schedule recommended by the Thai Government (i.e. four visits). Among those who did not conform, 56% made their first visit before the 6th month of pregnancy but did not complete the subsequent three visits. Forty-four percent made the first visit after the 6th month of pregnancy; 57% of women attended one ANC clinic only. A small proportion, 8.5%, went to three or more ANC clinics.

Women sought care for minor ailments such as nausea, dizziness or headaches at various health centres, including private health clinics, community health centres and hospitals. In addition, during pregnancy, more than one third of the women studied (37%) sought care from at least one traditional caregiver, among whom 77% received care from TBAs and 23% sought care from masseurs. The most common reason was to have massage and abdominal manipulation (*taeng thong*) to relieve physical discomfort. About 32% wanted reassurance that they and their babies were safe and healthy; only 16% mentioned receiving care from traditional caregivers to ensure an easy birth.

A number of women perceive that they or their spouses had a responsibility to prevent or cure symptoms. Traditional caregivers play some role in preventing or curing the symptoms. This includes spiritual performance to ward off a demon which may cause repeated abortion, or drinking blessed water to cure severe vomiting. Herbal medicines are also used, e.g. *yahorm* and *yadom* for nausea and *yahmong* and *namman-nuat* for swollen feet. A piece of blessed areca nut can be eaten to cure severe vomiting. Family members are consulted to ensure that no "potent or strong" medicines are eaten, as they may harm the woman or an unborn child, and medicines prescribed by a doctor to treat other symptoms, such as stomach pain or headache, may not be taken if the woman or her relatives evaluate them as "too strong".

Women's perceptions of the ability of doctors or nurses to prevent or cure varied. Some felt that doctors had the ability and knowledge to prevent or cure many symptoms, and had numerous medications to treat health problems; others felt they were unable to prevent or cure any symptoms. Although some symptoms are considered to be normal for pregnant women, particularly nausea and vomiting, most women believed that doctors or nurses can do something to stop the symptom (Table 3.4). Other women simply had confidence in doctors' ability and efficiency of curative measures: "Nowadays doctors are competent. They have good medicines.

They inject, give drip. They operate. They can do everything. They can help" (woman, aged 37, 6th pregnancy).

Technologies available at and after birth, such as the incubation of premature babies, the dilation of the cervix, and curettage of the uterus after abortion, were also perceived as curative aspects of care. Percentages of women who perceived that the symptoms were preventable or curable by doctors or nurses is shown in Table 3.4 above. Those who perceived that symptoms could not be prevented or cured biomedically held these beliefs in association with the causes of the symptoms. If a problem was "natural", such as nausea and vomiting, swollen feet, or pain, it was unlikely to be preventable: "If [I] have abdominal pain, it tells that [I] will be giving birth. If it [the baby] is going to be born, it will. You can't stop it. Don't have to prevent it" (woman, aged 40, 4th pregnancy). A number of women explained that swollen feet could be prevented by their own actions, such as raising their feet, using bandages to wrap around their feet and ankles, or not standing or sitting in one position for too long. They could also prevent vaginal bleeding by taking precautions in daily activities, not carrying heavy things, and not eating spicy or hot chilli food. Traditional forms of prevention such as having traditional birth attendants massage or manipulate their uterus (taeng kun), or having a traditional healer perform ritual ceremonies, could also prevent vaginal bleeding or a baby not moving for two days.

To assess women's perceptions of the benefits of ANC, women were asked to describe how antenatal care could help them and their babies. More than half of the women mentioned that attending ANC ensured the safety of both women and their babies; that women would be cared for by doctors; that doctors could detect their or their babies' abnormalities; that help could be given in time if this were the case; and that therapeutic abortions could be undertaken if necessary. Medication and medical technology were seen to be beneficial to their own and their infants' physical health. Attending an antenatal clinic would enable them to get proper medication if indicated, to get vitamins, to have physical check ups, blood tests, and injections, particularly tetanus toxoid. Some women said that having a blood test would enable them to know, too, whether they had a sexually transmitted disease. Attending ANC indicated their love for their unborn baby. Any vaccines they received would be transmitted to their babies: "Going there to [ANC] is good. I can get an injection, they said to prevent tetanus. I love my baby. Anyone who loves their baby has to have ANC." Thirty-one percent of women also perceived that ANC provided psychological benefits. It reassured them that they and their babies were healthy. They said that they were happy after attending a clinic and that they gained confidence in their pregnancies and outcomes. A small percentage of women (22.7%) also perceived the benefits of ANC as providing additional knowledge. They would be able to ask questions of health caregivers and to receive suggestions, to identify the expected date of delivery, and to be informed about their own and their babies' health.

However, 30% of women perceived that ANC only helped them in labour. They believed that attending a clinic would shorten the process of being admitted to a delivery room, or save relatives providing a history of the pregnant women's health at the time of admission. Some women said that attending ANC would prevent them from being blamed by health care personnel for not taking adequate care of themselves or their babies. These responses reflect women's negative attitude towards health care personnel in delivery rooms. Most hospitals in Thailand do not allow women's spouses or relatives to be with them during labour. The women are taken care of by nurses, midwives or obstetricians, and a number who had not attended any ANC but had delivered in hospital were dissatisfied with the quality of care (see Rice and Manderson, this volume). Some were reprimanded by health care staff for not attending antenatal clinics, and some felt consequently that they were not taken care of properly or appropriately when giving birth. Information from this group of women is passed to others and sets a precedent in which pregnant women perceive that lack of ANC attendance is associated with being scolded or reprimanded by health care personnel. A woman in her third pregnancy said:

> I want to have the delivery in a hospital. No one around here [TBAs] can help in delivery any more. They are too old, cannot see. Having delivery in hospital, I need to go to the [ANC] clinic. Otherwise, they [nurses] won't take care of me when I am in pain. Many women said sometimes they [the women] were left to deliver on their own. No one cared. Sometimes [we] were scolded: why didn't we have the [antenatal] care? I am scared of having to give birth alone.

BARRIERS TO ATTENDING ANTENATAL CARE

Women are required to make a number of ANC visits before giving birth. The number of visits is increased if they make the first visit during early pregnancy. As one elderly woman commented: "Now they [pregnant women] go to [ANC] clinics. During my time, we didn't have to. When we were pregnant, we'd just have a baby. No [ANC] care. *Hmor tamyae* massaged us if we were uncomfortable. Unlike now, [pregnant] women go to [ANC] clinics lots and lots of time, every month. Once a month".

The number of ANC visits required was seen as problematic. Some women did not have anyone to take care of their older children at home, others felt they could not stop working on the farm, where every worker was important. During early pregnancy, some women were too ill to travel. Others indicated that their health was satisfactory and they did not require care from doctors or nurses. Many women attend ANC only during their late pregnancy, for several reasons. In early pregnancy the conceptus is visualised only as a lump of blood, not a human being, therefore not in need of care. Signs of life, foetal movement or palpable foetal parts need to be recognised by the women before the first ANC visit is initiated. Further, health personnel do not provide much information about the baby's condition. Women may make the first visit after the fifth month of pregnancy.

Younger women, particularly, did not present at all to a hospital where antenatal care was available. The hospital environment and its bureaucratic processes were alien to them and they needed companions, such as their mother or other women, who had similar experiences, to go with them. This meant that at least two people needed to leave their home and work in order to attend the clinic. This problem increased with travelling time and costs.

An older group of women said that during their previous pregnancies, they had their first ANC visits later, in the 7th or 9th month of pregnancy, for various reasons. These were, that the baby was large and palpable, that there was no need to make "too many" ANC visits, and that the first visit had to be made during an odd month of pregnancy. The same patterns were repeated with subsequent pregnancies. Few women also mentioned that they did not have the money to cover expenses to attend ANC, for example, travel costs and food expenses. Some women mentioned that they were tired of waiting at hospitals and that they did not want to get up early to visit the clinics. Some women said that muddy roads and the difficulty of getting public transport during the rainy season would also stop them from travelling from home to the hospital. After the initial visit, 32.0% of women anticipated problems in attending again. These included having no money and having to work. Women also felt that because they were in good health, future visits were not necessary. Some women did not have social support, e.g. having someone to accompany them to the clinics, or to care for older children, or they had moved and attended clinics at other hospitals.

DISCUSSION AND IMPLICATIONS

Women's perceptions of susceptibility to and severity of illnesses during pregnancy need to be discussed in the context of Thai society and culture. Many studies have shown that people in various communities, both in industrialised and less industrialised countries, hold different perceptions of health and illness (Zola, 1973; Fabrega, 1974; Mechanic, 1974; Kleinman, 1980; Gray, 1985; Morgan, Calnan and Manning, 1985), and these do not necessarily extend to bodily processes such as menstruation, pregnancy, birth or menopause. These perceptions influence women's health care behaviour, which might range from caring for themselves, seeking care from traditional healers, seeking advice from others or seeking biomedical care, depending on changes in general health and contextual and situational factors.

The present study express such differences in pregnancy. Using five hypothetical symptoms, women were found to take a range of actions for the same symptoms. They might, for example, rest, care for themselves, use herbal medicine, seek care from traditional healers, or seek care from biomedical staff, depending on beliefs about the causes of each symptom. Nature, personal predisposition as a result of previous actions (*kam*), health status prior to pregnancy, activities, or merely personal status, may cause unusual symptoms.

The implications of these findings in public health are important since women's beliefs may have a bearing on delays in seeking help from health personnel. Studies in Thailand have shown that the majority of stillborn infants were macerated stillbirths, the condition of long term deaths (Prasartwanakit and Ratanapreuksachat, 1989; Toongsuwand and Suvonnakote, 1983; Suthipintawong and Tangpoonphonvivat, 1984). Babies moving less or the cessation of babies' movement is a good warning symptom of the death of infants (Hall and Chng, 1982). Due to their understanding of the significance of lack of movement however, women may wait for a long period before they visit a hospital. Sometimes it can be too late to save the pregnancy.

Not all beliefs are negative, of course. Women believe that when pregnant, they should avoid stress and refrain from alcohol, tobacco or similar substances: these encourage the concept of a healthy baby and are in line with biomedical advice. Belief in *kam* also plays a strong role in explaining not only their own behaviours but that of their spouses, as a way of minimising actions which might have a negative effect on the baby.

There is no restriction on the type of health care centre and the number of clinics which women can use during their pregnancies. They can continue to receive care from one sector during their pregnancy up to their delivery, or they can receive ANC from the private sector and deliver in public hospitals, or vice versa. A number of women visit more than one ANC clinic during their pregnancy, and the availability of biomedical personnel and medical technology may influence their decision to seek care in a hospital (Begum, Seguerra and Hasan, 1994).

Most field research studies mention problems such as distance, lack of finances or lack of help. These problems are particularly noticeable in terms of the initial visit. All of these factors point to a need to underscore the importance of pregnancy care offered by a nearby community health centre or private clinic as a prerequisite to later visits to hospitals. Some women are able to anticipate their problems in attending the clinics and it is suggested that avenues be opened to enable women to discuss appropriate solutions. It is also necessary for health caregivers to identify women who have problems at the time of their first visit, since it is found that the majority of those who do not conform to the schedule are those who attend an early appointment but fail to attend later appointments.

Some of the women in this study are from rural areas where there are community health centres, and normal pregnant women can attend such clinics. A formalised arrangement between hospitals and the community health centres can be established for high risk pregnant women. The program can be arranged in such a way that women attend community health centres for most of their pregnancy with occasional visits only to hospitals for initial risk assessment, standard pathology investigations, and for a final check-up prior to delivery. For some women this might reduce the problems of travelling, which has proven to be a barrier to attending ANC (see also Begun, Seguerra and Hasan, 1994).

About one third of women receive care from TBAs or masseurs. A number of studies in Thailand have indicated that TBAs provide good care to women during pregnancy, delivery, and postpartum (Boorapatt, Archeepsamoot, Saiyhudthong and Srisiri, 1986; Jirojwong, 1989; Songkhla Provincial Office, 1989; Jirojwong and Skolnik, 1991; Begum, Seguerra and Hasan, 1994). Available health care resources within communities need to be utilised. An existing training program for TBAs conducted by the Ministry of Public Health is likely to provide benefits to pregnant women. Regular supervision and recognition of TBAs by the government is seen as a positive approach.

This study indicates that women are more likely to receive benefits of ANC in terms of curative aspects rather than preventive aspects. Two factors are of importance here. The first is that an increasing number of women have given birth in hospitals over the past few decades (Thailand, Ministry of Public Health, 1980; Niyomwan, 1991) and this accounts for a decrease in the number of maternal deaths in the country (Muecke, 1976). This leads to an increasing proportion of women who have been exposed to curative biomedicine including obstetric care. In addition, an increase in the use of medical interventions, including operative obstetrics, has reduced the incidence of morbidity and mortality of mothers and of babies (Prasartwanakit and Ratanapreuksachat, 1989; Koranantakul, Jinorose, Akara-winek and Pinjaroen, 1990; Department of Obstetrics and Gynaecology, 1991). Exposure to the benefits of curative aspects of care during delivery, and the increasing use of technology during pregnancy and delivery, such as sonographs and operative delivery (caesarean sections), may have an indirect effect on women's perceptions of care during pregnancy.

ACKNOWLEDGMENTS

This study could not have been achieved without the support of Michael Skolnik. He has now completed one circle of life: "birth, ageing, illness and death". Because of his good *karma* in this life, he will be born again as a healthy and happy human being. I dedicate this paper to him.

ENDNOTES

1. Biomedical obstetric care was known in Thailand from the late nineteenth century, but the first recorded delivery of a birth in the royal family assisted by a biomedical trained doctor, Dr. Peter Gowan, took place only in 1967 (Nukoonkit, 1986). Home birth was regarded as the norm until the late 1970s. In 1971, about 11% of births were attended by biomedically trained health care personnel such as doctors, nurses, midwives or trained traditional birth attendants (TBAs) (Thailand, Ministry of Public Health, 1980).

2. Another variable which has been included in the model is a cue or trigger for appropriate action. Cues can be internal, such as perception of body states, or external, such as interpersonal interactions, the impact of media, or receiving a reminder card from a health care provider. Demographic, psycho-social and structural variables were also included in the model. However, only four HBM variables; susceptibility to illnesses, severity of the illnesses, barriers to attending ANC, and the benefits of ANC, will be discussed in this chapter.

APPENDIX 3.1: Samples of the questions used.

HBM Variable Assessed	Sample of Questions
Susceptibility to the illness	How much chance was there that you could have had swollen feet not higher than the ankles during your present pregnancy?
Severity of the illness	(a) If you had swollen feet during your pregnancy, how worried do you think you would be about it? (b) If you had swollen feet not higher than the ankles, what would you do to lessen your worry?
Benefits of ANC	(a) In what way do you think the doctor or the nurse can do to prevent swollen feet? (b) In what way do you think the doctor or the nurse can do to cure swollen feet? (c) To what extent does the antenatal care help you and your baby?
Barriers to attending ANC	(a) What made you make the first visit at the .... month of pregnancy? (b) During pregnancy, you will be asked to come to the clinic a few times. If you cannot come, what will be your reasons?

REFERENCES

Archananuparp, S. (1988a) Bot niyom Thai: satha nakarn karnpaet Thai naipartchubaan [Promoting Thai: current situation of the Thai medical care]. *Southern Regional Primary Health Care*, **3**, 20–25.

Archananuparp, S. (1988b) Bot niyom Thai: satha nakarn karnpaet Thai nai partchubaan [Promoting Thai: current situation of Thai medical care]. *Southern Regional Primary Health Care*, **3**, 19–21.

Begum, K., Seguerra, J., Hasan, I. (1994) *Birthing Choices: A Perspective from Southern Thailand.* Unpublished MTH dissertation. Brisbane: Tropical Health Program, The University of Queensland.

Boonyanurak, P. (1985) *Use of Prenatal Clinics by Pregnant Women in Thailand.* Unpublished DEd dissertation. New York: Columbia University.

Boorapatt, S., Archeepsamoot, S., Saiyhudthong, P., Srisiri, N. (1986) Karn yaem marnda lae boot lhaang klod kong rong pa ya barn Prachuap Khirikhan [The programme of maternal and child health visits during post partum period: Prachuap Khirikhan Hospital]. *Thai Medical Council Bulletin*, **15**, 97–101 (Thai).

Caldwell, J.C. (1981) Maternal education as a factor in child mortality. *World Health Forum*, **2**, 75–78.

Department of Obstetrics and Gynaecology (1991) Total obstetric data 1990, Hatyai Hospital. Unpublished manuscript.

Fabrega, H. (1974) *Disease and Social Behaviour: An Interdisciplinary Perspective.* Cambridge: MIT Press.

Fraser, T. M. (1966) *Fishermen of South Thailand: The Malay Village.* New York: Holt, Rinehart and Winston.

Golomb, L. (1985) *An Anthropology of Curing in Multiethnic Thailand.* Illinois Studies in Anthropology No. 15. Urbana and Chicago: University of Illinois Press.

Gray, D. (1985) The treatment strategies of arthritis sufferers. *Social Science and Medicine,* **21**(5), 507–515.

Hall, M., Chng, P.K. (1982) Antenatal care in practice. In *Effectiveness and Satisfaction in Antenatal Care,* edited by M. Enkin and I. Chalmers, pp. 60–68. London: Spastics International Medical Publications.

Hanks, J.R. (1963) *Maternity and its Rituals in Bang Chan.* Data Paper of The Cornell University Southeast Asia Program, No. 51. New York: Cornell University.

Health Association of Thailand. (1987) *Patitin sataranasuk Poso 2531 [Public Health Diary 1988].* Bangkok: Saha prachapanit (Thai).

Hern, W.M. (1975) The illness parameters of pregnancy. *Social Science and Medicine,* **9**(7), 365–372.

Jirojwong, S. (1989) *Types of Antenatal Care and Other Related Factors Associated with Low Birth Weight in Southern Thailand.* MMedSc dissertation. Perth: The University of Western Australia.

Jirojwong, S., Skolnik, M. (1990) Types of antenatal care and other related factors associated with low birth weight in Southern Thailand. *The Asia Pacific Journal of Public Health,* **4**, 132–141.

Jirojwong, S., Skolnik, M. (1991) Livebirth registration data in Hatyai: use of health care resources in a growing community. In *Proceedings of the 1991 Thai National Symposium on Population Studies* (Thailand, November 21–22, 1991), edited by The Population Council, pp. 83–100. Bangkok: 21 Century.

Kaetsingha, O. (1978) Karnpaet Thai kaab Karnpaet tawantok [Thai medical care and western medical care]. *Social Medical Journal,* **1**, 10–18 (Thai).

Kay, M.A. (editor) (1982) *Anthropology of Human Birth.* Philadelphia: F.A. Davis Company.

Khamparnya, T. (1990) Karn darmnern ngarn arnamai mae lae dek lae gnarn waang paen krobkrue tarm krob naew taang pra sarn paen parttana chonna bot 2533 [Maternal and child health and family planning services according to the framework of rural development co-ordination programme 1990]. *Family Health Journal,* **18**(1), 50–52 (Thai).

Khanjanasthiti, P. (1986) Maternal and child health care movement and the child mortality, morbidity. *Ramathibodi Medical Journal,* **9**, 124–130.

Kleinman, A. (1980) *Patients and Healers in the Context of Culture.* Berkeley: University of California Press.

Koranantakul, O., Jinorose, U., Akara-winek, W., Pinjaroen, S. (1990) Prenatal diagnosis at Songklanagarind Hospital. *Songklanagarind Medical Journal,* **8**, (January-March), 43–52 (Thai).

Laderman, C. (1983) *Wives and Midwives: Childbirth and Nutrition in Rural Malaysia.* Berkeley: University of California Press.

Laderman, C. (1987) Destructive heat and cooling prayer: Malay humoralism in pregnancy, childbirth and the postpartum period. *Social Science and Medicine,* **25**(4), 357–365.

MacCormack, C. (editor) (1982) *Ethnography of Fertility and Birth.* New York: Academic Press.

McKinlay, J.B. (1972) The sick role-illness and pregnancy. *Social Science and Medicine,* **6**(5), 561–572.

Mahamakut Rajvitayalai (1982) *Prasoort lae Arttha Katha. Matchimnikai Mulparnnas.* **1**(3). Bangkok: Siwaporn (Thai).

Manderson, L. (1981a) Roasting, smoking and dieting in response to birth: Malay confinement in cross cultural perspective. *Social Science Medicine,* **15B**, 509–520.

Manderson, L. (1981b) Traditional food beliefs and critical life events in Peninsular Malaysia. *Social Science Information,* **20**(6), 947–975.

Mechanic, D. (1974) *Politics, Medicine, and Social Science.* New York: John Wiley and Sons.

Morgan, M., Calnan, M., Manning, N. (1985) *Sociology Approaches to Health and Medicine.* London: Croom Helm.

Mosley, H. W., Chen, L. C. (1984) An analytical framework for the study of child survival in developing countries. In *Child Survival: Strategies for Research,* edited by W.H. Mosley and L.C. Chen, pp. 25–45. Cambridge: Cambridge University Press.

Muecke, M. A. (1976) Health care system as socializing agents; childbearing the north Thai and western ways. *Social Science and Medicine,* **10**(7–8), 377–383.

Mulholland, J. (1979) Thai traditional medicine: ancient thought and practice in a Thai context. *Journal of Siam Society,* **67**(2), 80–115.

Niyomwan, V. (1991) Sarup karndarm nernn ngarn arnamai mae lae dek pi ngob pramarn 2533 [Summary of maternal and child health services 1990]. *Family Health Journal,* **19**, 5–8 (Thai).

Noonsuk, C. (1980) Prapaeni kaewkaab karn kerd kong chaw paktai [Customs relating to births of the Southern Thais]. In *Chiwit Thai paaktai, vol. 4 [Life of the Southern Thais,* vol. 4], edited by C. Sukrakarn, pp. 51–74. Nakorn Sritammaraaj: Nakorn Sritammaraj Teacher College (Thai).

Nukoonkit, P. (1986) Development of nursing education in Thailand. Unpublished MEd dissertation, Bangkok: Chulalongkorn University (Thai).

Pimchaipong, R., Theepswang, J., Krisevatana, C. (1988) Birth weight of newborn infant: relation to maternal age, occupation, education and antenatal care. *Bulletin of the Department of Medical Services,* **13**, 489–495 (Thai).

Pongnikorn, S. (1989) The results of antenatal women referred to examination at district hospitals and local health centres in Lampang Province. *Bulletin of the Department of Medical Services,* **14**, 133–140 (Thai).

Prasartwanakit, V., Ratanapreuksachat, R. (1989) Obstetrical practice and perinatal outcome at Songklanagarind Hospital 1987–1988. *Songklanagarind Medical Journal,* 7, 21–29. (Thai)

Rajadhon, Phya Anuman (1961) *Life and Ritual in Old Siam: Three Studies of Thai Life and Customs,* translated and edited by W.J. Gedney, Westport: Greenwood Press.

Rice, P.L. (editor) (1994) *Asian Mothers, Australian Birth: Pregnancy, Childbirth and Childbearing: The Asian Experience in an English-Speaking Country.* Melbourne: Ausmed Publications.

Riley, J.N. (1977) Western medicine's attempt to become more scientific: example from the United States and Thailand. *Social Science and Medicine,* **11**(10), 549–560.

Rosenblum, E.H., Stone, E.J., Skipper, B.E. (1981) Maternal compliance in immunization of preschoolers as related to health locus of control, health value, and perceived vulnerability. *Nursing Research,* **30**(6), 337–342.

Rosenstock, I.M. (1974) Historical origins of the Health Belief Model. *Health Education Monographs,* **2**, 328–335.

Royston, E., Ferguson, J. (1985) The coverage of maternal care: a critical review of available information. *World Health Statistics Quarterly*, **38**(3), 267–288.

Songkhla Provincial Office. (1989) *Barnyai saruup changwat Songkhla 2530 [Summary of Songkhla Province 1989]*. Songkhla: Mongkol Karn Pim (Thai).

Suthipintawong, C., Tangpoonphonvivat, S. (1984) Causes of perinatal death in autopsy cases, Songklanagarind Hospital. *Songklanagarind Medical Journal*, **2**, 245–249 (Thai).

Suwanwela, N., Sookthomya, V. (1988) Prevalence of anemia in pregnant women at Hat-Yai Hospital. *Bulletin of the Department of Medical Services*, **13**, 673–680 (Thai).

Thailand, Ministry of Public Health (1972) *Public Health in Thailand: 1971*. Bangkok: Kurusapha Ladprao Press (Thai).

Thailand, Ministry of Public Health (1980) *Thailand Health Profile*. Bangkok: Samnark Kaw Panit Press.

Thailand, Ministry of Public Health, Family Health Division (1987) Plan and policy of the maternal and child health and family planning programme in 1988. Unpublished manuscript. Bangkok: Ministry of Public Health (Thai).

Thompson, V. (1967) *Thailand: The New Siam*. New York: Paragon Book Reprint.

Toongsuwan, S., Suvonnakote, T. (1983) Perinatal mortality survey: Siriraj Hospital, Thailand 1979. *Journal of the Medical Association of Thailand*, **66**, 93–98.

Zola, I.K. (1973) Pathways to the doctor-from person to patient. *Social Science and Medicine*, **7**(9), 677–689.

Zweig, S., LeFevre, M., Kruse, J. (1988) The Health Belief Model and attendance for prenatal care. *Family Practice Research Journal*, **8**, (Fall/Winter), 32–41.

CHAPTER 4

Use of Health Services by Filipino Women During Childbearing Episodes

Josefina V. Cabigon

In accordance with the global concern about women's welfare and development, the Philippine Government and particularly the Department of Health have been addressing the health of women. Data recently available indicate that in 1987–1993, more than two Filipino women died of maternity-related causes for every 1,000 live births (Philippines, National Statistics Office, Macro International Inc., 1994a), due to postpartum haemorrhage, hypertension, and septicemia. Of the estimated 8.8 million women married and at reproductive age in the early 1990s, 1,500,000 become pregnant annually, and of the estimated 6 million regarded at "risk" of pregnancy, only 3 million practise family planning (FP); the other 3 million represent the unmet need for FP. An estimated 155,000 to 750,000 abortions are induced annually. Among pregnant and lactating mothers in 1987, about 70% had adequate energy and protein intake and close to half suffered from iron-deficiency anaemia (Philippines, Department of Health, 1995).

Research in recent years has focused on child rather than maternal health, and in this context, the links between infant and child mortality and socioeconomic, environmental, demographic, cultural, biological and behavioural factors, have been identified (e.g. Engracia, 1983; Martin, Trussell, Salvail and Shah, 1983; Baltazar 1984; Adair, 1989; Guilkey, Popkin and Akin, 1989; Cabigon, 1990; Stewart, Popkin, Guilkey, Akin, Adair *et al.*, 1991). Most surveys concerned with women's health have concentrated on fertility and family planning, and the first detailed research aimed at identifying social and environmental factors with maternal mortality was undertaken with the 1993 National Demographic Survey and Safe Motherhood Survey.

The use of public and private health services during pregnancy, birthing and postpartum, including both traditional and biomedical health services, is particularly relevant to women's health. The combining of demographic research on the levels and patterns of use of health services, with ethnographic work on folk beliefs and practices observed during pregnancy, parturition and confinement, provides valuable insights into the health of women in the Philippines. It complements biomedical and epidemiological research into our thinking about women's health. Women hope for good health for themselves and their children: "Women...follow dietary and behavioural precautions to ensure a healthy pregnancy, safe delivery and rapid recovery, acting upon their own and others' beliefs regarding both physical changes

83

and metaphysical and ritual vulnerability" (Manderson, 1981:509). However, their ability to realise these goals varies considerably, and is influenced both by maternal health and economic status and by their understanding of the purpose and value of government health services. This chapter examines several areas for which relevant data are available, relating to (1) prenatal care; (2) postpartum care; (3) medical care for symptoms of reproductive problems; and (4) family spacing including contraception and abortion. It begins with a description of the levels and patterns of care in each area. It then looks at corresponding traditional beliefs and practices, the role of traditional birth attendants, and the prioritisation in health programs, public and private.

DATA SOURCES

This chapter mainly uses data from the 1993 Safe Motherhood Survey, the 1993 National Demographic Survey, and the 1992 Socio-Economic Survey of special groups of families.[1] All three draw on nationally representative samples. The sample of the 1993 Safe Motherhood Survey included all respondents (8,400) in the 1993 National Demographic Survey who had ever been pregnant. The sample of the 1993 Demographic Survey included 15,029 women of any marital status aged 15–49. The initial and larger national survey, the 1993 National Demographic Survey, and the later and smaller national survey, the 1993 Safe Motherhood Survey, were undertaken by the National Statistics Office in collaboration with the Department of Health, The University of the Philippines Population Institute and other government agencies concerned with women's health issues. Technical assistance was provided by the Demographic and Health Research Division of Macro International Inc. (Philippines, National Statistics Office, Macro International Inc., 1994a). The 1992 Socio-Economic Survey was carried out by the National Statistics Office and the National Economic and Development Authority-Integrated Population and Development Planning Project; its sample was 6,563 households and 39,197 individuals drawn from families belonging to the bottom 30% of the population as defined by national per capita income (Herrin and Racelis, 1994:17). These three data sources are primarily used to describe the levels and patterns of use of prenatal care and postnatal care. It is expected that the 1993 National Demographic Survey and Safe Motherhood Survey are consistent since the sample for the 1993 Safe Motherhood Survey is a subset of the 1993 National Demographic Survey sample. Further, the two surveys were conducted within the same year, the 1993 National Demographic Survey between April and June, and the 1993 Safe Motherhood Survey between October and December, and it is unlikely that respondents had changed beliefs and behaviour significantly during this period.

These data are supplemented by the 1993 Comprehensive Baseline Study on Family Planning/Maternal and Child Health undertaken in Tarlac,[2] one of the 73 provinces of the Philippines (Cabigon, Raymundo, Lusterio and Zafra, 1994); a qualitative study of industrial workers, mostly women, conducted in 1993-1994 in select regions of the country (Metro Manila, Southern Tagalog, Southern Mindanao,

Northern Mindanao) (Cabigon and Magsino, 1994), a 1994 study on abortion prevalence (Cabigon, forthcoming), and a 1991 study of the urban poor women in Metro Manila (Cabigon, 1992). These latter data sources are particularly valuable in the search for explanations of observed levels and patterns of health service use. Relevant findings of other researchers are also incorporated where appropriate.

PRENATAL CARE

Levels and Patterns of Prenatal Care

Available data sources at the national level consistently reveal a high overall level of prenatal care among Filipino women, a little over 90% based on the 1993 National Demographic Survey, Safe Motherhood Survey and Comprehensive Baseline Study, and a little over 80% among low-income families in the 1992 Socio-Economic Survey (Herrin and Racelis, 1994; Philippines, National Statistics Office, Macro International Inc., 1994b). By contrast — although the figures are not comparable — an earlier study found only 35% of mothers who were admitted as hospital emergency cases had received prenatal care (Sahagun, 1987).

In the recent data sets, most mothers made at least three prenatal visits (average number of visits is in fact a little above four), even going beyond the recommended number of visits by the Maternal and Child Health Program. However, the first prenatal visit usually occurs during a fourth month of pregnancy and a negligible proportion present for a prenatal check-up earlier (Philippines, National Statistics Office, Macro International Inc., 1994b). According to the 1993 Comprehensive Baseline Study, only about 21% of women receive prenatal care during the first month of pregnancy, primarily because women preferred to present later, when pregnancy was certain and there was no possibility of false pregnancy, for example, due to menstrual delay (Cabigon, Raymundo, Lusterio and Zafra, 1994).

Raymundo (1987, 1989) demonstrated that chances of pregnancy-related complications were lower among urban poor women who had received more than four prenatal visits, compared with women who had presented for care on three or fewer occasions. Similarly, the 1993 Safe Motherhood Survey indicated that among women without prenatal care, births ending in a perinatal death were twice as frequent as births surviving the first week of life (Philippines, National Statistics Office, Macro International Inc., 1994b).

All data sources for this chapter reveal the importance of education to pregnancy care. The higher the education of mothers, the greater the likelihood of presenting to a physician for prenatal care and the less likely the woman will seek prenatal care from a traditional birth attendant (Cabigon, Raymundo, Lusterio and Zafra, 1994; Philippines National Statistics Office, Macro International Inc., 1994b). In Metro Cebu,[3] Philippines, for example, Becker, Peters, Gray, Gultiano and Black (1993) illustrated that maternal education was the most consistent and important determinant of use of prenatal care and three other health services, viz. family planning, childhood immunisations and use of oral rehydration salts.

Traditional Beliefs and Practices

Cultural beliefs regarding health and illness have emerged as an important reason for non-use of prenatal services, as Sahagun (1987) demonstrated in a study of women admitted to hospital in labour and as emergency cases. In the in-depth interviews and focus group discussions I have conducted, however, traditional beliefs and practices did not affect women seeking prenatal care, rather, they supplement or are separate from biomedical understandings of pregnancy and birth. The following example is drawn from an interview I conducted with a traditional birth attendant in Tarlac, the province where the 1993 Comprehensive Baseline Study was undertaken:

Question: Some women observe certain practices when they are pregnant. What practices are common among pregnant women in your community?

Response: Pregnant women usually avoid eating foods that are black in colour. There is the common belief that expectant mothers who eat black foods will give birth to a dark skinned baby. Some keep themselves pretty and clean because they want their babies to be pretty or handsome.

Question: What advice do you usually give to your pregnant clients?

Response: I tell them to keep good personal hygiene and avoid excessive physical exertion to prevent the foetus from being harmed. I also tell them to avoid staying or sitting for a long time in the door, to facilitate delivery whenever it is the time for the child to come out.

The responses gathered from in-depth interviews and focus group discussions are more often proscriptions than prescriptions, with the underlying purpose of proper care of the baby in the womb (cf. Jirojwong, this volume). According to von Raffler-Engel (1994), the movement or kicking of the baby in the womb is a signal to the mother to tell her "I am here and I need care". She documents folk beliefs about the unborn in various parts of the world, which include (1) the need for kind treatment and care of the expectant mother, including satisfying cravings for food; (2) avoidance of funerals; (3) protection of the foetus from evil spirits; (4) avoidance of unpleasant maternal experiences or impressions, in order to prevent birthmarks; and (5) proscriptions and prescriptions affecting action, behaviour, and diet. The beliefs that exist in the Philippines fit into these five general categories. However, the beliefs that predominated in focus group discussions and in-depth interviews were that (1) pregnant women should avoid too many sweets; (2) they should avoid performing heavy work; (3) pregnant women exposed to a cold breeze or sleeping on an uncovered floor are likely to secrete blood with mucus during labour, and the child will be prone to colds; and (4) pregnant women should always look nice and tidy.

Even with the existence of modern prenatal care services, the role of traditional birth attendants (TBAs) is still essential during pregnancy. The evaluation of a pilot project in Bohol by Reynes (1986) disclosed that despite the intensive modern maternity services offered by the project to the community, the usual practice of consulting traditional birth attendants still prevailed during the 1976–1978 period of evaluation. Focus group discussions in the 1993 Comprehensive Baseline Study revealed supporting evidence of the importance of the traditional birth attendant in alleviating women's immediate fears associated with pregnancy.

> Moderator: Who are the persons usually consulted by pregnant women in your community whenever they have obstetric problems?
>
> Participant 1: Midwife in the health centre.
>
> Participant 7: The *hilot* [traditional birth attendant].
>
> Moderator: What types of prenatal services are provided by *hilots* which government midwives could not provide?
>
> Participant 3: Massaging of the abdomen at six to eight months of gestation.
>
> Participant 5: Whenever I feel uncomfortable with my pregnancy, I go to the *hilot* whom I can reach because there is no midwife in our health centre.

The importance of the *hilots* is understandable particularly in remote areas, where midwives could not reach all women daily, as most have catchment areas of two to three *barangays* (villages). The most knowledgeable and accessible person expectant mothers can approach when they have obstetric problems in these areas is the traditional birth attendant.

Role of Government Organisations

Parents want their children to grow up healthily and happily; hence, they take advantage of any opportunities for the sake of their children. This may play an important role in the high level of use of prenatal care among Filipino pregnant mothers. The 1993 Safe Motherhood Survey and Comprehensive Baseline Study reveal that by the early 1990s, women were increasingly using public health facilities, particularly the midwife at *barangay* health stations and rural health units. The components of prenatal care provided in these health facilities include examination and preventive services on weight, height, blood pressure, fundal height (abdomen measured), foetal heart auscultation (listening to baby's heart), leopold manoeuvre (checking baby's position), tetanus toxoid injection, and advice and information on diet, danger signs in pregnancy, breastfeeding, family planning and postpartum care (Philippines, Department of Health, 1993; Philippines, National Statistics Office, Macro International Inc., 1994b:36). These components are regarded as essential for the proper care of the unborn and in preparation for delivery and early mothering. Casual talks with some pregnant mothers in clinics, which I observed at clinics as part of the 1993 Comprehensive Baseline Study, indicated that mothers made considerable sacrifices to come from distant places to access the services offered in the rural health units.

Quantitative and qualitative data from focus group discussions with mothers and from the 1993 Comprehensive Baseline Study are consistent in indicating a high level of awareness of mothers that pregnancy and childbirth are potential health risks for themselves and for their children; hence they consider prenatal check-ups to be a routine activity for pregnant women, and families and others urge pregnant women to seek prenatal care. One of the traditional birth attendants I interviewed reported that one of her clients, whom she attended during a previous pregnancy, had experienced swelling of her feet during her next pregnancy, even at three months of gestation. This TBA had been trained by the Department of Health, understood the logic of referral, and in this case brought her client to the provincial health office for a medical check-up and treatment. In the sample villages of the 1993 Comprehensive Baseline Study, "go to the health centre" was common advice given to pregnant women by other mothers.

Awareness of the importance of prenatal care may be attributed to the campaigns of the maternal and child health program. Health policy is guided by the principles of equity, quality and access to health care in partnership with the people. Primary health care, with its focus on prevention and health promotion, is given priority. Its Maternal and Child Health Program covers the Expanded Programme on Immunisation, Women's Health and Safe Motherhood, Family Planning, Nutrition, Growth Monitoring and Promotion, and Control of Childhood Diseases (Philippines, Department of Health, 1993; Philippines, National Statistics Office, Macro International Inc., 1994b:36). The Department of Health has tapped all channels of communication in its campaign for health promotion and prevention from diseases. The former Secretary of Health, Dr Juan M. Flavier, and his successor, Dr Jaime Z. Galvez-Tan, have been given short but prime time on television to promote health programs, and priority programs are promoted by lasting, catchy and impressive slogans such as *alis disis* (disease prevention) and *patak* (immunisation including tetanus toxoid injection), which are used on the television and radio, in printed materials and by midwives and volunteer *barangay* (village) health workers.

According to Costales (1994), the high level of prenatal care, with about four visits during pregnancy, suggests that the Department of Health recommendation of three prenatal visits during pregnancy is achievable. There are however two related problems the Department has to deal with. The first is the small proportion of expectant mothers presenting for a prenatal check-up during the first trimester of pregnancy. As already noted, under the Women's Health and Safe Motherhood Program, the standard recommendation regarding the number, timing and content of prenatal visits is that all women have a minimum of three visits during pregnancy, with at least one visit in each trimester. However, most expectant mothers do not receive prenatal care during the first trimester. The second pertains to ineffective communication between government service providers and clients, even when services are adequate (Peters, Becker, Black, Gray and Logarta, 1991). Urban women are more likely to use private health care services than are rural women (ibid.).

Role of Non-government Organisations

Non-government organisations have played an important part in promoting women's health, particularly in the provision of prenatal care. There are around 50 such organisations in the Philippines. Women's Health Care Foundation was founded in 1980 and provides comprehensive health and information services related to reproductive health in strategic areas in Metro Manila, serving more than 35,000 clients from 1980–1994 (Women's Health Care Foundation, 1994:3). Woman Health Philippines, established in 1986 to promote Filipino women's rights to community health services and reproductive freedom, has been working towards a revitalised national population program in these areas. The Development of People's Foundation in Davao City[4] has addressed the health needs of urban poor women, including prenatal care, in Davao City. These non-government organisations have made unique contributions in the high level of prenatal care in the country.

PARTURIENT CARE

Levels and Patterns of Parturient Care

Home deliveries predominate. Most are attended by traditional birth attendants; midwives are the next most popular. Most home births are normal deliveries with healthy outcomes. As observed with prenatal care, higher educated women are more likely to be assisted by medically trained attendants.

Traditional Beliefs and Practices

One traditional birth attendant provided a vivid description of how she performs home delivery. She asks one of the household members to boil water in a big container and to keep the container on the fire until the birthing process ends. She prepares the linen, diapers, clothing needs of the baby, basin and her delivery kit. She checks the extent of effacement by inserting her fingers. She says that once the head of the child is about the length of the first dividing line of her middle finger from the cervix, the cardinal movements of labour start. She then instructs the woman to relax and to maintain deep breathing until the baby has fully emerged. If the delivery is normal, the birthing process is short. If the delivery is not normal, e.g. breech presentation, the effacement process takes a longer time. She claims that she has already performed two deliveries with breech presentation with healthy results.

In one delivery that I witnessed, the skill of the *hilot* was impressive. The cardinal movements of labour lasted just a matter of minutes and there was a cry from the newly-born child. The *hilot* used a sharpened bamboo-like material for cutting the umbilical cord. She placed the baby on a winnower turned upside down, symbolising the world, then lifted and dropped the winnower with the baby on it three times, reciting "Be strong and healthy to face the world".

In the Ilocos Region, the husband has to stay around during birthing, for it is his responsibility to bury the placenta. He is supposed to go directly to the selected place without turning back, and bury the placenta as fast as he can. The burial signals the end of pain experienced by the parturient woman, the end of any problems associated with the labour (e.g. depletion, loss of blood), and a fast recovery. Focus group participants offered further beliefs:

Moderator: What beliefs on birthing prevail in your community?

Participant 1: In our place, there is a common belief that putting squash leaves on the abdomen during labour facilitates the delivery process.

Participant 2: Touching the abdomen of the parturient by her enemy eases the delivery pain.

Participant 5: A parturient who drinks coconut water at the onset of labour is likely to experience normal and fast birthing.

Birthing position varies, and one of the traditional birth attendants said that it depends on the parturient's own preference as to whether she lies or squats. It is common, however, to lie down.

Traditional birth attendants interviewed vary in their responses as to the presence of others during birthing. Some do not mind as long as these people do not create noise, for their presence encourages the woman to face delivery courageously. Others allow only immediate family members who are interested in staying around, to ensure that the woman feels secure and relaxed during the delivery.

Government Policy

Philippines health policy is one of decentralisation, which considers home birthing as safe. A law states that only those finishing the midwifery degree can attend to birthing mothers. However, there seems to be no strict enforcement of this law, as indicated by the popularity of traditional birth attendants in home deliveries. In fact, the Department of Health has provided training to traditional birth attendants and some of those I interviewed showed me their delivery kits, lent by the Department of Health, which have to be returned once they cease to attend deliveries. One traditional birth attendant also showed me her records, complete with names, sexes, places and dates of deliveries.

POSTPARTUM CARE

Levels and Patterns of Postnatal Care

While the level of prenatal care is high, the level of postnatal medical consultations is much lower (about a third for the national average and about a half among low-income families). This is evident in all available Philippine data sources. Again, the government midwife is the most common postnatal provider. As observed with prenatal and parturient care, the higher the education of the women, the more she is likely to receive postpartum care (Cabigon, Raymundo, Lusterio and Zafra, 1994;

Herrin and Racelis, 1994; Philippines, National Statistics Office, Macro International Inc., 1994b).

Traditional Beliefs and Practices

During the postpartum the mother is regarded as vulnerable to "cold", resulting from the depletion of heat during childbirth. Throughout the region, there is similar emphasis on the proper care of the postpartum woman to restore her to a state of equilibrium (Manderson, 1981). Postnatal beliefs emphasise such vulnerability. The dietary and behavioural proscriptions and prescriptions during postpartum focus more on the health of the mother than the child. Recall that during the pregnancy the dietary and behavioural proscriptions and prescriptions are focused more on the health of the unborn than the mother.

Confinement of Filipino mothers normally lasts for a month postpartum. During the first nine days of confinement, several traditional practices are prescribed, and according to one traditional birth attendant, physical confinement for home delivering mothers is necessary. Almost all focus group participants were in accord that a woman postpartum should: (1) not take a full bath for the first five to nine days; (2) wear heavy clothing or be wrapped with blankets to prevent her exposure to *hamog* (harmful and cold wind); (3) tightly bind her abdomen to prevent profuse bleeding; and (4) wash her vagina with boiled guava leaves. On the seventh or ninth day, the woman takes a full bath. The full bath can be either plain warm water or warmed water boiled with herbs, usually guava leaves. In rural areas, the post-parturient should take a bath in a well-sealed room. This full bath day is the beginning of "mother roasting" for the purpose of "drying out" the womb (Manderson, 1981; and see Jirojwong, Townsend and Rice, and Whittaker, all this volume). According to Hart (1965) as cited by Manderson (1981:515), "mother roasting" can be observed in various forms in the Philippines such as: (1) lying beside a stove for up to 30 days after delivery; (2) squatting over a clay stove with live coals under an improvised tent; (3) sitting on a chair over hot water, stones, and burning twigs; and (4) "bathing" in smoke from smouldering leaves. The last two means were mentioned during the focus group discussions and in-depth interviews with traditional birth attendants in the 1993 Comprehensive Baseline Study. One of the participants in a focus group discussion reported that her mother subjected her to a series of "baths" in smoke from smouldering leaves once a week, from her first full bath and "roasting" on the ninth day to the end of her one-month confinement.

In addition to physical confinement, full bathing and roasting, the postpartum mother is massaged daily with coconut oil (all parts of the body, including the abdomen to remove unexpected blood clots) by the *hilot* for the first nine days of confinement. One TBA reported that the massaging of the post-parturient aims to: (1) regain lost health; (2) restore the uterus to pre-delivery position; and (3) make breast milk available for the baby.

Dietary precautions are essential to the recovery of the postpartum woman. Most participants in the focus groups stated that the postpartum woman is considered to have a cold stomach, hence she needs to take in plenty of chicken or fish broth with herbs (e.g. *malunggay*, a tree-like vegetable which is popular among the Ilocanos) during physical confinement starting right after childbirth. Green leafy vegetables are generally prescribed, as are rice, salt and spicy food, believed to build strength and restore harmony after birth. Certain other foods were proscribed to post-parturients; these include *gabi*, a root crop, and young squash leaves which are said to cause itchiness. In the Ilocos region, watermelon is also avoided because it is considered a cold food and it exacerbates the cold stomach of the postpartum woman.

Role of Traditional Birth Attendants

As mentioned earlier, TBAs perform the abdominal massage to revert the uterus to its proper pre-delivery position, and this is conducted for women who have given birth both at public and private health facilities. Most TBAs provide a child delivery "package" which includes nine days of postnatal care for the mother and the baby or until the mother has taken a full bath. This service includes: (1) the daily bathing of the baby and cleaning its navel; (2) massaging the post-parturient (all parts of the body); and (3) administering all the rituals for the full bath (bathing and roasting). For most mothers, the *hilot's* care is sufficient and they see little need for biomedical care, as typified in one focus group discussion.

> Moderator: What are the reasons for postpartum women not presenting for postnatal care?
> Participant 7: No time and money.
> Participant 9: No need because they feel healthy especially if they are taken care of by the *hilot*.

Role of Government Organisations

Postnatal visits at rural health units are supposed to include examination of the abdomen, breasts and internal pelvis, and advice on family planning, breastfeeding and baby care, although in fact most respondents are simply given information on breastfeeding and baby care, and have an abdominal examination. Very few have breast and internal pelvic examinations (Philippines, Department of Health, 1993; Philippines, National Statistics Office, Macro International Inc., 1994b:36).

The attention to the child rather than to the mother reflects the emphasis of earlier policies and programs, as well as the individual perspectives of medical practitioners, researchers and even mothers themselves. Emphasis has been on child survival, and it has only been from the late 1980s that maternal survival was given equal emphasis in program implementation and research. However, with at least 21 child survival programs (such as child immunisation, growth monitoring and deworming), local health administrators face the difficulty of providing the necessary attention to maternal care. After delivery, the prime motivation of mothers to go to the health centres, as perceived both by mothers and service providers, is to have their child immunised or checked (Cabigon, Raymundo, Lusterio and Zafra, 1994; Cabigon and Magsino, 1994).

REPRODUCTIVE PROBLEMS

According to the 1993 Safe Motherhood Survey (Philippines, National Statistics Office, Macro International Inc., 1994b:82–83), most women experiencing symptoms of reproductive health problems (uterine prolapse, urinary incontinence, vaginal discharge, urinary tract infection, dyspareunia, and menstrual disorders) did not seek medical treatment (see also Hull, Widyantoro and Fetters, this volume). Women were more likely to go to traditional healers (41%) for symptoms of uterine prolapse, than to a doctor, nurse or midwife (26%) (the remainder did not seek care). The three most important reasons given for not seeking care were: the problem experienced was not regarded serious, women were unable to seek care for resource-related factors such as cost, transportation and time, or they were embarrassed or frightened. The percentage of women with reproductive health problems experienced during the six months preceding the study, and not seeking any medical care, was even higher among urban poor women in Davao City (83%) (Sanchez and Juarez, 1994:64–65) than the national average (23%).

The perception that a given reproductive health problem is not serious, hence there is no need to seek medical treatment, features in the reproductive lives of many women. Some evidence of this comes from the focus group discussions in the 1993 Comprehensive Baseline Study:

Moderator: What do women in your community usually do if they have reproductive problems such as urinary tract infection, menstrual disorders, dyspareunia [painful sexual intercourse], or vaginal discharge?

Participant 2:   Those with urinary tract infection drink coconut juice.

Participant 5:   Women here usually do not go for medical check-ups unless the problem is really serious.

Participant 6:   Any health problem that can still be bearable and not seriously felt by the women is usually ignored. Herbal medicines are tried first.

Participant 9:   I agree, with life getting harder and harder, food for my family comes first before considering using the money for a check-up or medicine.

Economic considerations are common as most Filipino families still live below subsistence level (National Statistical Coordination Board, personal communication). Hence the alternative chosen is the least expensive — either self-treatment or no treatment at all.

Again the traditional birth attendant is the most common consultant for reproductive health problems in the community. One woman I interviewed was both a healer and a birth attendant. She prescribes herbs she found to be effective for some of her clients, e.g. drinking from the water boiled with guava leaves to cure urinary infections.

FAMILY SPACING

Contraception

The Department of Health aims to ensure: (1) family health management or empowering the family to become an active partner in health care; (2) integrated Family Planning/Maternal and Child Health services which respect the right of families to have children; (3) community health management or recognising people as important health resource; and (4) health care financing or realistically acknowledging the importance of money in the attainment of health aspirations (Galvez-Tan, 1994:i).

Four in ten women currently married, aged 15–49, use contraception. The four most common methods used (from most to least popular) are female sterilisation, pill, withdrawal and natural family planning, which includes the rhythm method. Use of contraception increases with education. Filipino women adopt family planning fairly early in the family building process, with one in five using family planning after their first child and one in four after their second (Philippines, National Statistics Office, Macro International Inc., 1994a).

Abortion

Abortion as well as the use of modern contraceptives has figured in the controversy between the Catholic Church and the current administration, and this has triggered interest in more accurate measurement of abortion prevalence, in undertaking wide-scale studies of attitudes and perceptions regarding abortion, and in studying the social and psychological background of women undergoing induced abortions. So far, data available on levels of abortion are inconsistent, primarily owing to different methods of measurement used. Valenzuela (1969) suggested that 30% of married women of reproductive age interviewed in Laguna had had at least one abortion. Flavier and Chen (1980) reported that 17% of the rural married women aged 15–49 years surveyed in five villages (barrios) in Cavite[5] province admitted to at least one abortion, some to two or more and a few to three or more. The 1979–1983 review of septic abortion at the Philippine General Hospital (Ramoso-Jalbuena and Ladines-Llave, 1989) revealed that 73% of 408 women who had had abortions cited financial reasons, already having too many children, or desired spacing of children, indicating that abortion was used by these women to avoid unwanted pregnancies. Seven of these died from complications of septicaemia. Financial reasons were also cited by most of the 35 women studied by the Institute for Social Studies and Action (ISSA), twelve of whom had repeat or multiple abortions (Marcelo and The Project Management Team, 1991). The 1993 Safe Motherhood Survey showed that of the early pregnancy losses, induced abortions comprised 7% for the nation as a whole, and 9% for Metro Manila (Philippines, National Statistics Office, Macro International Inc., 1994b). In contrast, my 1994 Study on Abortion Prevalence in Metro Manila, involving a regionally representative sample of 1169 women (single or married and aged 15–44 years), revealed a prevalence rate (proportion of women who have had one or more abortions in their lifetimes) of about 17% (Cabigon, 1995).

Further, one in six births in the five years preceding the 1993 National Demographic Survey were unwanted (Philippines, National Statistics Office, Macro International Inc., 1994a). Why are there unwanted pregnancies? Insights from women's perspectives come from the Sanchez and Juarez report (1994), in which the reported reasons included the last child being too young, economic difficulty of rearing another child, ideal family size being already met, and desire for more time for work. What happened to most of these accidental pregnancies? The 1993 Safe Motherhood Survey, as a follow-up survey, revealed that among those claiming to have unwanted pregnancies, eight in ten continued the pregnancy, 5% aborted the pregnancy, 14% tried to abort but failed, and 4% did "something" to resume their menstrual period (Philippines, National Statistics Office, Macro International Inc., 1994a). Chronic poverty, closely-spaced births and failure to use an effective contraceptive method all lead to abortion (Marcelo and Project Management Team, 1991; Sanchez and Juarez, 1994: Cabigon, 1995), methods of which include bitter herbal concoctions, tablets, repetitive hard abdominal massage by a traditional birth attendant until bleeding starts, and the use of catheter, suction or curettage (Marcelo and The Project Management Team, 1991; Philippines, National Statistics Office, Macro International Inc., 1994a; Sanchez and Juarez, 1994; Cabigon, 1995).

The above indicates that induced abortion is practised by some Filipino women despite it being illegal and taboo according to the Catholic Church. Abortion is a feature of the reproductive lives of many women. Further evidence is found in a study of women working for an industrial company, aimed at evaluating factors leading to continued company support to an industry-based family planning program in which the rising incidence of abortion emerged as a serious problem (Cabigon and Magsino, 1994):

> Last year, we had an abortion case almost every month. In fact, late last year I had to rush an abortion case to our hospital because the bleeding happened while she [the woman] was working; the foetus was almost in full term for that woman was then five months pregnant; it was a shocking experience for me to witness and I sympathised with the woman's predicament; aside from those abortion cases we witness inside the company, there are also plenty of them experiencing abortion outside because we keep a record of absentees and when the workers came back for duty, most of them gave abortion as the reason for being absent from work. (company nurse)

Government Response

What has the Philippine Management Program on Population been doing? As mentioned earlier, the level of current use of contraception and use of family planning services is quite high. However, withdrawal, rhythm or natural family planning has remained on par with the pill in terms of popularity (Cabigon, 1992; Philippines, National Statistics Office, Macro International Inc., 1994a). Accidental pregnancy, primarily due to high failure rates of these methods, stood out as the main reason for stopping use, followed by the desire for further pregnancy and the side effects of contraception (Philippines, National Statistics Office, Macro International Inc., 1994a). Withdrawal is the method most preferred by husbands. Most current users claim that the types of information provided to them by family planning service providers are biased towards how to use and benefit from the method, with less attention on complications or possible side effects (Cabigon, Raymundo, Lusterio and Zafra, 1994).

In recent years, the maternal and child health program has been greatly affected by the 1991 Local Government Code which passes the responsibility of health program implementation from the DOH central office to the local government units. The Philippine Management Program on Population recognises the close interrelationship between population, resources and environment, and is under the coordination of the Population Commission. The Department of Health Family Planning Program is under the Philippine Management Program on Population, but it has been essentially a health program. Its implementation was also transferred from the Department of Health central office to the local government units under the 1991 Local Government Code. Nonetheless, the Ramos[6] administration has strongly promoted the population program as a strategy for attaining sustainable development. Through the Department of Health, the population program provides information and services on the range of family planning methods and respects the right of every individual and couple to make their own choice, based on adequate information and according to their religious beliefs and convictions (Philippines, Department of Health, 1990). The primary goal of the population program is to improve family welfare through a focus on women's health, safe motherhood and child survival.

However, the high level of family planning use (40%) is not translated into substantial reduction of fertility, and Filipino women around 1991 still had an average of four children. More vigorous efforts by the population are indicated. For example, the widespread use of ineffective methods like withdrawal and rhythm or natural planning implies the need for these users to be apprised of basic knowledge of reproductive physiology to help them become successful users of such methods. To dispel rumours about the side effects of pills, IUD and sterilisation, there is a need for more balanced information on the use, benefit, contraindications and management of complications of methods. There is also a need for continuous follow-up of women who stop using modern effective methods. Availability, accessibility and affordability of maternal and child health and family planning services also remain important issues.

CONCLUSION

In seeking explanations of the observed patterns and levels of use of health services, I have focused on the cultural norms, beliefs and attitudes and explored how these have some bearing on observed patterns. Such data are mainly qualitative. They imply the need to study critically and analyse the use of health services from various perspectives, including to document the anthropological and sociological underpinnings of factors related to use of health services (see Kroeger, 1983). The analysis also implies that cultural practices and beliefs have some bearing on the use of health services. There is a need to examine this relationship further. The analysis indicates a need to encourage cooperation among the Department of Health, non-government organisations, and the community in increasing women's awareness of their right to health, and in encouraging them to use available health services (public and private) for their own health as well as for the health of their children.

ENDNOTES

1. Families living below the poverty line or within the bottom 30% of the national per capita income ladder.
2. Tarlac is one of the provinces of the Central Luzon Region.
3. Metro Cebu refers to Cebu City and its surrounding areas, which are other parts of Cebu province, one of the provinces of the Central Visayas Region.
4. Davao City is within Davao del Sur, one of the provinces of the Southern Mindanao Region.
5. Cavite is one of the provinces of the southern Tagalog Region.
6. Fidel Ramos as President of the Philippines, 1992–1997.

REFERENCES

Adair, L.S. (1989) Low birth weight and intrauterine growth retardation in Filipino infants. *Paediatrics,* **84**(4), 613–622.

Baltazar, J.C. (1984) *The Impact of Family Planning Practice on Neonatal Mortality.* Unpublished PhD thesis. Los Angeles: University of California.

Becker, S., Peters, D.H., Gray, R.H., Gultiano, C., Black, R.E. (1993) The determinants of use of maternal and child health services in Metro Cebu, the Philippines. *Health Transition Review,* **3**(1), 77–89.

Cabigon, J.V. (1990) *Philippine Mortality in Changing Time.* Unpublished PhD thesis. Canberra: Australian National University.

Cabigon, J.V. (1992) *Urban Poor Health Nutrition and Family Planning: 1991 Metro Manila KAP Survey.* Final Report. Quezon City: University of the Philippines Population Institute.

Cabigon, J.V. (1995) *Preliminary Findings on the Study on Abortion Prevalence in Metro Manila.* Paper for Press Release. Diliman: The University of the Philippines.

Cabigon, J.V. (Forthcoming) *A Study on Abortion Prevalence in Metro Manila.* Final Report to the Ford Foundation.

Cabigon, J.V., Magsino, E. (1994) *A Study on Factors Leading to Continued Company Support to an Industry-Based Family Planning Program, Philippines.* Final report to The Population Council. Diliman: The University of the Philippines.

Cabigon, J.V. Raymundo, C.M., Lusterio, C.R., Zafra, J.S. (1994) *A Comprehensive Baseline Study on Family Planning/Maternal and Child Health in Tarlac.* Final report to Japan International Cooperation Agency. Diliman: The University of the Philippines.

Costales, Ma. O.D. (1994) *Material and Child Health: Results of the 1993 National Demographic Survey.* Paper Presented at the 1993 National Demographic Survey National Seminar, 15 July, Manila Pavilion Hotel, Manila.

Engracia, L.T. (1983) *Infant Mortality and Health Services in Rural Philippines.* Paper presented at the 6th National Population Welfare Congress, 17 November, Philippine International Convention Center, Manila.

Flavier, J.M., Chen, C.H. (1980) Induced abortion in rural villages of Cavite, the Philippines: knowledge, attitudes and practice. *Studies in Family Planning,* 11(2), 65–71.

Galvez-Tan, J.Z. (1994) *Health Program and Policy Implications of the 1993 National Demographic Survey.* Paper presented at the 1993 National Demographic Survey National Seminar, 18 July, Manila Pavilion Hotel, Manila.

Guilkey, D.K., Popkin, B.M., Akin, J.S. (1989) Prenatal Care and Pregnancy Outcome in Cebu, Philippines. *Journal of Development Economics,* 30, 241–272.

Hart, D.V. (1965) From pregnancy through birth in a Bisayan Filipino village. In *Southeast Asian Birth Customs: Three Studies in Human Reproduction,* edited by D.V. Hart, Rajadhon, Phya Anuman and R.J. Coughlin, pp. 65–71. New Haven: HRAF Press.

Herrin, A.N., Racelis, R.H. (1994) *Monitoring the Coverage of Public Programs on Low-Income Families: Philippines, 1992.* Pasig: National Economic Development Authority — Integrated Population and Development Planning Project.

Kroeger, A. (1983) Anthropological and socio-medical health care research in developing countries. *Social Science and Medicine,* 17(3), 147–161.

Manderson, L. (1981) Roasting, smoking and dieting in response to birth: Malay confinement in a cross cultural perspective. *Social Science Medicine,* 15B, 509–520.

Marcelo, A.B., The Project Management Team (1991) *Attitudes and Perceptions Towards Induced Abortion: The Women, Professionals and the Public.* Paper presented at the ISSA Conference, 15 March National Engineering Center, University of the Philippines, Quezon City.

Martin, L.G., Trussell, J., Salvail, F.R., Shah, N.H. (1983) Covariates of child mortality in the Philippines, Indonesia and Pakistan: an analysis based on hazard models. *Population Studies,* 27(3), 417–432.

Peters, D.H., Becker, S., Black, R.E., Gray, R.H., Logarta, J. (1991) Quality of care assessment of public and private outpatient clinics in Metro Cebu, the Philippines. *International Journal of Health Planning and Management,* 6(4), 273–286.

Philippines, Department of Health (1990) *Summary Proceedings.* Manila: Department of Health.

Philippines, Department of Health (1993) *Strategy Paper for Philippines 2000.* Manila: Department of Health.

Philippines, Department of Health (1995) *Abridged Situational Analysis of Philippine Health Situation.* Unpublished Report. Manila: Department of Health, Family Planning Services.

Philippines, National Statistics Office, Macro International Inc. (1994a) *National Demographic Survey 1993.* Calverton, Maryland: NSO and MI.

Philippines, National Statistics Office, Macro International Inc. (1994b) *National Safe Motherhood Survey 1993.* Calverton, Maryland: NSO and MI.

von Raffler-Engel, W. (1994) Folk beliefs about the unborn child from around the world. In *The Perception of the Unborn Across the Cultures of the World,* W. von Raffler-Engel, pp. 31–63. Toronto: Hogrefe and Huber Publishers.

Ramoso-Jalbuena, J., Ladines-Llave, C. (1989) Septic abortion: a five-year review at the Philippine General Hospital. *NCRP Research Bulletin*, **41**(3), 357–378.

Raymundo, C.M. (1987) Risks of motherhood among the urban poor. In *Proceedings of the National Conference on Safe Motherhood* Manila, September 3–4.

Raymundo, C.M. (1989) *The Filipino Adolescents: Their Implications for Philippine Development*. Research conducted as part of the UP Center for Integrative and Development Studies (UP CIDS) and UNFPA Project on Population, Human Resources and Development, Quezon City, October.

Reynes, J.F. (1986) *Women in Transition: Patterns of Prenatal Care in Semi-Rural Philippines*. PSTC Reprint Series No. 86–105. Brown: Population Studies and Training Center.

Sanchez, R.D., Juarez, M.P. (1994) *Community-Based Research and Advocacy on Reproductive Health Among Urban Poor Women in Davao City*. Davao City: Development of People's Foundation.

Sahagun, G. (1987) Hospital maternal deaths: causes and implication. In *Proceedings of the National Conference on Safe Motherhood*, Manila, September 3–4.

Stewart, J.F., Popkin B.M, Guilkey D.K., Akin J.S., Adair L., Flieger, W. (1991) Influences on the extent of breastfeeding: a prospective study in the Philippines. *Demography*, **28**(2), 181–199.

Valenzuela, A.B. (1969) *Abortion in Filipino women*. Paper presented at the Third Conference on Population, December, Manila.

Women's Health Care Foundation (1994) Clinic activity highlights. *Balita*, **1**(1), 3.

PART II:

FROM HER WOMB . . . .

CHAPTER 5

Journey to the Land of Light: Birth Among Hmong Women

Patricia V. Symonds

My interest in the subject of birth first began to develop in 1979, during the practicum for a medical anthropology course at Brown University in which I observed and assisted at a Providence, Rhode Island health center that served the residents of a low-income, multiethnic enclave of the city. The questions that I formed after witnessing a Hmong woman give birth, and my abiding interest in their lives, were later to lead to an enduring research interest in the subject of Hmong women and birth. After I began my doctoral field research in 1988 in Northern Thailand, I was to witness many other births (one of which is described in this chapter as "The Case of Ntxawm") and to discover the complex layers of meaning that surround that life event from a Hmong woman's perspective.

Through close ethnographic observation of numerous childbirths (both in the United States and in Thailand), many interviews with Hmong women, and a more developed understanding of the cosmology that surrounds birth, I began to comprehend the expectations the Hmong have for women, their role in society, and their relationships with others, and how the expectations of Hmong women themselves shape their experience of pregnancy and birth, as they thread their way between the various social proscriptions they encounter and attempt to take control over their reproductive, economic and social life.

The Case of Mee

I first witnessed a Hmong woman giving birth in a hospital in the United States: she was a fifteen-year old girl named Mee. That morning, as part of my Master's research on adolescent pregnancy and its implications for the Hmong in America, I had begun to interview Mee, through an interpreter, at the home of her husband's parents, where she and her husband were living. After we had talked for about an hour, Mee told me that she was in labour and feeling uncomfortable. I was taken by surprise because she had given no indication that she was in pain.

I drove Mee and her mother-in-law to the hospital, and obtained permission to accompany Mee so that I and my interpreter could, with Mee's mother-in-law, observe the birth. When the nurse requested that Mee remove her clothing she protested at first, but at her mother-in-law's request she complied, donning the skimpy hospital garment. The mother-in-law then refused to give the physician permission

103

to rupture Mee's chorionic membrane or to perform an episiotomy, and Mee was not a participant in these discussions. If she gave any indication that she was experiencing discomfort, her mother-in-law was able to quiet her with only a few words. As her labor progressed, and the contractions became stronger, Mee moaned slightly until her mother-in-law placed her hand on Mee's arm, saying: "If you make a noise it will be dangerous; you will tell the spirits that the child is coming. It will also make the infant afraid to enter this world because its mother is afraid. You must not shame yourself or me by making sounds".

I was intrigued by the fact that this young woman was able to deliver her son without expressing pain or discomfort, and I wanted to know more about the cultural construction of pain by the Hmong, the meaning of the prohibition against crying out during labor, and the role of the mother-in-law in women's lives. I determined then that I would like to pursue my study of Hmong women and the meaning of birth further, possibly abroad.

During that early period of research in the United States, I learned that few of the Hmong women who visited the Providence health clinic spoke English, and very few sought prenatal care. All expressed apprehension about the medical procedures to be undertaken during their visits, even those as simple as having one's blood drawn or providing a urine sample. Above all, they expressed fear and resentment at the prospect of being given a physical examination by a male physician. It was only after the interpreter and I had become close friends that I began to understand why Hmong women subjected themselves to the western medical practices that they so feared: many who came to the health clinic, ostensibly for prenatal care, in actuality came in order to become eligible for WIC Program (Women, Infants and Children) food vouchers, and to ensure that their children would become United States citizens after they were born.[1]

Over the next few months, I became acutely aware of the concerns of many Hmong women, especially their fears that a physician might insist upon performing an episiotomy or a Caesarean section. I learned that any surgical procedure is thought by the Hmong to alter negatively the balance of the body in relation to its surroundings, and to produce negative implications for future births as well. I also discovered that the Hmong believe that one never recovers completely from the effects of anaesthesia. I also became familiar with the concerns of the medical providers who were treating Hmong women, in particular their questions as to why Hmong women admitted to the hospital refused to eat hospital food or to drink cold juice or water, and why others would not come to the clinic for prenatal care or arrive early enough in their labor to allow the child to be born in the hospital. With increasing frequency, Hmong women were arriving with newborn babies already in their arms.

As I was to discover, the key to these puzzles about Hmong women and birth was to be found in the nexus of Hmong cosmology and beliefs that surround the idea of physical and spiritual well-being, or health, especially as they pertain to pregnancy. My initial interest in birth led me to study its relationship to Hmong cosmology and to undertake my doctoral research on this subject (Symonds, 1991). From January of 1987 to May of 1988, I undertook an ethnographic study of a

Hmong village I called Flower Village in the hills of Northern Thailand. Flower Village is populated with White Hmong (Hmong Dawb or Meo), and is situated in the northernmost province of Chiang Rai. This village was chosen because it is relatively traditional, located 20km from the main road and with few outside contacts, and relatively large, with 58 households at the beginning of my research. All data were collected in Hmong, recorded on a tape recorder and translated afterwards. My research involved participant observation, informal ethnographic interviews, and a formal questionnaire.

HMONG COSMOLOGY

The Hmong practice ancestor worship. They divide the universe into two different worlds, the World of Light and the World of Darkness. The former is the material world of the living, the latter the metaphysical spirit world where the pool of ancestors resides. These worlds are interconnected through the ongoing cycle of marriages, births and deaths (see also Nakayama, this volume).

     At the time of her marriage, it is said that a woman's soul changes its allegiance and residence from that of her own family, lineage and clan to that of her husband's, and this concept bears great influence on the life of every Hmong woman. Girls are treated as outsiders within their own families, because as a consequence of the patrilineal descent system, it is understood that they are only temporary family members. At the time of death, a person's soul (female or male) is transferred from its physical body to the Land of Darkness, where it becomes genderless or dual-gendered. These souls must be honoured or "fed" at designated times for as long as they are remembered by living generations. If they are neglected, it is said that they will be wrathful and will bring calamity and sickness upon the living.

BECOMING A WOMAN

The chief life goal for both Hmong women and men is to marry and have children, since marriage and reproduction ensure the continuation of the patriline. The first step toward women's realisation of this goal is the onset of menstruation. The age of menses falls between the ages 15 and 16 for 75% of the women in Flower Village. This is also the approximate age at which 60% of them marry, and at which 50% give birth for the first time, suggesting that the timing of these three major life events is closely correlated. The onset of menses *(cov khaubncaws)* is therefore considered a time of major transition in the life of a young girl, referred to as *ua poj niam*, or "being/doing a woman" (see also Rice, this volume). Although there is no formal ritual recognition of menses and it is seldom discussed among women, it signals the end of childhood. A girl who has begun to menstruate is no longer referred to as a child *(tus menyuam)* and is instead described as a young woman *(hluas nkauj)*. She is eligible to be married and to begin reproduction.

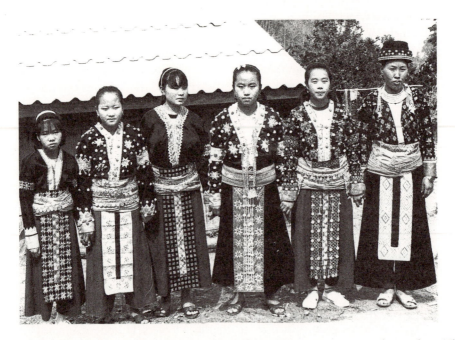

FIGURE 5.1 Young women at the onset of menses are anxious to marry and reproduce. They wore highly decorative clothing — especially the aprons (*sev*) which cover the genitalia and back. They signal "We are ready". (Photo: P. Symonds).

Menstrual blood is not considered polluting by the Hmong in my study (cf. Rice, this volume), and few restrictions are placed on a menstruating woman. Because the concept of physical health or well-being is predicated on the belief that the body must be kept in equilibrium, various traditional remedies are applied to maintain the body in a harmonious state. Like pregnant women, menstruating women are believed to be in a state of coldness (a belief widely shared throughout South and Southern Asia) and must therefore keep themselves physically warm and eat only warming foods, although unlike parturient women, they are not waited on and cooked for during this time.

Because menstruating women are believed to be in a state of disequilibrium, they are said to be vulnerable to illness and advised to exercise extra caution during this time. In addition to having to guard over their physical health, they are also considered vulnerable to spirits, in particular those found along pathways and/or near streams and other bodies of water (see also Rice, this volume). The following myth, related to me by a Hmong shaman in Flower Village, illustrates this concept of the vulnerability of women during both menstruation and pregnancy:

> Long ago Siv Yis looked down from his cave above and saw three very wicked brothers killing people, cutting off their heads and eating their bodies. He decided to do something about it and went down to where they lived to meet

them. He introduced himself and chatted for a while and asked where they lived. He was told they lived in a cave near by and he was welcome to spend the night. He refused, but made plans to meet them the next day. "Would you like me to bring along a beautiful girl?" he asked. The three brothers were delighted. On his return to his cave Siv Yis formulated a strategy for dealing with the wicked brothers. At the appointed time the next day he changed himself into a beautiful girl with beautiful clothes. He then appeared at the appointed place. "Where is Siv Yis?" the wicked brothers asked in surprise. "He cannot come today. Tomorrow, if possible, he will come. He said if anyone of you think I am beautiful and if you wish, one of you can marry me", she said. The wicked brothers talked together and decided that she was indeed very beautiful and that the oldest brother would marry her. They took her home to the cave, and their parents, who were most happy to have a daughter-in-law to help in the house and to produce children for their lineage. The young woman said to her future husband, "Bring me a very large pig and place several large pans around the cave, and I will cook for a party for our wedding". The brothers brought a very large pig into the cave which they sacrificed and butchered and put in the pots, which they had arranged around the cave. The daughter-in-law waited until there was a lot of fat in each pan and then upset it in the cave and set fire to it all. The wicked brothers and their parents were burned to death. The daughter-in-law escaped quickly to the outside and prepared to return home. Then she noticed the younger brother had hidden outside of the cave and escaped the flames. "Why did you kill all of my family?" he stormed. The daughter-in-law quickly turned back into Siv Yis and answered, "You and your brothers are wicked. You kill and eat people. You, too, should be killed, but you have been saved, and I cannot kill you now, but you will live forever in a hole in the earth". The young wicked brother answered "I will not kill and eat people any more, but if young menstruating girls and pregnant women walk over the holes in the ground in which I live, or over springs or lakes which I visit, I will enter into them and cause them trouble".

If a young menstruating woman experiences severe cramps, or a pregnant woman experiences spotting or other complications, she is said to have disturbed the surviving wicked brother of the story.

COSMOLOGICAL ASPECTS OF BIRTH

The birth of the first child signals a major transition for a Hmong woman, and is one of the few areas in life where she experiences empowerment and through which she earns her niche in a new family. Still, it must be stressed that her role is a limited one, especially in the area of ritual or spiritual work. Although, for example, women are allowed to become shamans, they cannot call in the souls of the newborn nor guide them back to the World of Darkness. Neither are women allowed to honour or "feed" the ancestors at New Year's celebrations, visit grave sites, or prepare sacrificial animals, all important ritual acts.

The Calling in the Soul Ceremony: The Journey to the Land of Light

The Hmong hold that a child's soul does not enter its body until three or more days after the child's birth when a naming ceremony, known as "Calling in the Soul", has been conducted by the oldest male paternal relation (usually the grandfather). Prior to that time, the child is not considered a human being because it is believed that women give birth to a physical body devoid of human qualities and spirit. Full of celebratory percussion and noise, the atmosphere surrounding the naming ceremony contrasts sharply with the silence that surrounds the actual birth of the child, as we saw in the case of Mee. The noise created by the men signals to the spirit that it has survived the journey to the Land of Light and that the child's body is ready to receive it. Men alone are given license to call in the spirits because it is said that the presence of women would frighten them away.

When a person dies, it is said that three souls, or life essences, leave the body. At the time of death, a person is no longer considered gendered because it is the body, the vessel which holds the soul, that is believed to provide a person with gender. One of these three souls *(ntsuj duab)* stays with the bones in the grave, but the second soul *(ntsuj nyuj)* goes to the land of the ancestors where it lives in a village in a household that is similar to the one it left behind, and where the social structure is said to be the same as that on earth, i.e., with the same lineages and clan groups. There it fuses with its spouse's soul to create a single, unified or dual-gendered pair. Thus, when a widow or widower dies, she/he joins her or his deceased spouse to create a dyadic spirit.

This dual-gendered pair can influence the lives of their descendants for good or for ill and as such they are venerated and fed by their descendants as a single unit. In this concept, we see one of the reasons why an unwed woman is considered socially anomalous and feared at the time of her death. It is believed that she will always be alone, and that any debts she may have incurred in this life will not be repaid because she has not produced offspring to repay these debts for her. Neither may she return to her natal lineage because she is considered "unlucky".

The third soul *(ntsuj tsov kab or ntsuj noog)* travels to the spirit world where it will be judged by a deity, and will then await another body in which to return to earthly life. Ideally, the soul will reincarnate into a human body that is of the opposite gender from the one she/he inhabited in the most recent life. This third soul, then, is a continuing cosmic entity which alternately occupies the body of a male or a female.

When a woman first goes into labour, the chosen soul is instructed by the chanter that it is time for its rebirth, and it then waits at the gates of the ancestral village to obtain the aforementioned "mandate for life", the paper that will allow it to return to earth (Thao, 1984). For the Hmong, a soul is believed to be part of the "ancestral mass" (Lemoine, 1972a), a pool of souls that belongs to the descent group, and each of these souls requires a human body in which to be reborn. One soul has already been reborn into the infant as soon as its bones begin to grow in the uterus. The seed is said to be provided by the father, and the blood and fat through the egg provided by the mother, reflecting the bone/flesh dichotomy also reported for the

Green Mong by Radley (1986). The second soul is believed to be acquired from the "wind" at the very moment the child takes its first breath.

It is said that the child's third soul does not enter body until the time of the naming ceremony on the third day, or soon thereafter. If an infant were to die before the third soul had been called in, her/his body would be disposed of in the forest without ceremony because it would not yet be considered a full human being, or Hmong person. As mentioned earlier, at dawn on the third day, the oldest male member of the lineage opens the small spirit door located directly across from the family altar *(Xwm Kab)*. This spirit door is opened only for ritual purposes, in this case to coax the newborn child's soul *(tus plig)* to return to earth, the Land of Light, in order to inhabit the child's body.

In this sense, males are considered ultimately responsible for the birth of the social being or the creation of the social individual. The Hmong believe that the child, the product of the union of the egg and the seed, is nourished by and grows inside of a woman's body, where it resides for "ten moons", but it cannot properly be said to belong to the mother. As mentioned earlier, the uterus is called "the house of the child", or "the house for the child", *lus tsev tus menyuam,* and it is believed to be merely the vessel or "basket" in which the seed grows (see also Chindarsi, 1976). And in this way, although women are acknowledged to be the producers of the physical body of the child, it is men who are considered the reproducers of social life in Hmong society.

CONCEPTION

Because the human body is considered the site for souls or life essences, the conception of a child is much celebrated, marking the creation of a new vessel through which ancestral souls will be able to re-enter the material world and be incorporated into the lineage. A confirmed pregnancy, which provides a vessel for the soul of a departed ancestor, is a very important event.

The Hmong believe that conception occurs when the egg *(lub qe)* of a woman and the seed *(tus qab)* of a man meet, and begin to grow. The seed is said to be produced in the testicle *(noob qes)*, during intercourse. The egg is then produced inside the uterus *(lus tsev tus menyuam)* at about the time a woman menstruates. Thus, according to Hmong, the most fruitful time to conceive is just before or during a woman's menses. The planting metaphor, which analogises rain and menstruation, is used in a Hmong saying about the ideal time to conceive: "It is better to plant the seed when it is raining or about to do so". During this time, the Hmong say that a woman is "blooming" and consequently more "open" to conception.

The seed is said to be produced inside the male's body during intercourse whereupon it travels inside the woman's body to meet the egg. The Hmong believe that if the egg is stronger than the seed, the egg will eat the seed and it will die; then, the egg will leave the body and the woman will not conceive. If, however, the egg and the seed are of equal strength, the seed will become planted inside the egg; combined they create an infant. The child receives its sustenance while in the uterus from its mother's blood and fat. Once the seed, which according to the Hmong possesses all of the human attributes which are provided by the man, is planted in the egg and begins to grow, the placenta or "shirt" of fine material begins to take shape around the developing body. Hmong foetal development theory posits that the first attribute a child develops is its eyes, followed by its head and neck, bones, internal organs and stomach. At three months, the Hmong believe that the sex of the child can be determined according to the following formula: if a female egg has been produced and the husband has slept on the right side of his wife, the baby will be a girl. If the husband has slept on the left side of his wife, the baby will be a male child.

PREGNANCY

Because of the importance of producing offspring for the patriline, families take great interest in observing how long it takes for a young wife to become pregnant, although it is not unusual for a woman to become pregnant even before her marriage has taken place. After marriage, mothers-in-law keep a vigilant eye on their daughters-in-law for any increase in their consumption of sour food which the Hmong believe is the first sign of pregnancy. During this time, a young woman's in-laws also observe her behaviour to assess whether she has been trained properly by her own mother, whether she works sufficiently hard in the fields and whether she is humble. For example, if she is complimented on her sewing skills, a good Hmong women is expected to engage in culturally-sanctioned self-deprecation, denying that it is good work.

   If a woman should become pregnant, and the pregnancy progresses normally, an offering is promised to the ancestors in a ritual for the birth of a healthy child. Throughout pregnancy, until the moment that labor pains are felt, women continue to work in the fields, to plant, weed, and harvest rice and other crops, and to perform their usual domestic duties such as feeding the live stock and chickens and cooking and caring for their other children if they have any. Although a pregnant woman does not for the most part receive any dispensation from her regular chores, if a task requires heavy lifting or extensive reaching she is encouraged to ask for assistance. Pregnant women are also advised to be cautious around water, and to avoid crossing rivers or streams. They must take precautions not to step over the strings that are used to leash or tie animals such as pigs or horses, an action which is believed to cause the umbilical cord to become twisted. And they are not allowed to walk far by themselves in the woods or gardens for fear that they might be frightened by something which would result in soul loss and physical illness.

WHY WOMEN GIVE BIRTH

The women in Flower Village frequently related the following story about why women give birth. It involves the reversal of sex roles as an explanation for how men and women struck a bargain in the ancient past as to which of the sexes would give birth:

A long time ago Hmong men used to give birth to the babies of the lineage. It was difficult and painful for men to do as they only had a small hole for the child to come out of. This caused them to labor for seven days and seven nights. One day a man delivered a child as small as a grasshopper. The man killed and ate a cow in order to replenish his strength and then, because he was too lazy to carry the infant on his back, he tied it to his shin. Then, he went off to the field to join his wife who was already working there. As he walked along, he came upon a chicken. The chicken saw the baby and pecked it off the man's shin and ate it. The man started to cry and continued to do so until he reached the field where his wife was working. "Why are you crying?" his wife asked. "Because the chicken ate my baby after I laboured painfully for seven days and seven nights", he answered. "Stop crying," said his wife, "from now on why don't I have the babies? The hole I have is bigger and if I open my legs the child could be as big as a small stool we sit on. Then the chicken will not be able to eat it. But, if I do this you must kill me a chicken to eat every day for a month after I give birth and I must stay at home eating chicken that you have prepared for me, regaining my blood and strength." The man agreed and from then on women gave birth and men killed chickens for them to eat and cared for them for a month after the birth of each child.

As this story illustrates, the Hmong believe that women are more suited to give birth than men because of their physiology but that men were once also able to do so, if less skilfully, bravely and quietly. The story also reveals that giving birth is a task laden with importance and meaning for the Hmong, and how the process of giving birth creates a change in the physical state as well as the spiritual state of women, underscoring the significance of the postpartum period.

DIET DURING PREGNANCY

There are no dietary prescriptions or proscriptions during pregnancy; women are allowed to eat whatever they desire at this time because it is believed that if they do not, the child will be scarred or marked in some fashion. For example, if a pregnant woman has an urge to eat chicken and there is no chicken available, the child's ears may become notched or chicken-like as a result. Similar beliefs concerning pregnancy and food cravings are shared in other Southeast Asian cultures, for example, areas of the Philippines where it is believed that, if left unsatisfied, such cravings can result in miscarriages (Hart, Coughlin and Rajadhon, 1965). Laderman (1983), in her research on birth in Malaysia, also found that people believe unsatisfied cravings may produce problems for the foetus.

At approximately the seventh month of pregnancy, a ritual called "doing the spirits" *(ua neeb)* is performed to ensure the safety of the foetus at birth. At this time, the shaman reiterates an earlier promise to provide a sacrificial animal to the ancestors if a healthy child is born. Two joined paper dolls are placed in front of the pregnant woman who is seated on a small stool behind the shaman. The pair of paper dolls is then cut apart and burned to signify the successful separation of the mother and child, since it is said that if the child is very strong and the mother tired and weak from the birth, the child may steal the mother's soul and cause her death.

If the baby dies at birth, the woman will attempt to become pregnant very soon thereafter, because the loss of the child represents the loss of a place and a body for the ancestral soul. It is believed that the soul has returned to the land of the ancestors to await the birth of a body it finds more suitable.

Older lineage members, including mothers-in-law, in recognition of the fact that when they die they too will need bodies in which to be reincarnated, encourage their daughters-in-law to continue to produce children throughout the span of their reproductive lives. An additional reason for this encouragement is that grandchildren will eventually care for and feed their deceased grandparents as ancestral spirits.

THE CASE OF NTXAWM: THE POSTBIRTH EXPERIENCE

The supreme importance of the male lineage is reaffirmed at the time of birth, even though, ironically, the occasion appears to be a woman-centred one because of the conspicuous absence of men during the actual period of labor and birth. However, immediately following the birth, the husband enters the scene to undertake his ritually prescribed task of burying the placenta and from that point on the "birth" of the child becomes a cultural event overseen exclusively by the male members of the patriline, as we will see in this case study.

Burying the Birth Shirt

Ntxawm had just given birth. Next to the main housepost *(ncej dab)*, where the household lineage spirits are said to reside, Ntxawm's husband carefully buried the infant's "birth shirt" or placenta. This act is always undertaken with great care because it believed that a child's health may suffer if insects or animals are allowed to dig up and eat any of the placenta. Ntxawm's husband then collected the effluvium from the birthing process, and went outside to wash the sarong she had worn during the birth in a wash basin. He then dug a small hole in the ground and poured the blood into it, covering it over carefully. This task is almost always carried out by the new father in order to protect the new mother and child. It is believed that if the spirits found the blood, they would desire more, something that might make both mother and child sick.

Ntxawm's mother-in-law boiled water and beat an egg and some pepper into it, and gave it to Ntxawm to eat in order that she might regain her strength and produce good milk for the child.

Postpartum Diet and Proscriptions

The Hmong believe that it is very important for the mother and child to be kept warm during the month following the birth, especially for the first three days (when the child has yet to acquire a soul). When a child is born, the mother of the child is said to be in a "cold" state and her body must therefore be returned to its proper state of balance (for an overview on the practice of mother roasting in the region, see Manderson, 1981). With the exception of an occasional papaya, which is believed to produce good strong milk, she is not allowed to eat any fruit or vegetables, which are considered "cold" foods capable of causing the blood to congeal; it is believed that if her blood were unable to flow out freely, a woman might suffer from a multitude of sicknesses in her old age. Therefore, Ntxawm was not permitted to drink cold water. Nor could she eat the rice that is made for the family each morning, since the everyday rice has cooled by midday and is served cold at both midday and evening meals. Instead, either Ntxawm's husband or mother-in-law cooked fresh, hot rice for her at every meal. Each day, her husband killed one of the family's chickens, or bought one for her in the valley or from another Hmong family in the village. The chicken was boiled with special green herbs and freshly cracked white pepper, which are believed to remove any stale blood that continued to flow out of her body, in order that she might remain strong and that her uterus, *lub tsev tus menyuam* (literally translated as "the house of the child"), might be cleansed and made ready for the gestation of her next child. The Hmong consider the fat and blood of chicken particularly nourishing for a postpartum women, since it both replaces the fat and blood believed to have provided nourishment for the child during gestation, and also provides breast milk for the child over the next several years.

Ntxawm stayed at home to rest with her son for thirty days, all the while eating a special postpartum diet to regain her strength and to speed her body's return to its formerly "balanced" state. Throughout this period, she was not permitted to visit the houses of other families because she was in what is referred to as a "new" *(tshiab)* state. It is believed that a woman in this state might bring harm to people in other households, harm for which her family would be held responsible and for which they would be required to pay damages. In the event that her family refused to pay such damages, her soul would be required to return as a slave after her death in order to work off this debt in the household of those who were harmed. To warn others of her condition, her husband wove together out of pieces of bamboo *(caiv)* a taboo sign, and placed it outside of the house to warn people outside the family that they should not enter the house. It also served to warn anyone who was ill that there was a newborn child in the house and that they should not enter. Pregnant women are also forbidden to visit the household of a young mother, since the Hmong believe that an encounter with a pregnant woman may diminish the milk supply of the new mother. Anyone who is permitted to enter the house must remove their shoes and leave their bags outside.

Various proscriptions about washing were also observed, for example, Ntxawm bathed herself in warm water, although typically she washes only in cold water. She refrained from washing her hair until a full month had elapsed, since this too is believed to cause illness. Her mother-in-law gave the child his first bath, heating the water in a pan on a tripod placed over the fire.

Certain proscriptions about breastfeeding are also observed. Hmong women, for example, do not begin to breastfeed their children immediately after birth.

Traditionally, they are advised to wait for a day or two until they begin to produce milk and they consider colostrum to be unhealthy for the child to drink. Ntxawm washed the colostrum away, and, like the placenta, it was carefully disposed of out of fear that if an animal ingested the colostrum the child would become ill. If the child cried during the first or second day following the birth, another lactating woman from the lineage was asked to feed the infant. The breast milk of lactating mothers is regarded as a very powerful medicine, dangerous if used incorrectly, and a number of taboos attach to it as a consequence of these beliefs. For instance, lactating women who have recently given birth are not permitted to cook out of fear that the milk might accidentally become mixed with the family food.

The first three days following the birth are the most dangerous for a child, because the soul has not yet inhabited her/his body. It is believed that a soul cannot inhabit the child's body before the child has been provided with a name during a formal naming ceremony. During this period, Ntxawm and her child lay in front of the fire to keep warm.

The case study of Ntxawm's birth illustrates several important facets of the Hmong birth process that explain why Hmong women were experiencing difficulty adjusting to the atmosphere of western hospitals. In these examples of the various taboos that surround pregnancy, birth and the postpartum period, it is clear that Hmong women would resist the idea of going to a hospital or clinic for prenatal care, birthing, or postnatal care, because if they were pregnant they would bring harm to women who are nursing, and, correspondingly, after the birth, they might bring harm to people who are ill or to pregnant women. Hmong women recognise that if they were to stay in the hospital for the birth, the effluvium and "birth shirt" would not be saved for proper burial, and that they might be urged to have surgery they consider unnecessary and dangerous, to begin breastfeeding immediately after the birth or to eat proscribed foods. Another factor is the importance of privacy and modesty: Hmong women would never by choice be treated by a man for gynaecological purposes, and a woman in labor usually gives birth alone, never in the presence of an unknown male (see also Rice, 1993, 1994).

PRIVACY, THE BIRTH SHIRT AND THE POSTPARTUM DIET

Although a woman's husband is not typically present for the child's birth, he is nevertheless held responsible for the important post-birth task of burying the placenta and cleaning and removing the birth detritus; shame is attached to the neglect of this duty. In many societies the disposal of the placenta is similarly ritualised in the Turnerian sense of that term, i.e. "prescribed formal behavior for occasions not given over to technological routine, having reference to beliefs in mystical beings or powers" (Turner, 1967:25). Many cultures share the Hmong belief that a person is connected to the placenta for life, for example, in some Southeast Asian cultures, the placenta is thought to be the child's twin; in others, it is believed to have sympathetic magical powers (Hart, Coughlin and Rajadhon, 1965).

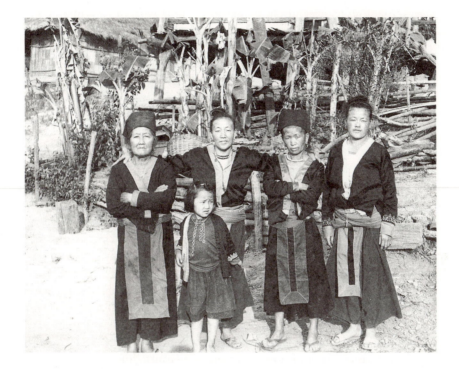

FIGURE 5.2 After marriage older women still cover themselves with the *sev*, but they are not decorated, merely practical. (Photo: P. Symonds).

For the Hmong, there are several important symbolic associations surrounding the placenta and its disposal. The amniotic sac in which a foetus develops is considered analogous to the shell of a chicken's egg. Once the child has been born, the amniotic sack is buried along with the placenta which has gradually grown around the child. The placenta is attached to the mother via the umbilical cord or *txoj hlab ntawv*, which the Hmong call the "life line" or "encircling paper" in an interesting parallel with the "mandate for life", the paper which the soul must collect in the land of the ancestors before returning to the earth.

Together, the amniotic sac, the placenta and a small piece of the umbilical cord which remains attached when the cord is cut at birth are known collectively as *lub tsov tus menyuam* or the "birth shirt". If the infant is a male, the birth shirt is buried beneath the main post of the house because in Hmong cosmology the main post of the house is believed to be the connecting link between the earth and the ancestral spirits. In accordance with the rules of patrilineal descent, the son's "shirt" is buried at his family's home because he will remain with his family throughout his life where he will be held responsible for the spiritual duties of the lineage, whereas the "shirt" of the daughter will not remain part of her natal lineage because, as mentioned earlier, the Hmong practice exogamy.

Like the effluvium from the birth, a child's birth shirt is buried with great care. First it is wrapped in leaves and placed flat in the hole with the umbilical cord on top of it. It must be covered carefully so that animals cannot ingest it, which might cause the infant to vomit food or to become afflicted with skin or other diseases. At this time, a woman who has not yet given birth to a son is allowed to ask *Kab Yeej*, the Goddess of Birth, to send her a son at the time of her next confinement; when her husband buries the placenta, it must be turned inside out and a promise made to sacrifice a pig if the requested son arrives.

At the time of her or his death, every Hmong individual is admonished to return to the place of her or his birth to retrieve the birth shirt which must be worn on the return trip to the land of the ancestors (Lemoine, 1972b; Tapp, 1989). Without this birth shirt, Hmong say, one cannot be reborn as a human being. The placenta, then, is not only essential for a child's physiological development, it can also be described as her/his "spiritual clothing" to be worn on the journeys from the other world to this one and the return. The burial of the placenta can thus be understood to be a ritual creation or recreation of the cosmos, one that carries great meaning for the Hmong. It represents both the individual's birth and rebirth. In this way, the buried placenta becomes the transitional object around which the liminal states of birth, death and rebirth can be said to revolve.

Another facet of Hmong culture that is revealed through a close study of birth is that a post-parturient woman is given a diet high in both protein and fat, and these meals are typically prepared for her by her husband. Because childbirth is viewed as an act that depletes a woman's body of both blood and strength, it is prescribed that she follow various traditional dietary prescriptions or risk vulnerability to disease in later life. Of particular interest, because it is in striking contrast to everyday life in Hmong culture, is the idea that all the decision-making concerning birth appears to rest squarely in the hands of women. It is one of the few areas in Hmong women's lives in which they experience increased status and empowerment. As we have seen, husbands are required to cook their wives' meals, in a reversal of the ordinary household roles in which it is men who make decisions and women who cook the meals. During this month-long period, women not only eat first, but they also eat meat, a prestige food because of its expense and limited availability. In addition, a woman who has given birth is allowed special privileges in that she is required to rest, is kept warm and comfortable at all times, and is not allowed to work in the fields.

The conceptual paradigm of hot/cold foods and body temperatures, and the belief in women's postpartum "vulnerability" has been reported for most of Southeast Asia (e.g. Hart, Coughlin and Rajadhon, 1965; Mougne, 1978; Manderson, 1981; Laderman, 1983). Several authors, for example, report that the Southeast Asian understanding of hot/cold foods is derived from the influence of Indian Ayurvedic humoral traditions, but I suggest that for the Hmong the influence is that of traditional Chinese medicine, a system that asserts that each person is possessed of two opposing vital forces, or *ch'i*, in her or his body. These two opposing qualities are cold (*yin*) and hot (*yang*) and they must be kept in equilibrium if optimum health is to be maintained (see Chu, this volume). In the postpartum period, the Hmong believe that a woman has been depleted of heat, and must therefore eat only those foods that will serve to increase heat, while avoiding foods that would produce a cooling effect. Throughout South and Southeast Asia, chicken is considered a heat-building food *par excellence*, which provides some background as to why the woman in the story recounted above specifically requested that she be fed a chicken a day. Although the Hmong believe that a postpartum woman must be kept physically warm, they do not, however, follow the tradition of lying by the fire, or "mother-roasting" as it is called, a practice common throughout Southeast Asia (Hanks, 1963; Hart, Coughlin and Rajadhon, 1965; Muecke, 1976; Mougne, 1978; Manderson, 1981).

The case study of Ntxawm also illustrates the undisputed belief in the value of breast milk in Hmong culture. Although the Hmong do not include dairy products in their diet, breast milk is highly regarded as the food that sustains life in newborns and young children. One of the debts for which wife-takers must pay during the negotiations for bridewealth is breast milk, as well as the food to be provided for the woman during her lifetime, a clear illustration of the connection between Hmong women's physical contribution to the community through her ability to give birth and the continuity of life in Hmong culture.

DIVISION OF LABOR

The story about why women give birth also suggests that women willingly chose to take on the burden of childbirth, thereby freeing up men to attend to the spiritual and cultural aspects of birth. If a women is unable to give birth she has failed in her foremost responsibility to the ancestors and the male lineage. Thus, spinsterhood is considered perhaps the worst fate a woman can have, one which causes her own and her family's loss of face. In addition to its purpose as an economic and social network of clans, marriage is also valued for its spiritual dimension: the continuation of the male lineage by providing ancestors a means by which to return to earth, the Land of Light. Consequently, there is great social stigma attached to childlessness, and a childless woman (one who has a "dry egg" or *lub qe quav)* leads a very difficult life. She is regarded as unfortunate, unlucky, and unfulfilled in this life and, perhaps even more importantly, in the next life as well. Childless women regard their lot as unlucky and often express their desire for a better reincarnation, for example, I once heard a childless woman say: "When I reach 120 years old [a Hmong synonym for death] and I return to this world, I want to return as a pig or chicken so that I can have many children".

Having been given or having "accepted" the burden of physically bearing children, Hmong women must also bear responsibility for infertility and failed births. If a woman has experienced numerous miscarriages, ectopic pregnancies or still births, it is said that she has committed some past act which is unacceptable to the soul. Repeatedly failed pregnancies are considered the soul's punishment for wrongdoing, and the woman is held responsible for her own childless state (Lemoine, 1972a). When a woman experiences difficulty conceiving, she first consults with traditional herbalists from her own village. If their remedies prove unsuccessful she may seek out women in other villages who possess special knowledge of fertility-enhancing herbs. Since women are considered responsible for a couple's inability to conceive a child, it is incumbent upon the woman to seek out help for this condition. For example, one woman in Flower Village who had been married for several years had been unable to conceive, despite all the rituals performed and herbal medicine prescribed. Then her husband died in an accident. The Hmong practise levirate so the young widow was soon married to her deceased husband's younger brother, at which time she immediately became pregnant and gave birth to a boy. The Hmong attributed her success to the rituals and the herbal medicine, not to the change of husband, although in confidence several women told me that they believed that infertility could result if the seed of the man were not "strong enough".

In these and related examples, we see that the dominant ideology, although often supported and given voice by women, is contradicted in their underlying subdominant voice. This is demonstrated by the clear differences between the responses women give in the presence of men (or women who represent male influence in their lives, such as their mothers-in-laws) and those they give when they are alone or in very informal situations with other women. For example, when asked what would happen if there were no men around to perform spirit calling rituals, women reply that they are capable of doing it themselves. Men, on the other hand, state that women do not have the knowledge to perform such rituals.

BIRTH CONTROL

In addition to the issues surrounding her ability to conceive and give birth, every Hmong woman must deal with the personal consequences of deciding to limit reproduction. Many Hmong women told me that birth control pills or injections leave them feeling weak, with a poor appetite and unable to work in the fields. They find that they must stay home and rest just as they rest during the postpartum period and, in addition, they claim to feel depressed and to be afflicted with what is known as *nyuab siab,* a difficult liver. Hmong women experience the added fear that if they refuse to produce more children for the lineage, their husbands may opt to take in junior wives, and although there are times when the taking of a second or later wife is necessary and even desirable for women, it is not the solution that most women prefer. It may be that the effects of social pressure to produce children, and subsequent feelings of depression, manifest themselves in the form of liver distress, the physical organ that provides an idiom for the expression of emotion in Hmong culture (Kleinman, 1988).

As we have seen, heirs are considered necessary to ensure one's well being in the afterlife as well as in this life: having sons is considered more important than having daughters because only sons are able to care for the family altar and feed the ancestors, thereby ensuring the continued prosperity of the lineage and household. If a married couple is childless, there will be no one to care for them in old age or to feed the ancestors. As mentioned earlier, if a couple has daughters only, a son-in-law may join the household of his wife's family, but this solution is not looked on as favourably as others. However, in spite of the importance placed on having sons in Hmong society, great value is placed on having an equal number of sons and daughters. In exchange for giving its daughters in marriage, a family is compensated with "bridewealth" (*nqe mis nqe hmo*, silver) that is exchanged for a future daughter-in-law who will continue the family line by giving birth to children. In this way, both sons and daughters ensure the continuity of the lineage; sons by fathering lineage members and daughters by bringing in bridewealth, which is used to obtain wives for the remaining sons. As mentioned earlier, a childless woman is regarded as unfortunate, unlucky, and unfulfilled in this life, but perhaps even more importantly in the next life as well. Consequently, women who do not produce sons sometimes encourage their husbands to take junior wives, because they too need descendants to feed them and to provide bodies in which they may be reincarnated after death.

Thus far, the Thai Government's efforts to encourage people in the valleys to avail themselves of birth control methods have met with a great deal of success, but they have met with considerably less success with minority highland groups such as the Hmong. Researchers have suggested that these groups continue to have many children because only large families provide enough children to work in the field, or that large families continue to be viewed as status markers for both women and men. Although these suggestions are valid, the ideological and cosmological components which serve to control women's reproduction remain unexplored. Hmong women are, as we have seen, reluctant to use any form of abortion or birth prevention because the spirits of lineage members are waiting to be reincarnated and because preventing conception might deny a soul its opportunity for rebirth. Although Hmong women have knowledge of emmenagogues or abortifacients, they are seldom used. Even after a woman has given birth to several children and believes that her family is complete, or that she would like to space the births of additional children at greater intervals, she is under considerable constraint by lineage members not to practice birth control of any kind. When I asked women in the village, in the presence of their mothers-in-law, whether they practiced birth control, I was almost always told no. If, however, I were to visit these women later on when they were alone or with other women, they would sometimes confide in me that they were trying one or another method, another example of the subdominant voice of women.

A factor that further complicates the issue of fertility regulation, as noted at the outset of this chapter, is the fact that Hmong women traditionally marry when they are quite young, at the beginning of their reproductive life cycle, and they continue to give birth until menopause (cf. Rice, this volume). Because of this long reproductive life cycle, it is not at all unusual for a mother-in-law to be pregnant at the same time as her daughter-in-law; both are believed to be performing their duty: to produce children for the family and the lineage in addition to producing children who will provide for their own reincarnations. As stated earlier, the Hmong also believe that a woman must give birth to more children than her own mother or mother-in-law if she is to fulfil her destiny. If she does not, she will not have paid all of her earthly debts and will not be able to be reborn as a male (Kunstadter, Kunstadter and Ritnetikul, 1990).

BIRTHING

Even though the Hmong believe that pregnancy makes women more vulnerable to spirits (a belief which suggests that pregnant women are in a liminal state, somewhere in between the spirit world and the everyday mundane world) and there are some taboos and proscriptions surrounding this life event, pregnancy is nevertheless considered a normal physical condition. As already noted, pregnant women consequently experience little deviation from their daily chores and routine. On occasion, children have even been born in the field house, but women in labor usually attempt to reach their own homes where the household spirits reside and where they will feel protected. If, however, the infant is born either in the field or on the way home from the fields, and the woman is alone, she cuts the umbilical cord with her knife and carries both the child and the placenta home. The placenta, as previously mentioned, is then buried and the woman remains at home to eat the prescribed postpartum diet for one month.

Ideally, as we have seen in the case of Ntxawm, Hmong women are expected to give birth alone. If this is not possible, a woman may request the presence of her mother-in-law or another woman of her choosing. Regardless of the presence or absence of others, women in labor are expected to exhibit a nearly herculean degree of stoicism, especially in view of the fact that the Hmong do not make use of pain killers to relieve the pain of labor. As one woman explained, "We do not show how we feel".

MIDWIVES

Although there are no formally trained midwives, there are women who are knowledgeable about pregnancy and birth who know, for example, how to turn babies in utero if they are in a breech position, something that many western-trained gynaecologists no longer feel competent to do. Not every village has a resident midwife, but these women are well-known and are frequently called upon when problems occur in nearby villages. Knowledge is passed on by older midwives. A midwife who lived in a village a substantial distance from Flower Village, explained that she had given birth to only one child; it was a difficult birth and both she and her child had come very close to dying. Her mother-in-law became frightened and sent for a woman in a nearby village who was known to be highly skilled with difficult deliveries. When the midwife arrived, she rotated the child which was in the breech position and she delivered a healthy son. The midwife later taught her these techniques so that she could help other women in her own village. In addition to these midwives, any women who has previously given birth may offer her assistance to young mothers who request or require it. In addition, when problems occur during labor and birth, a shaman may be called in to perform what is known as an *ua neeb* ritual in an effort to "see" what is creating the trouble for the young mother. She or he will then suggest appropriate measures to assist the woman in the birthing process.

CONCLUSION

The social requirements for being a good Hmong woman are to work hard in the fields, feed the animals, cook food for the household, embroider skilfully, and bear many children in silence. Without this last ability, to bear children, her lot is a poor one in this life and the next. The highest reward for being a good Hmong woman is equality in the land of the ancestors (as a dual-gendered soul) and possible rebirth into the body of a male in her next lifetime.

As illustrated in this chapter, a Hmong woman's reproductive health is related closely to her social status as an outsider in her natal family or lineage, and her reproductive health, especially her fertility, is a form of commodity in that it represents the well being of her new family's lineage. Fertility is further categorised or nuanced in Hmong culture as a Hmong woman's ability to have a son, and then to continue to have many more children (more children than her mother-in-law and equal numbers of boys and girls are two of the prescribed goals). Thus, a woman who desires to control her own reproduction through the use of birth control is socially discouraged from doing so, through the influence of a pervasive cultural discourse which suggests that in so doing she would also be upsetting the state of cosmological equilibrium that must be maintained through the continued and prolific reproduction of her husband's (and, in effect, her own) lineage.

In addition to the pressure placed upon her through this cultural discourse, in the form of traditional stories, taboos and proscriptions about physical and cosmological well-being, a woman's behaviour is also closely monitored by her husband's family, as we saw in the role of the mother-in-law during Mee's labor. There are, however, signs that the force of this traditional social discourse is weakening, as evidenced by the fact that when I spoke with young women alone, without the presence of mothers-in-law, many acknowledged that they were experimenting with some form of birth control.

As we have seen, a Hmong woman's social status as an outsider in need of her husband's clan to sustain herself economically, socially and cosmologically, places her in a circumscribed and liminal state from the moment of birth to the moment of death. The cultural discourse that surrounds her demands two things: her good behaviour socially, if she is to be supported economically; and her good behaviour as a procreator, some of which is within her power, i.e. through the practice of birth control, and some of which is not, e.g. being infertile. A woman's fertility is said to result from good behaviour and her infertility from misdeeds, therefore the concept of infertility as a biological condition rooted in purely physical causes (without social stigma) does not exist for the Hmong. Intentionality is ascribed to it, and social stigma attaches to it, thereby threatening the woman's social, economic, and spiritual status. Infertility is thus a fate truly to be dreaded because of the consequences that attach to it, and whatever power a Hmong woman has rests squarely upon her ability to give birth.

ACKNOWLEDGMENTS

For funding research that informs this chapter I would like to thank the Watson Institute for International Studies at Brown University. I am also grateful to the National Research Council of Thailand for permission to conduct field work in their country, and members of the Tribal Research Institute of Chiang Mai University for their kind cooperation. Thank you also to Ntxhi Vang for her assistance with translations of Hmong stories cited in this chapter. Thanks to Dr. Vichai Poshyachinda for his insightful comments and support during my field research. My sincere gratitude to the following people who helped during the field work period: John and Asue Hobday, Usaneeya Perngparn, and Cornelia Kammerer. Thanks to Lenore Manderson and Pranee Liamputtong Rice for careful readings and suggestions for this chapter. *Ua tsaug ntau* to all Hmong who have assisted me in my research. As always, special thanks to Alan E. Symonds for his patience, love, and support.

ENDNOTE

1. The Women, Infants and Children (WIC) Program is a special supplemental food program funded under the Federal Nutrition Program in order to provide adequate nourishment for low-income mothers and their children. It is administered by the U.S. Department of Agriculture's Food and Nutrition Service and operated by individual states.

REFERENCES

Chindarsi, N. (1976) *The Religion of the Hmong Njua*. Bangkok: Siam Society.

Hanks, R. (1963) *Maternity and its Rituals in Bang Chan*. Data Paper No 51. Ithaca: Cornell University Southeast Asia Program.

Hart, D.V., Coughlin R.J., Rajadhon, Phya Anuman (1965) *Southeast Asian Birth Customs: Three Studies in Human Reproduction*. New Haven, Connecticut: HRAF Inc.

Kleinman, A. (1988) *The Illness Narratives: Suffering, Healing and the Human Condition*. New York: Basic Books.

Kunstadter, P., Kunstadter S.L., Ritnetikul, P. (1990) Demographic variables in fetal and child mortality: Hmong in Thailand. *Social Science and Medicine*, **36**(9), 1109–1120.

Laderman, C. (1983) *Wives and Midwives: Childbirth and Nutrition in Rural Malaysia*. Berkeley: University of California Press.

Lemoine, J. (1972a) *Un Village Hmong Vert Du Haut Laos*. Paris: Ecole pratique des hautes, Centre National de la Recherche Scientifique.

Lemoine, J. (1972b) L'initiation du mort chez les Hmong. *L'Homme*, **XII**, 1–3.

Manderson, L. (1981) Roasting, smoking and dieting in response to birth: Malay confinement in cross cultural perspective. *Social Science Medicine*, **15B**, 509–520.

Mougne, C. (1978) An ethnography of reproduction. Changing patterns of fertility in a northern Thai village. In *Nature and Man in Southeast Asia*, edited by P.A. Stott, pp.68–106. London: University of London, School of Oriental and African Studies.

Muecke, M.A. (1976) Health care systems as socializing agents: childbearing the north Thai and western ways. *Social Science Medicine*, **10**(7–8), 377–383.

Radley, H.M. (1986) *Economic Marginalization and the Ethnic Consciousness of the Green Hmong (Moob Ntsuab) of Northern Thailand*. Unpublished PhD thesis. Oxford: Oxford University, Department of Anthropology.

Rice, P.L. (1993) *My Forty Days: A Cross-Cultural Resource Book for Health Care Professionals in Birthing Services*. Melbourne: The Vietnamese Antenatal/Postnatal Support Project.

Rice, P.L. (editor) (1994) *Asian Mothers, Australian Birth: Pregnancy, Childbirth and Childrearing — The Asian Experiences in an English Speaking Country*. Melbourne: Ausmed Publications.

Symonds, P. V. (1991) *Cosmology and the Cycle of Life: Hmong Views of Birth, Death, and Gender in a Mountain Village in Northern Thailand*. Unpublished PhD thesis. Brown University, Department of Anthropology.

Tapp, N. (1989) *Sovereignty and Rebellion: The White Hmong of Northern, Thailand*. Singapore: Oxford University Press.

Thao, Xoua (1984) Southeast Asian refugees of Rhode Island: perceptions of illness. *Rhode Island Medical Journal*, **67**, 323–330.

Turner, V. (1967) *The Forest of Symbols*. Ithaca: Cornell University Press.

CHAPTER 6

A Baby is Born in Site 2 Camp: Pregnancy, Birth and Confinement Among Cambodian Refugee Women

Kimberley Townsend and Pranee Liamputtong Rice

> The act of giving birth to a child is never simply a physiological act but rather a performance defined by and enacted within a *socio-cultural* context (Romalis, 1981:6, our emphasis).

Birth and its process in Cambodia, as elsewhere in Southeast Asia, is subject to and characterised not only by personal but also social and cultural rules. Birth is perceived as a critical life event and thus warrants correct behaviours and the careful preparation and management of the new mother and those around her. This persists from pregnancy to the puerperium, although practices are most strict and adhered to most diligently during the postpartum period. Manderson (1981:517) argues that many of these aspects of childbirth practices have not changed in Southeast Asia despite the fact that "childbirth has been medicalized and subsumed within a Western health care system". In a similar vein, Sargent and colleagues (1983:77) have noted these persist with Cambodian women who have been re-settled in the United States. They state that "a review of practices prevalent during pregnancy and the puerperium suggests that this refugee population manifests persisting concern with humoral pathology and an enduring reliance on indigenous practitioners, while selectively using available cosmopolitan health services in the urban setting". Rice (1994) also notes that for many Cambodian women living in Australia, adherence to tradition is common when they experience ill health and when they give birth, holding close familiar practices in their new living environment.

In this chapter we will show how Cambodian women make sense of the birth process while living in a harsh environment as refugees in a Thai-Cambodian border camp. We will describe the experience of giving birth and the cultural beliefs and practices surrounding birth. This chapter is based on interviews regarding childbearing and childrearing among Cambodian women in Site 2 refugee camp in Thailand. Interviews were conducted with 31 Cambodian women, a *Kru Khmer* (Cambodia traditional healer) and a maternal and child health nurse. All interviews were conducted in early 1993, before the camp was closed at the end of May 1993.[1]

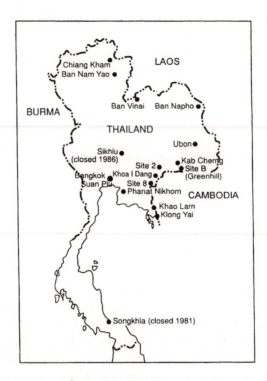

FIGURE 6.1 Refugee camp sites along the Thai-Cambodia (Kampuchea) border and in other parts of Thailand. Source: Feith (1988:28).

CAMBODIAN WOMEN IN SITE 2

Site 2 Khmer refugee camp was formed late 1984/early 1985, when Vietnamese troops overran the border bases of the Khmer People's National Liberation Front (KPNLF — a Cambodian resistance group). An estimated 100,000 or more civilians who were followers of the KPNLF sought refuge in Thailand. As a consequence a number of border encampments were set up. Many of these were later merged into Site 2 camp. The camp was situated about four kilometres from the border (see Figure 6.1).[2] In 1986 there were about 130,000 Cambodians in Site 2 (Soffer and Wilde, 1986); by early 1992, prior to the repatriation program begun on 30 March 1992, this population had increased to 218,282. Of these, 55,322 were women over 16 years and there were 21,643 female headed households (FHH). The average number of children per family was 2.26 and of FHH, 2.03. However, at the time of this study, there was a great shift in the number of camp dwellers. At the end of March 1993, the population of Site 2 was only 29,003. Women over 16 years numbered 6,509 and there were 2,120 FHH. The average number of children per family was 2.25 and of FHH was 1.98. By the end of May 1993, all Khmer had been repatriated to Cambodia.

The condition of the camp was relatively poor.[3] The camp did not have electricity, wells or running water. People lived in small bamboo huts, crowded together, on dirt floors. Food rations were given to women and young children. Healthy men did not receive food rations. However, they could get half-rations by working in the camp. One ration comprised 7 kg of rice, 500 gm of vegetables, and 500 gm of dried salted fish per week. Supplementary foods were available for malnourished people and pregnant women (Soffer and Wilde, 1984; Feith, 1988).[4] The Site 2 camp was divided into six smaller camps, all located within the same compound, for logistical purposes (named Ritysen, Sanroe, Nongchan, Ampil, Dangrek, and O'Bok). The camps were then divided into sections and sub-divided into allotments for administrative reasons.[5]

Maternal And Child Health Centres

There were several Maternal and Child Health Centres in Site 2. The centres were involved with antenatal care, postnatal care and child-spacing. The voluntary organization which operated these centres in Site 2 was called YWAM — Youth With A Mission.

When a woman was four months pregnant, she was asked to attend for prenatal care. The midwife checked for anaemia, blood pressure, and oedema. The midwife tested the women's urine to ensure she had not developed diabetes. A test for eclampsia was also performed. The midwife measured the fundal height to make sure that the baby was growing. At this antenatal appointment an extra rice ration was given to the woman to supplement her diet. She was then expected to return monthly. In the fifth month the midwife listened for the baby's movements and heartbeat. From the 28th week the woman was expected to attend twice a month and from the 36th week weekly. At the first visit the woman was given 14 iron tablets a week and one folic acid tablet a day. She also received two tetanus injections during pregnancy: the first at the first antenatal visit, the second at the 32nd week of pregnancy. One of the most important jobs of the midwife was to take a thorough and accurate history during the antenatal visits to identify those women at risk of complications.

After giving birth the mother received iron and folic acid for one month. The baby was given an injection of BCG to protect against T.B., an oral vaccination against polio, a vaccination against measles, and oral vitamin K against the clotting of blood. The midwife also gave the baby ointment to protect against "staph". The midwife claimed that some babies were infected with gonorrhoea in the birth canal and this ointment prevented further infection.

During the baby's first month, he/she was given a weekly check up. After this a monthly check up was given. The baby's weight was plotted. If the baby was not gaining weight then the mother was given vitamin B and a dry pack of food to help stimulate breastmilk production. If the baby was less than 2.5 kg when born, the YWAM provided the baby with a hat and cotton mittens, booties, a nightie, and a fleece blanket. YWAM also provided "poor" women in the camp with a sarong and short pyjamas after giving birth. After giving birth the KWA — Khmer Women's

Association — provided the mother with a mosquito net, mat and blanket for the baby. The MCH (Maternal and Child Health) program also provided the women with a yellow card which enabled the baby to receive a rice ration and UNHCR repatriation benefits of US$25. This card also contained the baby's birthweight and vaccination programs.

The midwives working at the MCH clinic were traditional birth attendants who had received some limited training through YWAM. There were one to three MCH midwives for every section in the camp. It was their job to help deliver the babies of those women in the section which they were responsible for. Hospital midwives, on the other hand, were given a one year training program through the ARC (American Refugee Committee). The teachers were Khmer and there was a Khmer program director. After this course they were eligible to take the UNBRO (United Nation Border Relief Organization) standardisation test. The hospital midwives could go out to women's homes and deliver. However, for complicated cases women had to deliver in the hospital.

The Women in the Study

The social backgrounds of the 31 Cambodian women who participated in this study are set out in Table 6.1 and are summarised as follows. All women were Buddhist. Their ages ranged from 18 to 57, with the mean age of 34 years old. The majority of the women were married (27) and four were widowed. Most women considered themselves as being "pure Khmer". Most were born in country towns. Only one woman was born in Phnom Penh, the capital city, and one in a border town in Vietnam. Most women had minimal education: nine had no formal education at all. Most women had several children. Many women stated that they had lost a few children during the Pol Pot regime; one 40 year old women for example, with 9 children lost 3 during the Pol Pot regime, another with 10 also lost 3 children during the regime. Most women mentioned that they lived with their husband and children in the camp,[6] and some also had siblings and parents living with them. Most women had lived in Site 2 for at least 10 years. Only 1 worked as a medic; the rest had no employment.

KHMER HERBAL MEDICINES

The Khmer traditional medical system derives largely from Ayurvedic medicine. It also incorporates Chinese and cosmopolitan pharmaceutical medicines (Sargent, Marcucci and Elliston, 1983; Sargent and Marcucci, 1984). Herbal medicines play an important role in Khmer health care, particularly for common physical illnesses and women's reproductive health, including menstrual irregularities and childbearing.

Information from a *Kru Khmer* (traditional healer) at Site 2 indicates that women must take a variety of herbs to maintain their health and to ensure safe delivery. During pregnancy a medicine called *Tnam Raksacoir* is taken. This medicine

TABLE 6.1   Sociodemographic characteristics of Cambodian women.

Sociodemographic Characteristics		Number	Percentage
Age:	Less than 20	1	3.23
	20–30	11	35.48
	31–40	14	45.16
	41–50	3	9.68
	Over 51	2	6.45
Marital Status:	Married	27	87.10
	Widowed	4	12.90
Birth Place:	Battambong	11	35.48
	Banteay Meanchey	3	9.68
	Svey Rieng	1	3.23
	Kompong Thom	3	9.68
	Prey Veng	2	6.45
	Kandal	4	12.90
	Kompong Chhnang	1	3.23
	Phnom Penh	1	3.23
	Kompot	1	3.23
	Kompong Speu	1	3.23
	TaKaeo	2	6.45
	Vietnam border town	1	3.23
Ethnicity:	Pure Khmer	30	96.77
	Chinese Khmer	1	3.23
Religion:	Buddhist	31	100.00
Education:	High school	2	6.45
	Primary (<2 years)	7	22.58
	Primary (>3 years)	9	29.03
	Primary education in camp	2	6.45
	None	11	35.48
Number of children:	1–3	15	48.39
	4–6	7	22.58
	7–9	4	12.90
	10 and over	5	16.13
Years in camp:	1–5	7	22.58
	6–10	3	9.68
	Over 10	21	67.74

comprises a mixture of five types of wood. A *Kru Khmer* gathers the wood from the mountain. He cuts the wood up into small pieces and dries it in the sun. The pregnant woman then must cook the wood to drink as a tea. This herbal medicine is supposed to help the mother and baby have good health, increase the mother's energy level, and ensure the birth is easy, quick and relatively painless. The mother must take this medicine from her fifth month of pregnancy until she gives birth.

During confinement four types of herbal medicines should be taken. *Tnam Koun Kchey* is made from over 80 kinds of wood and leaves. These are cut into small pieces, dried in the sun, mixed together, and put into bags for the women. The women must put two or three grams of this mixture in a pot and cook to drink like a tea. One pot should last about four to five days. This medicine is reported to help increase the mother's health and energy after giving birth, increase her appetite, help her to sleep, and help her not to worry or become depressed. It is also said to help stimulate breastmilk production. The mother can use this medicine for up to one year.

Tnam Kadow is made from over 70 different types of trees. Again, the *Kru Khmer* cuts the wood into small pieces, dries it and gives it to the woman to cook as a tea. She must put two or three grams of medicine in a pot. This medicine is to be taken for one to three days after giving birth. She must drink only one pot. This medicine helps to "flush out" lochia and any retained placenta in the uterus. It is also said to help protect the uterus from infections and to make the body warm. *Tnam Tek Dos* comprises a mixture of five kinds of wood and leaves, dried, mixed together, cooked and drunk as tea to help lactation. *Tnam Tois* is made from eight types of roots, again dried, cooked and drunk as a tea if a women experiences *toah* (see Rice, 1994) from eating or doing something which makes her ill or causes loss of appetite, if she feels nausea or pain, or loses lots of breastmilk. She must drink one or two pots, one pot lasting about three days.

Interviews with the women revealed an even greater variety of herbal medicines used during pregnancy and confinement, although they could not give full details of the mixtures. Women said their parents and husbands sought and prepared the medicines for them so that they would regain their health rapidly (see Tables 6.2 and 6.3).

PREGNANCY AND PRENATAL CARE: WOMEN'S PERCEPTIONS

All women interviewed received prenatal care provided in the camp. Most women commenced routine check-ups when they were four months pregnant. However, a number did not attend until the fifth or sixth month of their pregnancy. Women attended prenatal care for several reasons. Firstly, they felt that they needed to be assured about their own health as well as the health of their foetus and were told that if they attended prenatal care, they would receive vaccination against tetanus which would protect their foetus. They also needed to be assured about the "unseen" outcome of their pregnancy and possible problems which might arise during delivery. If complications occurred during delivery, they would then get help in time; attending prenatal care, women felt, would lessen their worries a great deal. Some women also sought prenatal care in the hope of obtaining some medication to lessen symptoms of illness, including nausea.

Since the midwives were traditional midwives, they had knowledge about turning the foetus into the "right" position, particularly in the case of breech

TABLE 6.2   Herbal medicines used during pregnancy.

Name of Herbs	Beneficial Effects	Preparation Method	Length
Tnam Sleak Kor	Deliver quickly; lessen childbirth pain	Use the wood from the tree named Dam Kor, chop and cook in boiling water, and bathe every day between 7 and 8 am	From 7 months to birth
Tnam Koun Ngea	Deliver quickly; lessen childbirth pain	Take the bark from Goyaya, Dam Trobak Prey, boil the herbs with water, and drink as tea	From 7 months to birth
Tnam Chun Toel Pong Moun	Deliver quickly	Gather wood from the mountain, cut into small pieces, dry in the sun, boil with water, drink as tea	From 5 months to birth
Tnam Chroy Po Leay	Make the baby strong so it will survive	Boil with water, and drink as tea	From 7 months to birth
Tnam Preas Krap	Deliver quickly	Gather herbs from the forest, boil with water, drink as tea or bathe with the herbs	From 7 months to birth
Tnam Chi Krohom	Prevent white colour on the skin of the baby after birth	Wash the herbs, dry in sun, cut into small pieces, cook with water, and drink as tea	From 3 months to birth
Tnam Trop Bak Prey	Prevent childbirth pain	Boil with water and drink as tea	From 5 months to birth
Sork Ton Say	Reduce childbirth pain; deliver quickly	Clean the wood, dry in the sun, boil with water, and drink as tea	From 7 months to birth
Tnam Pois Tom	Deliver quickly; improve the baby's/mother's health; increase breastmilk	Cut many kinds of wood into small pieces, dry in the sun, boil with water, and drink as tea	From 5 months to birth

presentation. Women felt quite comfortable with the care provided by traditional midwives, both because the midwives had some basic knowledge about western medicine which might help them if problems arose, and because they spoke the same language and shared cultural norms.

However, women also had a second incentive to attend prenatal care as this enabled them to receive supplementary food. An extra rice ration would be given to a pregnant woman. Most women were malnourished before they became pregnant, and accepted their need for extra food stuffs for the sake of their foetus. By attending prenatal care women also received a card which would entitle them to receive extra food rations for the child when born. This was crucial since there were no other legal means to obtain food rations without the card.[7]

CHAM NGU CHAN KOUN: HEALTH DURING PREGNANCY

Twenty-four of the 31 women reported being ill during pregnancy. Common symptoms reported included nausea, dizziness, vomiting, tiredness, loss of appetite,

TABLE 6.3   Herbal medicine used during confinement.

Name of Herbs	Beneficial Effects	Preparation Method	Length
Sork Tonsay	Clean out childbirth blood and uterus	Mix the herbs with water, black pepper and garlic, and drink as tea	1 month
Tnam Bi Ban	Increase appetite; make the body strong	Mix the following herbs: Bat Plil, Kreil Sua May, Dom Angkrong, Dam Sdok Sdua; boil with water and drink as tea	1 year
Than Srot Sboun	Prevent uterus from dropping	Use wood of Dam Down Preas, boil with three glasses of water until water is reduced to one glass, and drink as tea	1 year
Tnam Choeun Pleung	Flush out contents of uterus to make the body strong	Cut herbs into small pieces, clean, boil with water, and drink as tea	5 months
Tnam Cheam	Flush out contents of uterus for good health	Mix two kinds of herbs gathered from the forest, cut into small pieces, dry in the sun, boil with water, and drink as tea	5 months
Tnam Chea Sung Krohom	Flush out contents of uterus	Mix the herb with garlic, black pepper, husband's urine, and drink	Once, immediately after birth
Tnam Cham Not	Protect the uterus after delivery when performing hard work	Boil the herbs with water, and drink as tea	3 months
Tnam Sboun	Shrink the uterus to its normal size	Mix the herbs with alcohol and drink	1 month

palpitations and trouble sleeping. Some women also reported having headaches, fever, chills and swollen calves. The other women reported no ill health at all during pregnancy. A common cause of illness in pregnancy, according to the women, was *chum ngu chan koun*, literally illness "due to the power of the foetus". In this understanding, the foetus is more powerful than the mother, and because of this imbalance the mother becomes sick. Women believed that this was a natural part of pregnancy, which any pregnant woman would experience, and therefore, most women did not seek help: "I did not take anything or do anything. I just waited until it passed" (Chantou Noun). However, when the women attended prenatal care at the MCH clinic, they were, as noted above, routinely given iron tablets, folic acid tablets and Vitamin B complex. Women believed that these tablets helped to alleviate their symptoms. Those who experienced particularly poor health would also ask for vitamin injections from the MCH midwives, which they believed worked faster than tablets and improved their health sooner. All medication was provided free of charge at the centres.

DIETARY AND BEHAVIOURAL PRECAUTIONS DURING PREGNANCY

Although pregnancy is perceived as a natural event which most women experience, Cambodian women observe certain culturally determined restrictions to protect the foetus. According to the women interviewed, a healthy pregnant woman can eat most of the food that she also consumes when not pregnant, but she should increase consumption of fruit, vegetables and meat. Women believe that consuming more "sweet" food will help to increase their appetite and hence increase energy. A pregnant woman needs energy and strength to nourish the foetus for nine lunar cycles. Coconut is particularly desirable since not only is the juice sweet and so increases energy, but also because coconut meat is white and will help the foetus to have light skin, considered especially beautiful (cf. Cabigon, this volume).

There are certain food stuffs that women believe have harmful effects. These include spicy food, oily food, "hot" food such as chillies, pepper, fermented fish called *prohok*, scaleless fish such as cat fish and eel, and certain kinds of vegetables such as egg plant, taro, sweet potato, and garlic. Burnt rice should not be eaten, as it is "black" and will make the skin of the foetus dark. Western medicines such as aspirin, and alcohol of any kind, should not be taken since they are perceived to be "hot", can damage the foetus, and may result in miscarriage (cf. Manderson, 1981).

A number of behavioural prescriptions and proscriptions also pertain. Even though a woman may carry on with her daily chores, she must take things more easily. She should walk and perform tasks less vigorously. She should not perform heavy physical activities requiring large amounts of energy, such as carrying heavy loads of water and chopping fire woods, should not reach for high objects or travel long distances, and she must make sure that she will not fall over during pregnancy: any of these activities may result in miscarriage. In addition, a pregnant woman must not sit or stand in the middle of the doorway, on the staircase or on the rice-pounding machine, since these actions may cause an obstructed labour. She should not wrap a *kroma* (a piece of cloth used for a variety of purposes by most Cambodians) around her neck, since this may cause the umbilical cord to tie around the infant's neck. She must eat quickly and stop before everyone else is finished eating whether or not she is full; she must wake up before her husband rises, and perform various activities quickly so that she will give birth quickly. A pregnant woman should also not eat while lying down, as this can make the foetus lazy, causing it not to descend and resulting in a difficult and long labour (cf. Cabigon, this volume).

In general, women believe that if they do not follow these practices they will experience "bad luck" and difficulties during the birth. To further ensure well-being many women consult a *Kru Khmer* (traditional healer) for protection. The *Kru Khmer* makes a belt from cord and metal for the woman to wear from the time of pregnancy until after giving birth. This cord will protect the woman and the foetus, ensuring the woman remains healthy and prevents miscarriage or prenatal death. In addition, if a woman becomes pregnant without marriage she must ask the *Kru Khmer* to perform a ceremony to prevent the relatives from becoming ill, since it is believed that ancestral spirits may become angry and punish family members for the wrong doing.

BIRTH

Twenty-three of the 31 women in the study gave birth in their own homes within the camp. Most gave birth with the assistance of one of the midwife/traditional birth attendants from MCH centre whose duty it was to assist women in the sections for which they were responsible. Four women had a hospital midwife assist in giving birth at their home.

Women chose homebirth for several reasons. Most were familiar with homebirth in Cambodia, since they came from rural areas where modern health care and hospital services were scarce or inaccessible. Traditionally, birth is always managed at home, with a *Chmop* (traditional midwife) assisting the delivery.[8] Although within the camps hospital services were accessible, home birth was nevertheless encouraged; women quickly took up the option. Women felt that they were "healthy enough" to give birth at home. If they had not had any complications in pregnancy, they believed that the birth would not be complicated either. However, since a midwife from the MCH Centre would come to their home at the time of delivery, they were also confident of help if any complications occurred.

Some women said their labour was far too quick to get to a hospital. By the time they knew that they were in labour, they were already in second stage, and hospital birth was neither possible nor necessary. In addition, women with older children felt that they should give birth at home since there was no one to take care of the children, and so they could continue to some extent to look after the children at least during early labour. Some women gave birth at home due to their husband's wishes: "My husband did not want me to go to the hospital because he could not care for me there. He was too ashamed to take care of me in public" (Nary Rim).

TOAH AND DIETARY AND BEHAVIOURAL RESTRICTIONS

During the puerperium, which lasts for 30 days, Cambodian women are particularly cautious about their diet. In general, women avoid consuming any kind of food which they have not already eaten before pregnancy, in case the food is "wrong" for their body and may cause ill health. This is commonly known as *toah mhoop* or *toah chamney*, indicated by diarrhoea, dizziness, fever, headache, and insufficient breastmilk in the new mother. It also causes diarrhoea in the newborn infant if the mother breastfeeds.[9]

Food stuffs believed to be particularly dangerous for postpartum women include spicy food such as hot curry and chillies; sour food such as guavas, raw mangoes, and pineapples; salt water fish such as *pla too*; potatoes and any fresh vegetables; the head of a pig; long-green banana (*chak ombong*); and fermented fish (*prohok*). In theory, Cambodian women should only consume certain kinds of food during the puerperium. Rice soup cooked with fresh water fish, dried in the sun for one week, is ideal. Chicken or pork soup cooked with banana flowers is also consumed to stimulate breastmilk production. The stomach of pig stuffed with black pepper cooked as a soup should also be consumed for 6 months postpartum, as it is believed to increase strength as well as stimulate breastmilk. No other type of meat is allowed since they are considered "wrong" for a new body and will result in *toah*. Women also eat large amounts of black pepper, salt, garlic with rice, and dry fish to increase breastmilk production. It is also a common belief, though not verified, that women should take their husband's urine and mix it with garlic, black pepper and traditional herbal medicines to drink once, about half an hour after delivery. Women say that this will make them younger and prettier.

Although fresh vegetables are taboo during the puerperium, vegetable soup is seen as beneficial and hot water is drunk in large amounts to increase breastmilk. Sweet food is also believed to be beneficial since it helps to increase energy, as women are believed to lose their strength through childbirth and need to build up their energy and strength in the first month after childbirth.

During the puerperium Cambodian women avoid many activities, as they believe that it is important for them to have a good rest, particularly in the first three days after childbirth. If it is possible women should rest for three months so that they may regain full strength and health before resuming their normal household chores and other duties. Only light housework can be undertaken during the postpartum period, and the main task women undertake is care of their newborn. Women avoid rigorous physical activities such as walking long distances, carrying heavy objects, chopping fire woods and pounding rice. These activities are believed to stop breastmilk production and cause prolapse of the uterus. Breaking this taboo will result in *toah* which will jeopardise the health of both the postpartum woman and infant.

TRADITIONAL CUSTOMS OF CONFINEMENT

Birth is seen as dangerous, but in many Southeast Asian cultures, women are regarded as much more vulnerable during the period after birth (Manderson, 1981). It is a crucial time for women if they wish to maintain their own good health and ensure the survival of their newborn. Most cultures therefore have practices which help women to pass through this vulnerable period. Cambodian women observe several traditional practices during the puerperium.

Ang Pleung

Ang pleung, known as "mother roasting", is practised in a number of Southeast Asian cultures (Manderson, 1981) and is similar to *yu fai* practised by Thai women (see Jirojwong, and Whittaker, this volume). Traditionally, a new mother lies on a wooden bed over a warm fire for a period of one lunar month.[10] While roasting she must keep her body warm, by wrapping the body in a blanket, wearing a long sleeved top and long pants, or wrapping a *kroma* around the head and ears.[11] On the first day of the *ang pleung* ritual a woman must sleep with her face turning toward the fire and place a pillow over her head. At the same time her hands are spread out with palms turning downward. While staying on the bed she must also keep silent. This ritual is believed to prevent blurring vision and a swollen face, and make her skin lighter.

Ang pleung is vital for the health of a new mother. Childbirth is believed to deplete body heat, thus causing humoral imbalance in the body. The "new body" is therefore vulnerable and susceptible to harmful agents. Regaining heat lost in the childbirth process is essential to recover good health and ensure good health in old age. Because of the lost heat, the "new body" is seen as cold and containing "old water" which is poisonous for the body. Heat from *ang pleung* makes the body sweat. The sweat is actually the "old water" of the body, and once it is expelled, the body can absorb "new water", so the body becomes hot and this helps to regain health. Making the body warm also helps to prevent *toah* after childbirth, which might lead to such symptoms as numbness, headaches, dizziness, pain in the abdomen, swelling of the body and face, and diarrhoea. *Ang pleung* also helps to flush out retained blood and placenta from the uterus. It is vital to clean out the uterus so it will be ready for the next child. It is believed that childbirth blood and retained placenta are poisonous and have ill effects on the health of the woman in old age. Heat from *ang pleung* also helps to dry out the uterus so it may return to its normal size sooner.

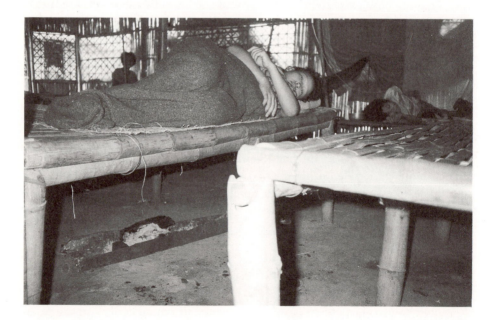

Figure 6.2 Women rests by the fire for *ang pleung* during her confinement. (Photo: K. Townsend).

During *ang pleung* a *Chmop* comes to massage the abdomen daily. During the first two weeks the *Chmop* massages twice, once in the morning and once at night. Thereafter, the massage is performed once at night time for the rest of *ang pleung* period, sometimes for two months if needed. The massage is believed to help "flush out" the contents of the uterus and to make the uterus return to its normal size.

The *Chmop* is invited to perform a ritual to mark the end of the period of *Ang Pleung*. The *Chmop* ties a white cotton string around the wrist of the mother and the baby and prays for good health and good luck. The mother washes the hands of the *Chmop* with powder and water and asks for forgiveness for bringing her into contact with lochia, blood and body substances in the process of birth. The *Chmop* is then offered some food. On the same day relatives, old people, neighbours and friends are invited to join the ceremony. Older people will be asked to pray for the good health of the mother and baby. Presents will be given to the newborn at the ceremony as well.

Ang pleung is traditionally practised for one lunar month, but women in the study indicated that their own observation varied. Most observed the ritual for three days and three nights immediately after birth, and then only at night times for two weeks. However, a number did this for a longer period (one to two weeks) and one practised *ang pleung* during day time and at night for two full weeks, then only at night time for a further two months.

Spong

This custom is known as "steam bath".[12] A basic and simple type of *spong* is with a hot rock. A rock is heated until it becomes very hot. It is then placed on the wooden bed where the puerperal woman spends time during the *ang pleung* ritual. A blanket is placed over the woman's body and the hot rock. Then a mixture of alcohol and *pon ley* (turmeric) is slowly poured onto the rock.[13] This creates steam, and the woman breathes in the steam slowly until the rock has cooled down.

A more elaborate *spong* involves using herbs. Several types of herbal medicines are boiled with water in a big pot. The hot pot is placed on the bed. The woman sits on the bed without any clothes on, and a blanket cover both her and the hot pot. The lid of the pot is opened slowly and the woman sits straight ahead, eyes open, and breathes in the steam until it has cooled down. *Spong* is believed to help sweat out "old water" in the body so that the body can absorb "new water", and this makes the woman have healthy and pretty skin, particularly on her face. It helps to increase the bodily strength and energy, and to protect against blurring vision, numbness, dizziness, headaches, fatigue and pain when the woman resumes work.

After *spong* the woman cleans her body with a mixture of herbs used to make *spong*, and warm water. If the water has cooled down, hot water is added to make the mixture quite warm. The herbal bath is also believed to prevent numbness, swelling, high blood pressure, and pain in the body. While bathing the woman also massages her breasts with *slukrey khoup* (lemon grass), which has grown for one year, to stimulate breastmilk.

After the *spong* inhalation and bath, the woman must massage her body with a mixture of alcohol and *poun ley* again to make her look prettier and younger as well as to protect against skin infection which could be caused by the heat of the *ang pleung* ritual.

Traditionally, *spong* is practised for one month postpartum; in the same period as *ang pleung*. Again, many women in the study practised *spong* for varying periods. Some said that they did it every morning for one week only, others performed *spong* every morning for two months. One woman said that it could vary from one to three months depending on how diligent their husbands were in heating the stone and helping to prepare the herbs. If a woman's husband is "too lazy", then she might do it for one month only. On the other hand, a woman can practise much longer, up to three months, if her husband is a "good man" and helps her to prepare the herbal bath. Women believed that the longer they practise *spong*, the better their health.

Sankat Tmor/Sankat Poo Wa

Another common postpartum practise is to heat a small rock over the fire while pouring water on the rock to create steam. The rock is then wrapped in a kroma or a blanket and placed on the woman's abdomen for a while. The abdomen is then massaged and the rock is placed back on again. Alternatively, *pon ley* (turmeric) is put in a pot and cooked in a clay oven. The pot of medicine is then placed on the woman's abdomen. This ritual helps to make the abdomen and uterus shrink to normal size. This ritual is performed for two weeks to one month postpartum.

RITUALS FOR THE NEWBORN

Not only the new mother, but also the newborn infant is vulnerable to all sorts of harmful agents. There are, therefore, several rituals to be performed for the survival and well-being of the newborn. *Poit sema*, for example, must be performed by a *Kru Khmer* within three days of birth to protect both the infant and the mother from bad spirits and ghosts. The spirits may make both of them sick; sometimes they may even take their lives. One informant gave an account of when a *Kru Khmer* makes a cross mark with *kambor* (betel) juice in each corner of the room and chants a *sutra* (magical words) for her. Within this perimeter no spirits are able to harm the newborn and its mother.

A knife or a pair of scissors is placed over the infant's head when sleeping, for a period of three months, to prevent the infant from becoming frightened. Fright may result in the loss of soul, which would in turn make the infant ill or prevent proper growth. At the time the mother takes a hot herbal shower she also takes her newborn with her. While bathing, the mother massages the infant's fontanelle with her mouth. This is to protect the infant from common cold, to prevent headaches and to ensure that the infant's nose does not get clogged. *Pon ley* is also used to massage the fontanelle for the same purpose. This ritual is performed for three months.

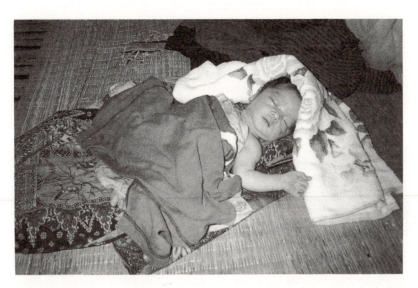

FIGURE 6.3 Young infant resting on the rattan matting of mother's bed during her confinement. (Photo: K. Townsend).

A small rock is dried over the fire until it is hot. It is then wrapped in a *kroma* or a blanket and placed on the infant's abdomen. A gentle massage is also performed at the same time. This is similar to the *sankat tmor* ritual of the mother. This ritual is believed to prevent the infant's abdomen from becoming distended, and to prevent diarrhoea and abdominal pains. Sometimes menthol oil is used to massage the abdomen, since menthol has the same "hot" properties as the hot rock. Diarrhoea can be prevented by dipping the mother's fingers in a mixture of water and salt, drying them over the fire, and placing them on the infant's abdomen. These rituals are performed for the first month only.

One woman explained how she cared for her male infant. She used her saliva to massage the infant's penis early in the morning during the first month postpartum. This is to protect the infant from getting a hernia when he becomes an adult male. There is no particular ritual for a female infant.

CONCLUSION

In this chapter, we have looked at beliefs and practices of birth of Cambodian women who were refugees in a Thai-Cambodia border camp. What is striking is the degree to which women maintain traditional birth practices following enforced migration. Although modern obstetric care was provided for mothers and their infants in the camp, and although the women utilised the care provided, most of them inclined toward their traditional practices and care when they had their babies. What can account for this? Although Cambodia has had contact with western medicine, mainly as a consequence of French colonialism, it was only accessible to the elite groups and urban dwellers. For those who lived outside main cities, "modern" biomedical care was scarce. Childbirth was traditionally managed at home with the assistance of *Chmop* (traditional birth attendants). Women are therefore more familiar with traditional birthing practices, and migration alone — perhaps especially when it is enforced — does not presuppose changes in behaviour.

However, given the accessibility of obstetric care in the camp, women believed that it would be an advantage to utilise it; some who had experienced poor health during pregnancy, needed medicine to alleviate their symptoms even though they believed that those symptoms were a "natural" consequence of pregnancy. Women also recognised the value of receiving antenatal care, given that this was the only way for them to receive an extra rice ration for the newborn; as Symonds (this volume) also illustrates for relocated Hmong women in the United States of America, use of government services can be very pragmatic. It is not surprising that most women adhered to cultural norms thereafter (at birth and during postpartum), since there was no manipulation in the system as in the case of antenatal care.

It is worth noting that the length of confinement practices, such as *ang pleung* and *spong* varied. Traditionally, *ang pleung* and *spong* rituals are observed for 30 days (one full month) postpartum. Some women, however, only practised these for three days and three nights; others for seven days at least. Why is there such a different length of confinement practices given that all women perceived the practices as critical for regaining strength, and for maintaining good health until old age? Since living conditions in the camp were poor, even though confinement practices could be followed, it may have been difficult for some women to have someone prepare a fire and a steam bath for them, particularly if they were widowed, divorced or if their husbands were living outside the camp most of the time. The collection of fire wood and fetching water from some distance are regarded as rigorous physical activities, and so women are not permitted to perform these tasks themselves. They had to rely on those who would help them, and confinement practices may have been foreshortened where women lacked adequate social support. But other women mentioned longer times for confinement practices, some for two months. For some, this related to their poor health after birth, and their perceived need for time to recover. The majority of women, in fact, arrived at the refugee camp in poor physical condition. This was partly due to their long and difficult journey from Cambodia. More importantly, all had lived through harsh conditions in Cambodia under the Khmer Rouge regime, where there was not enough food and medicines, and harsh forced labour. These conditions, and the poor conditions of the camp, meant that women found their health was even worse by the time they became pregnant. The process of pregnancy and birth, it was believed, further weakened their health. As a result, many women felt that they needed extra time to recover after birth to regain their health.[14]

Although the women interviewed adhered to a traditional diet, many mentioned that they also consumed "supplementary food" provided by the MCH midwife. This "supplementary food" included fruit and meat, proscribed foods during the puerperium in Cambodian culture. Women argued that since they were malnourished, they must take whatever was offered in order to improve their health. Women believed that when their own health was good, this would help their foetus to survive.

In sum Cambodian women have traditionally observed particular cultural beliefs and practices surrounding birth. This persisted even when they became refugees and lived in a refugee camp in a neighbouring country. Despite poor living conditions in the camp, women and their families tended to adhere to their cultural norms. However, many women acted pragmatically in ways contrary to traditional customs, in order to ensure their own and their infants' health and survival — a response to the circumstances of life in Site 2 Khmer refugee camp.

ACKNOWLEDGMENTS

We would like to express our thanks to all the Cambodian women who participated in the study. We were not able to maintain contact with them since the repatriation was finalised, but we wish them all well in Cambodia. We extend our thanks to Sou Thavy, our interpreter, who worked extremely hard for us during the difficult months of data collection. We hope that by now she has been accepted to join her father and settle in the USA. We also thank Jane Bell who led us to undertake this piece of research and introduced us, and lastly, we thank Rhonda Small and Professor Lenore Manderson who kindly read and commented on the paper for us.

ENDNOTES

1. All interviews were conducted by the first author (KT) while working as a Mental Health Co-ordinator for the Catholic Office for Emergency Relief and Refugees, with the assistance of Sou Thavy, a Khmer-born woman who was working as a medic at Site 2 camp. Data analysis and the writing of this chapter were undertaken by the second author (PLR). We are very grateful to Jane Bell for introducing us.

2. Site 2 Khmer refugee camp was located 75 km from Aranyaprathet town, along a road that parallels the Thai-Cambodia border, in the eastern part of Thailand. For security reasons, relief workers were not allowed to remain in border camps after 5 pm. Each day they travelled, mainly by vans or four-wheel drive vehicles which would take between 1.5 to 2 hours one way depending on the conditions of the road. In the rainy season, access to the camp was often inhibited.

3. Services provided in Thailand's refugee camps varied greatly between camps. Refugees in the border camps were given only basic essentials such as food, shelter and acute medical care. The Thai Government had the policy of keeping living standards at border camps well below those of the camps inside Thailand to encourage the return of border refugees to Cambodia and to discourage additional people from seeking refuge (Soffer and Wilde, 1986; Riener, 1987).

4. For more information about the life of Khmer women in refugee camps, see Mortland (1987), Moore (1993) and Ebihara, Mortland and Ledgerwood (1994).

5. At the time of the interviews, O'Bok camp was virtually empty since most people had been repatriated. However, women from all other camps were interviewed.

6. In reality, most men did not stay in the camp, particularly during the day time. They would go back to Cambodian territory and work as soldiers for the KPNLF (Khmer People's National Liberation Front). Since they did not receive any food rations from the camp, they had to rely on outside resources.

7. Several black markets sold food stuffs within the camp and there were some food stalls run by Thais outside the camp. However, not many women could afford this.

8. Even Cambodian refugee women who are settled in the U.S. still have *Chmop* deliver their babies at home. Sargent, Marcucci and Elliston (1983), for example, have observed home deliveries at which a *Chmop* assisted in Dallas.

9. There are at least four kinds of *toah: toah mhoop, toah sorsay, toah dam nak* and *toah toek sonsoem* (see Rice, 1994).

10. In some parts of Southeast Asia, roasting may extend to 40 days or longer. However, intense roasting may only occur in the first one to two weeks of confinement. See also Wilson (1973), Manderson (1981) and Laderman (1983) for Malaysia; Rajadhon (1965), Hanks (1963) and Mougne (1978) for Thailand.

11. The *kroma* prevents wind from entering the ears so that she will not get a headache and ringing in her ears.

12. Compare with *xong* in Vietnamese culture (Rice, 1994).

13. The mixture is varied. It can include water and salt or water and urine, if alcohol and *pon ley* (turmeric) are not available.

14. On the way in which personal and social circumstance influence the observation of birth rituals among Malay women, see Laderman (1983).

REFERENCES

Ebihara, M.M., Mortland, C.A., Ledgerwood, J. (1994) Introduction. In *Cambodia Culture Since 1975: Homeland and Exile*, edited by M.M. Ebihara, C.A. Mortland and J. Ledgerwood, pp. 1–26. Ithaca and London: Cornell University Press.

Feith, D. (1988) *Stalemate: Refugees in Asia*. Melbourne: Asian Bureau Australia.

Hanks, J. (1963) *Maternity and Its Rituals in Bang Chan*. New York: Cornell University.

Laderman, C. (1983) *Wives and Midwives: Childbirth and Nutrition in Rural Malaysia*. Berkeley: University of California Press.

Manderson, L. (1981) Roasting, smoking and dieting in response to birth: Malay confinement in cross-cultural perspective. *Social Science and Medicine*, **15B**, 509–520.

Moore, L. (1993) Among Khmer and Vietnamese refugee women in Thailand. In *Gendered Fields: Women, Men and Ethnography*, edited by D. Bell, P. Caplan and W.J. Karim, pp. 117–127. London: Routledge.

Mortland, C.A. (1987) Transforming refugees in refugee camps. *Urban Anthropology*, **16**(3–4), 375–404.

Mougne, C. (1978) An ethnography of reproduction: changing patterns of fertility in a Northern Thai village. In *Nature and man in South East Asia*, edited by P.A. Stott, pp. 68–106. London: School of Oriental and African Studies, University of London.

Rajadhon, Phya Anuman (1965) Customs connected with birth and the rearing of children. In *Southeast Asian Birth Customs*, edited by D. Hart, Rajadhon, Phya Anuman and R. Coughlin, pp. 115–204. New Haven: HRAF Press.

Rice, P.L. (editor) (1994) *Asian Mothers, Australian Birth*. Melbourne: Ausmed Publications.

Riener, L. (1987) Refugee politics: the Khmer camps system in Thailand. In *The Cambodia Agony*, edited by D.A. Ablin and M. Hood, pp. 293–331. Armonk, New York: M.E. Sharpe.

Romalis, S. (1981) *Childbirth: Alternatives to Medical Control*. Austin: University of Texas Press.

Sargent, C., Marcucci, J., Elliston, E. (1983) Tiger bones, fire and wine: maternity care in a Kampuchean refugee community. *Medical Anthropology*, 7(4), 67–79.

Sargent, C., Marcucci, J. (1984) Aspects of Khmer medicine among refugees in urban America. *Medical Anthropology Quarterly*, **16**(1), 7–9.

Soffer, A.D., Wilde, H. (1986) Medicine in Cambodia refugee camps. *Annals of Internal Medicine*, **105**, 618–621.

Wilson, C. (1973) Food taboos of childbirth: the Malay example. *Ecology of Food and Nutrition*, **2**, 267–274.

CHAPTER 7

Healers and Modern Health Services: Antenatal, Birthing and Postpartum Care in Rural East Lombok, Indonesia

Jocelyn Grace

The Alma Ata Conference of 1978, held under the auspices of the World Health Organization, laid down guidelines for achieving "Health for All by the Year 2000". These have had a strong influence on the planning of primary health care programs in many developing countries, including Indonesia. While one of its major recommendations was to involve traditional practitioners in the delivery of primary health care, the idea met with little enthusiasm on the part of national policy makers and modern practitioners in most countries (van der Geest, 1990). This is true of Indonesia, with the exception of the inclusion of traditional birth attendants in the area of maternal and infant health. The success of this strategy, however, has been limited by the lack of commitment and funding it has received. Lack of funding is a major problem in the delivery of primary health care services in rural East Lombok generally.

In Indonesia the Department of Health, as part of a broader program to improve the health status of the population, is attempting to reduce maternal and infant mortality in rural areas by providing antenatal and birthing services. Antenatal examinations are designed to improve the general health of pregnant women, and to identify high risk cases for appropriate medical attention throughout the pregnancy and at the time of delivery. All pregnant women who attend antenatal examinations receive supplementary vitamins (A and C) and iron, and tetanus inoculations (i.e. tetanus toxoid — TT) to protect the baby during the neonatal phase. Modern facilities and personnel are available for assisting deliveries. However these are not yet easily accessible to, or widely accepted by, the majority of the population. Consequently, the training of traditional birth attendants (*belian nganak*-S)[1] by government health staff was the most important intervention in the prevention of maternal and neonatal mortality during the 1970s and 1980s. In the 1990s however, the emphasis has shifted to the provision of trained midwives in every village, with the intention that they will gradually replace *belian nganak* (Sinung, pers. comm., 1992).[2]

In this chapter, I will describe the preferences of village women in East Lombok in respect to antenatal care, assistance during birthing and postpartum care, and the reasons which underlie them. Women's preferences and reasoning when choosing traditional and/or modern services can tell us much about which interventions will

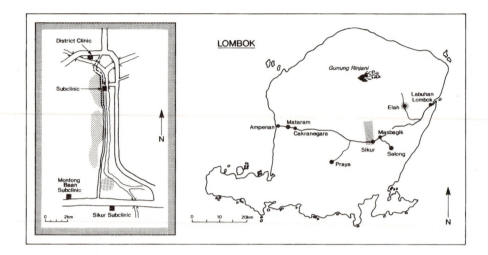

FIGURE 7.1   Map of Lombok.

be successful in improving maternal health. I will show that the underutilisation of antenatal care reflects women's lack of understanding of the purpose of this preventive health service, as well as its inaccessibility to many. In the area of birthing, the financial cost and inconvenience of government facilities and health personnel combine with social and cultural factors to create a strong deterrent to utilising these modern services, even in emergency situations. I set out to discover the general patterns of utilisation, and then to explain them by isolating the factors which combine in varying ways to determine the individual decisions women and their families make about where and when to seek treatment.

This chapter is based on doctoral research carried out between September 1989 and May 1992 in two neighbouring villages in the district of Sikur, East Lombok. Desaraja, where the district clinic (*puskesmas*) is located, was the site of preliminary research. The neighbouring village of Rajin was selected as the location for the major focus of this study (see Figure 7.1). Unlike Desaraja where the population is tightly clustered and almost all are within walking distance of the clinic, the residents of Rajin are spread out over a far wider area. This means that access to the clinic and subclinics is uneven, making it a more representative sample, and allowing for comparison on the basis of distance from health facilities.

A number of methodologies were employed, including structured interview series, semistructured interviews, and participant observation. The interview series were carried out in three of the village's nine hamlets — Rajin, Ajan and Wengkang. I was assisted for the major part of the research period by a young local woman who had recently graduated from high school. As many women in the village do not speak Indonesian, interviews were often conducted in Sasak, with my research assistant translating into Indonesian.[3]

LOMBOK

Official figures indicate that the maternal and infant mortality rates in the province of West Nusa Tenggara in Eastern Indonesia are the highest in Indonesia. Lombok as a whole has an official infant mortality rate of 125 per 1,000 and maternal mortality rate of 700 per 100,000 live births (Indonesia MOH and PATH, 1991). The regency of East Lombok has a higher rate of infant mortality than the other five regencies in the province, being perhaps as high as 200 per 1,000 live births (PATH, 1992). The major causes of maternal mortality are postpartum haemorrhage and infection, and a study conducted on the neighbouring island of Bali found that 66% of maternal deaths there occurred at home, and 30% in hospital (Fortney, Susanti, Gadalla, Sleh, Feldblum, *et al.*, 1988). In rural East Lombok the level of utilisation of the government health services for antenatal, birthing and postpartum care is relatively low. The majority of women still rely predominantly on care from *belian nganak*, and give birth at home.

Lombok is predominantly populated by people of the Sasak ethnic group, with small enclaves of Bugis, Balinese, and Javanese government employees. All Sasaks are Muslims, and Sasak society is patrilineal and patrilocal. The language spoken by commoners is related to, but distinct from, Javanese and Balinese; that spoken among the aristocracy (*halus* or high Sasak) is Balinese. Households are located in groupings called *gubuk* (S), formed around men related through the male line, with women marrying in and out. Village endogamy is no longer common but still many women live within walking distance of their natal family, and maintain close ties with women relatives. A woman will return to her parent's house if she divorces or is widowed, and she will often do so also if her husband is away for long periods. At the same time, women moving into their husbands' *gubuk* form cooperative social and economic relationships with each other.

In Rajin all residents are Sasak and consider themselves to be orthodox Muslims.[4] Rajin lies in the foothills of Mount Rinjani, in the central, most populated and well watered area of Lombok. Its good rainfall allows for two harvests of wet rice most years, a third in good years, in addition to dry season crops of corn, tobacco, soya beans and/or cassava. Over 90% of the population work in the agricultural sector, the majority as small landholders, sharecroppers and/or wage labourers. Both women and men carry out agricultural work, men ploughing and harvesting, women sowing and sometimes harvesting. Women also trade, produce handicrafts and work as non-agricultural labourers. Men work in industries such as brick-making, house and furniture building, handicrafts and transport.

Many households are landless, or have holdings too small to meet their basic needs. Wages are low and employment opportunities outside the agricultural sector limited, so many men migrate temporarily to other islands or to Malaysia to work. During their absence most women have to rely on their own income from agricultural labour, trading or handicrafts work, or resort to the hard and poorly paid labour of carting sand and stones for building.

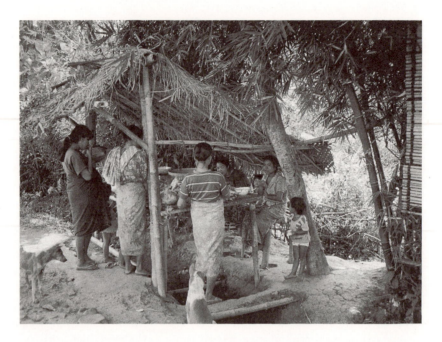

FIGURE 7.2   Women gather at a kiosk in the late afternoon, to shop and chat with their friends and neighbours, Rajin. (Photo: J. Grace).

Access to education and health services is very limited. Although primary schools are plentiful and relatively easy to reach, poverty prevents many children from attending for more than a few years, and limited employment opportunities for high school graduates gives poor families little incentive to invest in their children's education. Health facilities are less accessible than schools, and many residents of Rajin must travel by public transport to reach a subclinic or the district clinic. The fees for treatment during public sessions are low, but still represent a considerable expense for the poorest households when combined with the cost of transport, loss of income and other expenses.

MODERN HEALTH FACILITIES AND PRACTITIONERS

Clinic and Subclinic

Government health interventions designed to reduce maternal and infant mortality are offered through the district health clinic (*puskesmas*), the village subclinics (*puskesmas pembantu*) and the health posts (*posyandu*) (see also chapters by Jennaway, and Hunter, this volume). In 1991/92, there was only one clinic in the district, which had a population of 56,000 people, although a second clinic was being built and a Javanese woman doctor had already been employed to run it. Health personnel at the district clinic in Desaraja included a Balinese male doctor, so antenatal care was provided by two of the female nurses and the midwife. Antenatal examination sessions were held at the clinic twice a week, and once a week at some subclinics, including Sikur immediately south of Rajin. These sessions are always held in the morning, as clinics and subclinics are only open, and staff paid to work, until midday. Unfortunately in the morning women are also busy earning an income from agricultural labouring and trading.

Each village subclinic is staffed by a resident male nurse and an assistant, who because of their sex cannot carry out antenatal examinations. Some villages have a resident midwife as well, and Rajin was fortunate in receiving one toward the end of my research period. It had been planned that every village in Lombok would have one by the mid 1990s, but this did not eventuate because of a misunderstanding at provincial level which led to insufficient numbers of women nurses being trained in time (Sinung, pers. comm., 1992). While the subclinic nurses and village midwives are only paid to work in the mornings, they are expected to be available to treat patients privately at other times. When they do so, they are allowed to set their own fee, which is usually three to five times as much as the official fee of 300 rupiah for treatment during public hours at clinics and subclinics.[5]

All salaried health personnel have at least twelve years education, and most are in their twenties or thirties. Most in this district are Sasak. However, they rarely come from the villages in which they work, but from the district capital and villages on the main road. The slow and uneven development of infrastructure in East Lombok, particularly roads and schools, in part explains this. Only in the past five years have primary schools been easily accessible to the majority of the population in this village. Before that the only schools were in the central hamlet, Rajin. Few young people have been able to gain access to nursing, teaching and other government jobs even when they have the education to be eligible to apply for them. These jobs are difficult to acquire, usually involving large payments and/or good connections to secure.

In addition to antenatal care, the clinic is also responsible for training *belian nganak* (traditional birth attendants); again the midwife and female nurses do this work. The *belian nganak* are instructed on sterile birthing procedures, and given metal scissors for cutting the cord, alcohol for sterilising the scissors, a metal dish in which to do so, mercurochrome for treating the cord, and a simple hand-held scale for weighing the new born. They are told to refer women who are having difficult deliveries to the hospital in the regional capital, Selong (see Figure 7.1). *Belian nganak* are told to send women for modern antenatal care, in particular to encourage pregnant women to have TT injections, and to report deliveries. During her visit to the clinic, the *belian nganak* is given fresh supplies of alcohol and mercurochrome.

The clinic and village midwives and the nurses who train *belian nganak* often mentioned how difficult it is because they are old and lack formal education. However, the trained *belian nganak* who I interviewed all expressed great enthusiasm about the training they had received, and the equipment and medicines they now use. Unfortunately most received their training many years ago, and have been given little or no follow-up training. Only a few still continued to report births and replenish their supplies. Money is required to run such training sessions, as the staff must be paid extra, and *belian nganak* need to be given their fares and lunch. There seems to be no regular budget allocation for training, to increase the number trained or to improve the skills of those already trained.

The quality of services delivered at clinics and subclinics is dependent on available resources and the conscientiousness of the nurses and midwives. Ideally the village nurse should be available at least every morning to treat patients, and the village midwife should be able to offer antenatal care and assist women when birthing. However, in Rajin the subclinic was often unattended by the nurse, and the midwife was unable to examine pregnant women because the subclinic had no bed on which they could lie. The midwife felt she could not request one from the Health Department, and that it was up to the village to supply it. Six months after her arrival she was still waiting.

Health Posts and Other Outreach Activities

The village midwife is expected to give ongoing training and support to the registered *belian nganak* by supervising their deliveries, and, as discussed above, to be available on a private basis to assist deliveries when requested. In Rajin the village midwife found herself frustrated in carrying out ongoing training because *belian nganak* "forget" to call her when women are giving birth, and she does not feel comfortable in going to assist unless invited by the *belian nganak* or the family. She also felt it was difficult working as a village midwife and being expected to "go down" (*turun*) to the people. She said she would rather work in a clinic where she could just sit and wait for patients to come to her.

In addition to those trained by and registered with the clinic, a number of other *belian nganak* operate in Rajin. They continue to use only traditional methods and equipment during delivery (e.g. bamboo to cut the cord). When formal training sessions are held only those who are already registered are notified. The village midwife was in contact only with those who were registered, and she made no effort to bring or keep the list up to date in order to reach all women who regularly assist deliveries.

Health posts are held monthly in every hamlet of every village, and while the community is expected to initiate and run them, medical services are supplied by clinic staff. Setting up and carrying out less technical activities (e.g. weighing infants) on the day of the health post is usually arranged by the hamlet leader (*kadus*), the voluntary health workers (*kader*), and/or other willing residents of the hamlet. The clinic establishes a roster which enables them to supply staff, vaccines and equipment for immunisation to every health post. As there are seven villages in the district, with from five to ten hamlets in each, this stretches clinic staff, transport and equipment to the limit. While ideally antenatal examinations should be offered at health posts, resources do not allow for it, and even the most important and basic of the preventive service offered at health posts — immunisation — is inadequate in terms of coverage and quality. The physical distance between health posts makes transport a problem for both staff and women who wish to attend. In addition, the reuse of unsterile needles places those receiving inoculations at risk of contracting Hepatitis B, which is endemic in Lombok.

ANTENATAL CARE

Belian Nganak (Traditional Birth Attendants)

In Rajin all *belian nganak* are women, and are past the age of having children, usually between about 50 and 70 years of age. Most have had no formal education, and were taught their skills by their mothers and/or grandmothers. Many women seek their services from the time they first think they might be pregnant, and throughout the pregnancy. Women usually choose a *belian nganak* who lives nearby, who is related, or has been known by her husband's family for many years. It is less expensive and more convenient to be treated and attended by a *belian nganak* than to travel to a clinic or subclinic to see a midwife. In addition, the *belian nganak* speaks the same dialect and is of the same social class as her patients.

The role of the *belian nganak* is both clinical and ritual. She performs the rites and ceremonies which mediate the important life-cycle events of pregnancy and giving birth, carrying women through these transforming and dangerous processes.

> Ibu Nur lives near the eastern mosque in Rajin (hamlet), in a house with mud floor and bamboo walls, one among many in this poor and crowded *gubuk*. She is about 60, small and slim, and neatly dressed. Her husband is dead, but when living he worked as a farm labourer, and owned no land or cattle. She has never been to school. She earns her living making handicrafts, which many women in her *gubuk* do, working at home and selling to the kiosks in the main street. She earns a little extra as a *belian*. Ibu Nur learnt her skills by assisting her mother and grandmother, but did not become a *belian* in her own right until after they had died, about ten years ago. She is a *belian* for pregnant women and birthing, and she treats very young babies for colic, and infants for fever, colds and coughs. She attended training, first in Selong and later at the clinic in Desaraja, which she said she enjoyed very much because she learnt more about how to nurse well. If she has trouble with a delivery she sends the woman to the hospital in Selong.
>
> When treating pregnant women Ibu Nur warns them not to eat anything *keras* (harsh), which she believes causes miscarriage. This includes certain commercial headache powders and unripe pineapple. She also tells them to get a lot of exercise and to bathe in order to be healthy. Women who have suffered a miscarriage come to her, and she refers them to the clinic for an injection. She does not massage them, as she thinks it is dangerous.

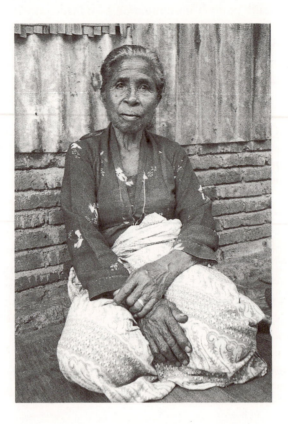

FIGURE 7.3   Ibu Nur, *belian nganak*, Rajin. (Photo: J. Grace).

Ibu Ramadan is the most popular *belian nganak* in Ajan. She is a portly, middle-aged woman in her fifties. Her home is among a group of brick and cement houses situated on the slope above the road. Inside it was clean and neat, but dark and empty of furniture. She wore a clean *kabaya* (top) and *kain* (sarong). Her teeth are red butts from chewing betel, but her mind was clear and she spoke coherently and with vitality. She has been married three times, and her present husband is a farmer, owning both rice fields and cattle. She has never been to school. Ibu Ramadan has been a *belian* for 14 years, taught by her mother and grandmother, and began practising while her mother was still alive. She treats women who are pregnant, assists with deliveries, and treats women for menstrual problems and after miscarriages. She received training in Selong in 1977. If a case is beyond her expertise, she sends the women to the hospital in Selong.

In treating women for illnesses associated with pregnancy, Ibu Ramadan massages the abdomen, for she believes such illness is caused by the baby being squeezed *(terjepit)* inside. She also uses massage to manipulate the uterus for contraception, and can reverse the procedure when the woman wishes to conceive again. She advises against eating foods which are harsh — pineapple, *jamu* (Javanese herbal tonics and remedies) and alcohol — as they can cause miscarriage. She gives no other advice to pregnant women in respect to their activities.

Ibu Setima is a slim, wiry little woman, with quick, lively movements and an animated and comic style of expression. Ibu Setima claims she is "about fifty". She lives in a house of brick and cement on the side of the hill, next to the narrow, winding road which connects Rajin with Ajan and Wengkang. Her clothes are simple, worn and grubby, and upon our arrival she produced great clouds of dust and dirt, wildly sweeping the front porch before putting down a mat for us to sit on. At thirteen Ibu Setima was forced to marry a man she did not like. She was divorced a week later and married the man she is still with today. He is a farmer, owning both rice fields and cattle, so by local standards they are quite well off. When younger, Ibu Setima worked in the fields, but now receives income only as a *belian*. She is the only *belian nganak* in her area, and so most women having babies in Wengkang and Dasan Paok (southern section of Ajan) call on her services. She also treats infants for common illnesses. She was taught by her mother, and began practising in her own right immediately after her mother died. She received training in Selong many years ago, and in Desaraja more recently. When a delivery is difficult, she sends the woman to Selong.

Women seeking relief from illness during early pregnancy are massaged around the area of the uterus, because Ibu Setima believes that the baby is sometimes squeezed *(terjepit)* and cannot move inside. She also uses massage when treating women after miscarriage, which she attributes to eating young (unripe) pineapple and carrying heavy objects. Her advice to pregnant women is not to move around a lot and not to jump, because this might damage the baby, causing it to be unhealthy or to suffer convulsions after it is born. She recommends that women avoid eating a fish called *keritaq* (S), which will make the sack which contains the baby too wide, causing it to have difficulty breathing, so it will not live long.

Women who live in the hamlet of Rajin, and those in Ajan who come from Rajin, participate in a ceremony held during the seventh month of pregnancy. However, most women in Ajan and Wengkang do not perform this ceremony, which they consider to be only for those of aristocratic status *(bangsawan)*. Many in Rajin and Ajan who hold this ceremony are not, in fact, *bangsawan*, but they live close to, and have been connected through patron-client relationships and marriage with *bangsawan* families. Women relatives and neighbours of the pregnant woman gather and prepare the necessary ritual dishes and food to be shared after the ceremony. The *belian nganak* is invited to come and perform the ceremony, which begins with her washing the pregnant woman's hair in coconut milk *(santan)*, then washing her abdomen with water, followed by coconut milk, then water again, while reciting Islamic prayers (*mantra*). The *belian nganak* is presented with a ritual food offering, as well as being given a kilogram of uncooked rice and a small gift of money (about 500 rupiah) (cf. chapters by Jirojwong, Cabigon, and Symonds, this volume).[6]

Modern Antenatal Care

The purpose of the antenatal care provided by the clinic is to monitor women's health and foetal growth, and to detect potentially problematic deliveries for referral to the hospital. During the first visit the woman is given a card on which her gynaecological history is recorded, and she is given a TT (Tetanus Toxoid) injection if she has not already had three in the past.[7] At every visit women are weighed, their blood pressure is taken, they are examined and are given iron and vitamin pills. Later in pregnancy, the midwife listens for the heartbeat and feels for the position and size of the baby. If the baby is in the wrong position, or its head appears to be too large for the size of the woman's pelvis, the delivery may not be straightforward and the midwife will advise the woman to go to the hospital for the delivery. An antenatal examination costs 300 rupiah, plus return fares, which range from 200 to 400 rupiahs.

I attended health posts almost every month in the three hamlets while living in Rajin, but rarely saw the nurse from Rajin subclinic in attendance, and on no occasion did I observe him or anyone else seeking out pregnant women. Those pregnant women who came to the health posts were given tetanus inoculations though, and sometimes vitamin C and iron tablets as well. One of the purposes of placing midwives in every village is to increase coverage of antenatal care. Rajin's village midwife could do no more than give TT injections and iron and vitamin tablets to pregnant women, because there was no suitably private place to conduct examinations, and the shortage of staff necessitated her helping with basic immunisation services.

Food and Behavioural Taboos During Pregnancy

Humoral medical traditions form the foundation of folk beliefs about illness and treatment throughout Southeast Asia (Manderson, 1981). Research on food taboos during pregnancy in Malaysia quite clearly show that they have their bases in this system of thought, being conceived of in terms of the categories "hot" and "cold". Laderman (1987) has documented the foods and medicines pregnant women avoid in Peninsular Malaysia are those considered "hot". They are believed to endanger the embryo, and later the foetus, which is said to require a cool environment in order to be healthy. Similarly, on the island of Madura in Indonesia, Niehof (1988) found that women avoided "hot" foods and drinks during early pregnancy for fear of damaging the embryo.

In Central Java, Geertz (1961) recorded that particular foods were also prohibited for pregnant women. However, in this case the explanations for avoiding these foods was not given in terms of "hot" and "cold", but more specifically with their supposed effects on the baby, or in causing difficulties during delivery. According to Hull (1986), many detailed descriptions have been made of the food taboos in Java, along with a variety of folk explanations which only occasionally refer to "hot" or "cold". There appears to be no clear and consistent application of humoral theory to folk explanations of food taboos during pregnancy in Java. Similarly in Rajin, there is a rather fragmented and inconsistent set of beliefs about "hot" and "cold". Some healers speak in these terms, others do not. Old and middle-aged people categorise foods this way, while the young regard these beliefs as old-fashioned — *cerita orang tua* ("old people's stories").

Neither the *belian nganak* nor the pregnant women interviewed on the subject of taboos during pregnancy referred to "hot" or "cold" foods. Two thirds of these women did not consider any foods taboo during pregnancy. Those who did, named the same foods the *belian nganak* had. Pineapple was most commonly mentioned to be avoided during early pregnancy for danger of miscarriage.[8] Women continue to carry on their activities as normal while pregnant, including working in the fields, but refrain from doing heavy work such as carting water or other heavy objects on their heads. In the past, men were not allowed to cut their hair for the length of their wives' pregnancies, but this taboo is no longer observed.

Food and behavioural taboos during pregnancy are often cited as the cause of nutritional deficiencies in pregnant women in traditionally-oriented societies (Hull, 1986). It was, therefore, important that they be investigated in the course of this research. However, my approach to this subject was "normative" (Hull, 1986:238). That is, I recorded only what women and *belian nganak* said about food taboos during pregnancy, which may not necessarily be what they do. Nevertheless, it seems reasonable to conclude that food and behavioural taboos during pregnancy have little or no biomedical significance for maternal and neonatal health in the village of Rajin.

CONTEMPORARY PRACTICES IN SEEKING ANTENATAL CARE

The pregnant women interviewed ranged in age from fifteen to forty, and Table 7.1 gives a breakdown of their formal educational status and age, in relation to their geographical location. While this is a small sample, the slight variation in distribution of educational status between Rajin and Ajan/Wengkang is representative of those populations. The greater number of pregnant women in their teens in Ajan/Wengkang compared with Rajin is considered by educated villagers to reflect the generally lower level of formal education in the former. However, all the teenagers who were pregnant had at least some primary school education, one lower high school. All women in Ajan/Wengkang with no schooling were over the age of thirty, reflecting the fact that government primary schools were built several years earlier in Rajin than Ajan and Wengkang.

The number of women seeking traditional and modern antenatal care in each geographical location is represented in Table 7.2. Of the pregnant women interviewed just over half had visited a *belian nganak*, and the clinic or a health post. However, half as many women in Ajan/Wengkang visited a *belian nganak* in early pregnancy compared with Rajin, and the same is true in respect to seeking antenatal care at the clinic. A third of the women interviewed in Ajan/Wengkang had attended a health post, so at least half the women in both locations had received TT inoculations. These trends reflect, in part, the easier access for women in Rajin to both the clinic and *belian nganak*. Rajin is closer to Desaraja, and has cheaper and more frequent public transport. Rajin's population is also more tightly clustered than Ajan/Wengkang's, so all women there have quick and easy access to a *belian nganak*.

TABLE 7.1 Age, education and location of women seeking antenatal care.

	Ajan/Wengkang	Rajin	Total
Age			
15–18 years	4	0	4
19–22	3	4	7
23–26	1	7	8
27–30	2	4	6
31–35	4	0	4
36–40	1	0	1
Total	15	15	30
Education			
No schooling	6	1	7
Some primary	7	10	17
Lower high	2	4	6
Total	15	15	30

TABLE 7.2 Antenatal care and location.

	belian nganak yes/no	Clinic yes*/no	Health Post yes*/no (**)
Ajan/Wengkang	6/9	6/9	11/2 (2)
Rajin	10/5	11/4	4/5 (6)
Total	16/14	17/13	15/7 (8)

*This includes women in early pregnancy who stated their intention to seek antenatal care.

**Not necessary because they received TT at the Clinic.

The educational status and forms of antenatal care utilised by the pregnant women interviewed are compared in Table 7.3. Women with no formal education have the lowest attendance at the clinic for full antenatal care, but the majority attend health posts for TT inoculations. Interestingly, many of those with no formal education had not visited a *belian nganak*. Almost all those with some primary school education visited a *belian nganak*, and almost half had been to the clinic. The highest rate for seeking antenatal care at the clinic was amongst those with the highest educational status. Educational status is also a factor in the higher rates for seeking antenatal care at the clinic among women in Rajin compared with Ajan/Wengkang. The earlier introduction of both primary schools and health posts in Rajin means that women there have had longer exposure to general education, and contact with health personnel, than in Ajan/Wengkang.

TABLE 7.3   Antenatal care and education.

	belian nganak yes/no	Clinic yes*/no	Health Post yes*/no (**)
No schooling	1/6	1/6	5/2
Some primary	13/4	11/6	7/4 (5)
Lower high	2/4	5/1	2/1 (3)
Total	16/14	17/13	14/7 (8)

*This includes women in early pregnancy who stated their intention to seek antenatal care.

**Not necessary because they received TT at the Clinic.

TABLE 7.4   Visiting healers compared with seeking modern antenatal care.

	Visited a *belian nganak*	Clinic yes*/no	Health Post yes*/no (**)
Yes	16	11/5	7/3 (6)
No	14	6/8	8/4 (2)
Total	30	17/13	15/7 (8)

*This includes women in early pregnancy who stated their intention to seek antenatal care.

**Not necessary because they received TT at the Clinic.

TABLE 7.5   Frequency of visits to antenatal clinic.

	Follow-up Interviews	Second Series of Interviews
None	3	10
One/two	4	5
Three/four	3	5
Five or more	1	10
Total	11	30

Of women who did and did not visit a *belian nganak* in early pregnancy (Table 7.4), the former group showed a higher rate of attendance at the clinic for antenatal care. The number of women going to health posts was the same for both groups, however when combined with those who sought antenatal care at the clinic, twice as many women who had visited a *belian nganak* received TT inoculations as those who did not.

Of 17 women who had sought antenatal care at the clinic, the majority had been only once or twice at the time they were interviewed. Eleven of these women were interviewed again after their babies were born, and the number of times they received antenatal care at the clinic is shown in Table 7.5. In the second series of interviews, women with children under the age of five were also asked about antenatal care during their last pregnancy. Of the ten women in this latter group who had not sought antenatal care, seven had received TT inoculations at a health post.

While the majority of women interviewed had received two or more injections during their pregnancies (one having had five), very few knew the purpose of the *suntik ibu hamil* ("pregnant woman injection"). Women know of an illness that causes many babies to die within a week of being born, but do not associate the injections for pregnant women with that illness.[9] While many receive tetanus inoculations, far fewer receive full antenatal care. This is partly because the TT injection is more easily accessible, free of charge, and available at health posts, but also because injections are positively perceived.[10] Antenatal care, on the other hand, has no similar attraction and involves expenditure of money and time. Most women have not been informed of its benefits, and so do not feel inclined to seek it out. Many of those who do, act on the advice of their *belian nganak*, but most attend only once or twice.

BIRTHING

Belian Nganak

The first time a Sasak woman gives birth she returns to her mother's house and is cared for by her mother and other women relatives and friends. For the second and consecutive births, she remains in her own home and is usually helped by her husband, female relatives by marriage, (e.g. mother-in-law), friends and neighbours, and if they live close enough, her mother and sisters. The *belian nganak* is called in when the labour begins. She will give the woman herbal medicines to help with the delivery, and recite *mantra*. *Belian nganak* assist the delivery of the baby by massaging. The perineum is never cut, and if there is a tear the wound is left to heal without being stitched. Women usually give birth in a sitting or squatting position, although those women assisted by a midwife, and also by some of the trained *belian nganak*, now lie down during delivery. It used to be customary for all containers in the house to have their lids removed, and all the windows and doors to be open during the labour, to ensure an easy parturition.

The *belian nganak* stays with the woman throughout her labour, assists the delivery, cuts and treats the umbilical cord, waits for the placenta to deliver, and cleans up. The placenta *(adik-adik)*, considered to be the baby's younger sibling, is washed and wrapped in white cloth and newspaper, and buried in the yard of the house. If the baby is a girl, the *adik-adik* will be buried under the eaves of the house, if a boy away from the house. This is so daughters will stay close to home and their mother when they grow up, while sons will leave the home and wander farther afield. When the placenta is buried a piece of bamboo is positioned connecting it with the air above ground so that it can breathe, and a light is placed near it at night for a week after it has been buried (cf. Paton's account of birthing in Central Java, 1988; and Symonds among Hmong women in Thailand, this volume).

Those *belian nganak* who have not received Health Department training continue to use traditional methods — bamboo to cut the cord, *kunyit* (tumeric root, known to have antiseptic properties) to treat the stump. Those who have been trained by Health Department personnel are taught to use scissors when cutting the umbilical cord, alcohol to sterilise them, and mercurochrome on the end of the cord to prevent infection. However, none of the trained *belian nganak* interviewed had received, or still had, all these items. Two used mercurochrome and alcohol, and regularly replenished their supply with the midwife at the clinic. The other used to use them, but had run out and did not go to the clinic, so had reverted to using *kunyit.*

In addition to whether *belian nganak* have received training, it is important to consider how much of what they were taught was retained and/or implemented. Ibu Nur, Ibu Ramadan and Ibu Setima all received their training many years ago, and only two had received further training. This is reflected in their different understanding of the use of equipment. Ibu Ramadan no longer uses alcohol and mercurochrome, and explained that the round dish she was given was for washing the scissors in warm water, an inadequate method of sterilisation. Ibu Nur referred to "cleaning" the scissors, and indicated that she used alcohol to do so. All three said they travelled to the clinic to report births, but the clinic midwife said that only two of them did so, and that most *belian nganak* report irregularly if at all. She felt this was not surprising given that most *belian nganak* are old, poor, live a considerable distance from the clinic, and do not receive money for transport.

Modern Birthing Services

Women who choose to have their delivery attended by a modern midwife can do so in the regional hospital or birthing clinic, at the district clinic, or in their home. At the hospital in Selong they pay 50,000 rupiah if the delivery is normal, plus the nightly rate for a bed which ranges from 600 rupiah for 4th class, to 3,500 rupiah for 1st class. Additional procedures and medicines cost extra. The government-run birthing clinic (*Balai Kesehatan Ibu dan Anak*) in Selong costs about the same as the hospital, but educated women told me they preferred it because it is cleaner, less crowded, and the quality of care is better than the hospital. For government employees and their families the use of government health facilities and the cost of medicines are subsidised. This is not the case for the general population. Having the delivery assisted by a midwife, either in the clinic or at home, costs from 15,000–25,000 rupiahs, depending on what the family can afford to pay. In cases of problematic deliveries, midwives must send women to the regional hospital, as they do not have the expertise or equipment to deal with such cases.

TABLE 7.6   Preferred place for delivery.

	Home	Hospital	Total
Plan to deliver	29	1	30
If able to afford hospital	23	6	29
If problem with delivery	20	9	29

Women's Preferences and Beliefs

Almost all pregnant women interviewed planned to give birth at home (see Table 7.6), both because they could not afford the hospital, and because they preferred to be at home and be cared for by their husbands, mothers and other family members and friends. They also said that it is not usual or normal (*biasa*) to go to hospital. None of the eleven women reinterviewed after giving birth had any difficulty, and had delivered with the assistance of a *belian nganak* after labours ranging from a half hour to nine hours.

In addition to the expense and inconvenience of going to the hospital or clinic in the regional capital, fear is a major deterrent for many women, although they were unwilling to admit this. My research assistant felt that many who said they could not afford to go really meant they were afraid, and according to her and others, including the clinic and village midwives, women fear episiotomies and suturing. The village midwife confirmed that many women are cut and stitched, a procedure she considered to be almost always necessary during a woman's first delivery. This implies that episiotomies are routine in the hospital and with midwife-assisted deliveries.[11]

In cases of serious difficulty during birthing, the outcome depends on how quickly a woman receives appropriate medical attention. The clinic midwife is often called by a *belian nganak* or the family when a problem arise, but it is often too late and she can only advise them to take the woman to hospital. Trained *belian nganak* all said they refer problem cases to the hospital. The decision for a family as to whether to follow this advice or not is difficult, however, given the cost of transport, treatment and medicines involved (50,000–400,000 rupiah, plus 15,000 rupiah to hire transport). While poor families can obtain a letter from the village head (*surat miskin*, literally "poor letter") which exempts them from the cost of a bed, it does not affect fees charged for medical procedures and medicines. According to one of the doctors at the hospital in Selong, patients with *surat miskin* are rare — only two or three per month.

For most of the poor, the cost of care in the regional hospital is prohibitive even in emergencies. Two or three caesarean sections are performed each year at the hospital in Selong, and given the high maternal mortality rate in East Lombok, and its population of over 750,000, this suggests that the referral system is not working (Brooks, pers. comm., 1992).[12] Ibu Nur told us there were still many who, rather than go to the hospital when a problem arises, prefer to seek the services of a famous old *belian nganak* in Central Lombok. Ibu Nur tells of one of her patients who,

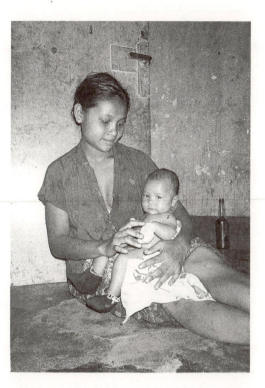

FIGURE 7.4   Young mother with her infant, Wengkang. (Photo: J. Grace).

after four days in labour, refused to go to the hospital because she was afraid of being cut and stitched. Her family took her instead to the *belian nganak* in Central Lombok who delivered the baby, but it was already dead. The point Ibu Nur was making was that because of the women's fear, the family had delayed in seeking help outside the village, and had then made the wrong decision in not taking her to the hospital (cf. Laderman's example, 1987:159–164).

Belief in sorcery or black magic (*ilmu hitam*) also explains why many women favour *belian nganak* over midwives and doctors in difficult deliveries. Most people believe that obstructed labour is due to black magic, and only a healer (*belian*) can deal with this problem. A doctor is powerless, as the appropriate *mantra* recited by a *belian* is necessary to counter the spell to allow the baby to be born. An educated woman friend told me that often doctors at the hospital, unable to overcome a birthing problem, are astonished to see the baby deliver normally after a healer has recited *mantra*. Many families will call in a *belian* known to be able to deal with black magic, before considering taking a woman to the hospital in Selong.

Few women consider midwife-assisted or hospital births, and the referral system for high risk pregnancies and birthing difficulties does not guarantee that women will go to hospital. As already noted, fear of standard episiotomies, social discomfort in dealing with modern practitioners, the expense and inconvenience of travelling to Selong, and the prohibitive cost of medical procedures and medicines all deter families from complying with referral to the regional hospital. There seems little point in identifying high risk pregnancies if such women are unable or unwilling to seek modern medical attention.

POSTPARTUM CARE

What happens during the period immediately after the birth and the week which follows is critical to the survival of both mother and baby. Once the placenta has delivered and bleeding is only moderate, the woman is past the most dangerous stage. Should the placenta not come away from the wall of the uterus, however, she is in danger of dying from loss of blood, and will need medical intervention quickly to remove the placenta, stop the haemorrhage, and replace lost blood. Less critical complications such as infection, may occur more slowly, and the *belian nganak* will be called on to treat them. If the perineum tears, the *belian nganak* puts mercurochrome (or *kunyit*) on the wound to prevent infection, reapplying it each day until healed. The *belian nganak* comes back every day after the birth also to treat the baby's umbilical cord. Her visits continue until the cord has fallen off and the wound has healed, usually four days to a week after the baby is born.

Manderson (1981) and Laderman (1987) have written in detail about traditional postpartum treatment of women in Malay society. They include roasting or smoking women, and specific restrictions on food and activities designed to protect the woman from the "cold" condition produced by giving birth, and to redress the balance between "hot" and "cold" in her body. This treatment takes place during a confinement period of a month to six weeks after delivery, when the woman and neonate are not allowed to leave the house. Cross-culturally there is considerable similarity in postpartum treatment, not only in Southeast Asia but also in other societies with humoral medical traditions (Manderson, 1981; see various chapters, this volume).

In the past women in Rajin were confined to their homes for forty days after giving birth, but this practice is no longer observed. Now a woman must remain inside only for the first three to five days, sitting with her knees drawn into her chest to facilitate the flow of blood out of the uterus. During interviews with *belian nganak* and women who had recently given birth, no mention was made of women being "cold" after delivering, nor of any treatment designed to heat her body. However, *belian nganak* gave women herbal medicines to drink during and after labour, and these may well be considered "hot" or "cold", given the humoral tradition which underlies folk healing practices in Rajin.

After one week, when the baby's cord has healed, a ceremony is held during which the *belian nganak* washes the baby's hair with coconut milk, and receives gifts and thanks for her role in the delivery and treatment of the newborn. Unlike the ceremony held in the seventh month of pregnancy, this one is performed in all hamlets, but not by those who give birth in the hospital or with the assistance of a midwife. The *belian nganak* receives a special ritual food called *beras pati*, and her cash payment. The payment given to the *belian nganak* for assisting the delivery and giving follow-up care is not fixed, and depends on how much people can afford. For poorer families it may be as little as 2,000 rupiah, and for the better off as much as 5,000 rupiah plus two kilograms of uncooked rice.

In the follow-up interviews the eleven women described the treatment they and their babies received postpartum. Several reported having been given injections before and immediately after the delivery. They did not know what they had been injected with, but said it was to make the delivery easier, and the woman's recovery faster. These injections were given by subclinic nurses who had been asked to come by the women's husbands. The subclinic nurses later told me that the injections are vitamin B complex, given to make the women "stronger". For the visit and injections, they are paid between 3,000 and 5,000 rupiahs, depending on the number of injections.

Of the eleven newborn babies, only one had its umbilical cords treated by a subclinic nurse, when she came to give the mother an injection (vitamins). The rest were treated on a daily basis by the *belian nganak* who attended the birth, two of whom used mercurochrome, the third *kunyit*. None of these babies' cords had been treated with any unsterile substances (e.g. dirt, chalk, ash) according to their mothers, although this practice still continues to a degree.[13]

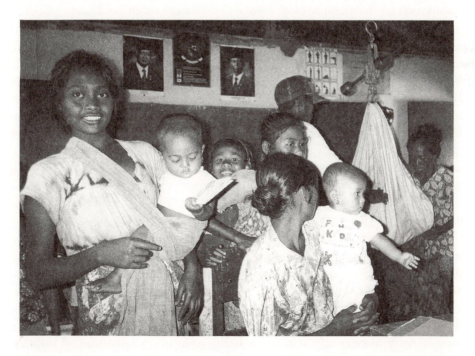

FIGURE 7.5 Women attending a health post (*posyandu*) with their friends, Wengkang. (Photo: J. Grace).

CONCLUSION

In rural East Lombok *belian nganak* remain the vital link between the majority of women and modern antenatal, birthing and postpartum care. Poverty, inaccessibility, lack of information and therefore understanding, are the major reasons why modern health facilities and services are under-utilised. Most women do not take full advantage of preventative care during pregnancy, and do not automatically seek modern medical attention when experiencing serious difficulty during delivery. Sasaks are very conscious of differences in social status, and many do not feel comfortable in seeking treatment from modern practitioners. *Belian nganak*, on the other hand, speak the same language, literally and metaphorically, and have always been available to deal with the anxiety and dangers of pregnancy, birthing and illness. Combined with their convenience and affordability, these factors strongly favour them over nurses, midwives and doctors.

While traditional birth attendants receive some training from the Health Department in sterile birthing procedures and follow-up care, the quality and frequency of that training and other outreach activities is inadequate to achieve substantial and ongoing positive results. Funding is lacking, and so clinic staff receive little incentive to carry out training and outreach activities. This combines with the negative attitude common among clinic staff and health officials towards traditional birth attendants because they are old and uneducated. The result is a general lack of commitment to taking full advantage of the position of *belian nganak* as trusted practitioners for the majority of women of childbearing age in rural East Lombok.

The antenatal interventions designed to reduce the risk of maternal and neonatal mortality are rarely and poorly understood by the women at whom they are directed. Health personnel from the village up to provincial level, when asked about the difficulties they face in overcoming health problems in East Lombok, immediately allude to women's ignorance and lack of formal education. However, observations at many health posts suggest that health staff do not offer explanations of the services they deliver, and voluntary health workers and women attending do not ask them questions. The health staff remain apart and aloof, conversing together and with educated residents of the hamlet, but rarely interacting more than superficially with the uneducated women who attend. While physical interventions are carried out, health education is neglected, and the attitude of many health staff seems to be that uneducated women are too ignorant to understand.

Women make rational, pragmatic decisions on the basis of what they know and understand, who they trust, and what they can afford. Given information which would enable them to understand how health interventions may reduce the risks to their own and their newborns' health, and given the physical and financial means to do so, they will increasingly accept them. However, a major obstacle is the lack of resources for the delivery of health services in rural areas. Were antenatal care made available in every subclinic and at health posts in the more isolated hamlets, the coverage would increase substantially. Were more money spent on training *belian nganak* and voluntary health workers, birthing procedures would become safer, and information would be disseminated far more widely and rapidly. Were emergency medical services in hospital free or subsidised for the poor, women's reluctance to use them would be reduced.

Belian nganak play an important role in women's lives in rural East Lombok. They are healers, and the rituals they perform and take part in are important aspects of the social, cultural and spiritual lives of Sasak families. There is no reason why women cannot continue to deliver their babies at home among family and friends, with the assistance of *belian nganak*. The risks of maternity can be greatly reduced by delivering comprehensive antenatal care, thorough and ongoing training for *belian nganak*, and easy access to medical intervention in emergency cases. The village midwife can play an important role by continuing the training of *belian nganak*, offering clinical support, and by acting as a link to emergency medical services outside the village. However, it would be a great shame if the significant event in women's lives of giving birth was taken out of their and their families' control, and placed in a context that was socially and culturally alien to them.

ENDNOTES

1. Indonesian words appear in italics, and Sasak words are further identified when first used by (S).

2. Sinung, K. (1992) UNICEF representative for the province of Nusa Tenggara Barat. Personal communication.

3. The relevant interview series for this chapter include one with pregnant women, and another with women with children under five years of age. There were thirty women interviewed in each series, fifteen in the central hamlet of Rajin (population approximately 2,000) and fifteen in the middle and southern most hamlets Ajan and Wengkang (with a combined population of approximately 2,000). The women interviewed were selected by a process of networking, taking into account geographic and socio-economic representativeness. A follow-up series with some of the pregnant women after they had given birth, was also conducted. Information about the services provided by *belian nganak* and clinic staff were collected during indepth interviews and through participant observation.

4. The majority of Sasaks adhere to the orthodox form of Islam, known in Lombok as *Waktu Lima*. There are still small pockets of the population who have not yet been converted to orthodox Islam but follow a syncretic form known as *Wetu Telu* (S), based more on customary law (*adat*) than religion.

5. Three hundred rupiah equals 15 cents (US). One day's income from agricultural labour, or handicrafts work for women, is 1,200 rupiah.

6. Koentjaraningrat (1985:352) mentions the ceremony in the seventh month of pregnancy in his description of Javanese religious rites. However, he describes only the *selamatan* or feast and other public aspects of it. Laderman (1987:360) gives a more detailed description of the ceremony performed in the seventh month of a woman's first pregnancy in Malay society. It involves the woman being bathed in "cold" lime juice and water, and both the pregnant woman and the traditional midwife having rice paste painted on their foreheads.

7. Many women who already have children do not have cards, and do not know whether they have received TT injections or not. In such cases they are given the inoculations.

8. In Dharma's *Indonesian Medical Plants* (1987) unripe pineapple is classified as an abortifacient.

9. When carrying out research the following year in another area of East Lombok I discovered that women there avoid having the TT injection, believing that it made the baby grow large, and so caused a difficult delivery. Even my research assistant, twice trained as a voluntary health worker, did not know the purpose of the injection, and had assumed it was to make delivery easier.

10. There is a large body of literature on the subject of the perception and use of injections in developing countries. The topic was discussed at length by van der Geest (1982), while Reeler's article (1990) offers a more recent overview of research on the misuse and abuse of injections in developing countries. In the Indonesian context, Hull (1979) and Sciortino (1992) describe the perception of injections in central Java, and their use by government health staff. Elsewhere I have described at length beliefs and uses of injections with respect to curative treatment of infants in this same village (Grace, 1994).

11. It is extremely unlikely that episiotomies are really necessary that often, and those who are inexperienced will often cut too soon and too often because they are afraid the perineum will tear. A small tear heals more quickly than a cut because of the ragged edges, but a small cut can avoid a large tear, which is desirable.

12. Mark Brooks was a consultant with World Bank Third World Health Project for Nusa Tenggara Barat and Kalimantan Timur, Jakarta.

13. The application of unsterile substances to the umbilical cord is the major cause of neonatal tetanus.

REFERENCES

Dharma, A.P. (1987) *Indonesian Medical Plants.* Jakarta: Balai Pustaka.

Fortney, J., Susanti, I., Gadalla, S., Sleh, S., Feldblum, P., Potts, M. (1988) Maternal Mortality in Indonesia and Egypt. *International Journal of Gynaecology and Obstetrics,* **26**, 21–32.

Geertz, H. (1961) *The Javanese Family: A Study of Kinship and Socialization.* New York: The Free Press of Glencoe.

Grace, J. (1994) Utilization of Curative Health Services for Potentially Life-threatening Infant Illnesses in Rural East Lombok, Indonesia. Unpublished paper given at the *ASAA conference,* Murdoch University, Perth.

Hull, V. (1979) Women, doctors, and family health care: some lessons from rural Java. *Studies in Family Planning,* **10**(11/12), 315–325.

Hull, V. (1986) Dietary taboos in Java: myths, mysteries, and methodology. In *Shared Wealth and Symbol: Food, Culture, and Society in Oceania and Southeast Asia,* edited by L. Manderson, pp. 237–258. Cambridge: Cambridge University Press.

Indonesia MOH and PATH (Ministry of Health and Programs for Appropriate Technology in Health) (1991) *Plan of Action: Child Survival-Plus Two (CSP2) Project, Lombok Island, West Nusa Tenggara Province, Indonesia — October 1990 to September 1993.* Unpublished Report. Mataram, Lombok: Indonesian MOH and PATH.

Koentjaraningrat (1985) *Javanese Religion in Javanese Culture.* Singapore: Oxford University Press.

Laderman, C. (1987) Destructive heat and cooling prayer: Malay humoralism in pregnancy, childbirth and the postpartum period. *Social Science and Medicine*, **25**(4), 357–365.

Manderson, L. (1981) Roasting, smoking and dieting in response to birth: Malay confinement in cross-cultural perspective. *Social Science and Medicine*, **15B**, 509–520.

Niehof, A. (1988) Traditional medication at pregnancy and childbirth in Madura, Indonesia. In *The Context of Medicines in Developing Countries*, edited by S. van der Geest and S. Whyte, pp. 235–252. Dordrecht: Kluwer Academic Publishers.

PATH (Programs for Appropriate Technology in Health) (1992) *Child Survival-Plus Two (CSP2) Project, Lombok Island, West Nusa Tenggara Province, Indonesia.* Baseline Survey, Draft Report. Mataram, Lombok: Indonesian MOH and PATH.

Paton, V.A. (1988) *Mbah Cipta's Gift: Healing in a Central Javanese Village,* Unpublished PhD thesis. Nedlands, W.A.: Department of Anthropology, University of Western Australia.

Reeler, A.V. (1990) Injections: a fatal attraction? *Social Science and Medicine*, **31**(10), 1119–1125.

Sciortino, R. (1992) *Caretakers of Cure: A Study of Health Centre Nurses in Rural Central Java,* Amsterdam: Vrije Universiteit Press.

van der Geest, S. (1982) The illegal distribution of western medicines in developing countries: pharmacists, drug pedlars, injection doctors and others. A bibliographic exploration. *Medical Anthropology*, **Fall**, 197–219.

van der Geest, S., Speckmann, J.D., Streefland, P.H. (1990) Primary health care in a multi-level perspective: towards a research agenda. *Social Science and Medicine*, **30**(9), 1025–1034.

CHAPTER 8

Women as "Good Citizens": Maternal and Child Health in a Sasak Village

Cynthia L. Hunter

> The body is . . . directly involved in a political field; power relations have an
> immediate hold upon it; they invest it, mark it, train it, torture it, force it to
> carry out tasks, to perform ceremonies, to emit signs (Foucault, 1977:25).

In 1973, the Minister of Home Affairs pointed out in a letter to regional governors
that the time had come for all Indonesians to accept responsibility and "become
involved in national development" (Sullivan, 1983:148). Economic development in
Indonesia is equated with reconstruction and modernisation, incorporating policies
of social engineering. Development is associated with notions about mental, moral,
and spiritual development. The state takes on the role of indoctrinating, guiding,
managing and mobilising civil society to serve the needs of the state.

Married women were singled out as a group with a crucial role in this new
approach. This resulted in the initiation of the Applied Family Welfare Program
(*Pembinaan Kesejahteraan Keluarga* – PKK),[1] a movement which is meant to reach
women at every level of society, including the village level. The official conception
of women's status and function as "good citizens" is marked by women's customary
roles as homebound childbearers and rearers, and loyal supporters of their husbands
(Sullivan, 1983, 1994).

Being a good mother is established in particular ways and the practices of
motherhood in contemporary Indonesia have a village and state dimension. The
techniques and desire for power and knowledge by which the state organises its
population to secure its control, welfare, and productivity are what Foucault calls
"bio-power" (1978:143). Family planning and the concept of "family" are part of a
state ideology and practice, which relate more to population control and the practice
of state power than they do to women's reproductive health. This chapter discusses the
discourses utilised in the representations of Indonesian women in the dimension of
maternal and child health. I describe the linkages between state imperatives through
the mechanism of PKK, and village practice as it exists in an East Lombok rural
mountain village. These are explored here as they are played out at the *posyandu*
(Integrated Village Health Service Post).

My understanding of the contemporary state framework in which policies and
programs are created and presented to society has been facilitated by examining the
state-populace discourse. Certain "keywords" (van Langenberg, 1986, 1990)[2] express

the ideology of the New Order in Indonesia in the areas of power, accumulation, legitimacy, culture and dissent. The centralised state in Indonesia exercises dominance in social control, in management of the means of production, in the control of reproduction, in the distribution of resources, and in cultural production (van Langenberg, 1986:4). The notions of *pembangunan* (development) and *pancasila*[3] are embedded in the government's aims to create and maintain a prosperous Indonesian nation. This discourse provides a linkage between a centralised establishment and the diverse ethnic communities. The close ties between the bureaucracy, the military and the ruling government party GOLKAR, and the gradual encroachment of the arm of government into villagers' lives by way of development programs[4] and civics education (Morfitt, 1981; Watson, 1987), ensures the state can increase its opportunities to gain social control and promote its commitment to equality (Morfitt, 1981; Dick, 1985) through the social justice of *pemerataan* (equity or equalisation). The redistribution of resources to all Indonesians provides the welfare and collectivist rationale for state intervention at all levels of society. These keywords are the basis of the interactional discourse between the system of the state and civil society. The exercise and implementation of the state as a separate entity from government is best described by what Foucault refers to as "governmentality", a complex form of institutional power, procedures and analyses which formulates a whole series of specific apparatuses and knowledges into a legitimate governmentalised administrative state (Burchell, Gordon and Miller, 1991:103). Foucault says that this governmentality has developed because of a political economy approach in which the state must deal with its population. The problems and techniques of government have become the only political issue. In my analysis I will refer to keywords which have particular relevance for notions of "citizenship" and women's relations with the state, although notions of "citizenship" incorporated through exploitation are as true for men as women at village level.

WOMEN IN DEVELOPMENT POLICY

The participation of women in national development became law in 1974 (Undang-undang Nomor,[5] Tahun 1975, cited by Sullivan, 1983:148) and was built into the second Five Year Development Plan (1974–79, *Repelita II*). The central aim was defined as the improvement of living standards such as housing, and social welfare services including expanded infrastructure, more equitable distribution of benefits, and increased employment opportunities. The state was to increase funding at the same time as it was expected communities would develop their own self help efforts, which, it was felt, would give people greater self-confidence and self-determination to build a better society. To create policy programs the government enlisted the support of women's organisations, particularly the *Kongres Wanita Indonesia* or KOWANI (Indonesian Women's Congress), the umbrella organisation for most of the women's associations. Members are predominantly upper and middle class, the wives of government employees, professionals, religious leaders and intellectuals, plus women working in these fields. The leaders of these organisations were enlisted to propagate two major state programs among women: *Keluarga Berencana* or *KB* (Family Planning Program) and *Pembinaan Kesejahteraan Keluarga* or *PKK* (Applied Family Welfare Program) (Sullivan, 1983, 1994).

Pembinaan Kesejahteraan Keluarga (PKK) (Applied Family Welfare Program)

The 1974 legislation specified the links between PKK and the state, and institutionalised PKK units in villages and urban kampungs as components of the Village Social Committees (LSD, now LKMD or Village Public Security Councils). Policy directives for the most fundamental development programs begin in the family, "because that was the most fundamental social institution that formed the roles, values, attitudes, and behaviour patterns on which fruitful development depended" (Sullivan, 1983:148). A woman was considered to be the central crucial agent of a family, her position incorporating five major roles: as a loyal backstop and supporter of her husband; as caretaker of the household; as the producer of future generations; as the family's prime socialiser; and as an Indonesian citizen. These government-defined roles emphasise women, not as equals alongside men, but as subordinates in a patriarchal state system. As well as these five major roles, women also had responsibilities for the spiritual, moral, mental and physical welfare of their families in line with the meaning of economic development. They were responsible for producing good future citizens, and learning to be good citizens themselves.

The PKK was supposed to help women meet these obligations, by encompassing appropriate ideals, information, guidelines, and by training them in their application. Suryakusuma (1991, cited by Warren, 1993:245) refers to "State Ibuism" (*Ibu* being both the word for mother and the respectful term of address for women) to describe the New Order's construction of womanhood as simultaneously instrumental and dependent. Women serve their families, their communities and the state. There is no recognition of them as independent political and economic participants. Suryakusuma (1991, cited by Warren, 1993:245) and Djajadiningrat-Nieuwenhuis (1987:46,50) similarly argue that the New Order gender ideology represents a fusion of traditional Javanese elite (*prijaji-*Jv) values and western middle class ones.

Elements of patriarchy become visible because the program theorists, the senior officials, development planners and key administrators are mostly male. The practitioners are exclusively female, the leaders and rank and file of the national women's movement. The government selects certain women to be leaders at various levels of the movement corresponding to the major levels of the state administrative hierarchy. In reality, the women chosen achieve office by virtue of their husband's position, e.g. *Ibu Desa* (the wife of the village head).

Organisational Structure of PKK

The mechanism for activating PKK ideals is composed of the PKK's own internal organisational structure and the state's civil administrative framework, "mediated" by the *Persatuan Istri Karyawan dan Karyawati di Lingkungan Departmen Dalam Negeri* or PERTIWI (The Union of Wives of Male Employees and Female Employees in the Department of Home Affairs). At the central government level PKK is aligned with the central bureaucracy via the PERTIWI leadership executive, the *ex-officio* head of which is the wife of the Minister of Home Affairs. The Bureau of Village Development, in Home Affairs, which has regional offices, advises PKK executives at various levels on general administrative and technical matters. The provincial level PKK leaders are female relatives of the provincial governor and often hold high regional positions in PERTIWI as well.

At the lower levels of the structure, at the *kabupaten* (district) level, the Bupati's wife is *ex-officio* head of both PKK and PERTIWI. Below this, at the *kecamatan* (sub-district) level, the camat's wife who is also a member of PERTIWI, is titular head of PKK. At the village level, the village head's wife or a close relative is titular head; at the hamlet or administrative ward level the wives of each of the hamlet heads are the heads of PKK.

DEVELOPMENT ORGANISATION IN THE VILLAGE

PKK in the Village

The *Lembaga Ketahanan Masyarakat Desa* or LKMD (Village Public Security Council) consists of ten sections including the PKK and health and family planning. All adult village women are eligible to be members of PKK and address the following ten principal programs:

1. the creation of good relations within and between families
2. correct child care
3. the use of hygienic food preparation techniques and close attention to nutrition
4. the securing of total family health — in physical, mental, spiritual and moral spheres
5. care that clothing is suited to its proper functions — protection, morality, modesty
6. intelligent use of house space to meet needs of hygiene, privacy, entertainment, etc.
7. the development of family attitudes appropriate to the modernisation process — planning for the future
8. the preservation of emotional and physical security and a tranquil environment in the home
9. effective basic housekeeping, calculated to maximise order and cleanliness, and
10. effective household budgeting.

This list indicates numerous female responsibilities but no rights. It is a list which emphasises *pemerataan* (equity) and *stabilitas* (stability). It is assumed that women will identify with national objectives but there is no mention of what they might gain in the *pembangunan* (development) process, nor is there any indication of a change in status. In fact, a contradiction arises. The ability of most married women to further national development by following the formula precisely presupposes a level of economic development and patterns of resource distribution which have not been reached. Sullivan (1983:155) suggests that the "male planners" and "well off" women who drew up the 10 point program "are unaware that they may constitute far distant *ends* rather than efficacious *means* for the majority of Indonesian housewives". This program could, theoretically, be considered as "development on the cheap". Women are already trying with what little resources they have to meet basic requirements. The government actually does not have the funds available to effect such measures.

Thus, the practical implementation appears unworkable, and the reception of these efforts by lower class women is questionable. The agriculture-based first Five Year Plan victimised many rural women, who lost their share of agricultural production to new technology. According to Sullivan (1983:156), their displacement resulted in "a real drop in importance and status in home and community as they became that much more dependent on their menfolk to sustain their families" (see also White, 1976; Stoler, 1977; Manderson, 1980). According to Hull (1979), there is a firm official stamp on the belief that women's place is in the home, not in the fields nor in any other influential sphere of economic activity (cf. Alexander, 1987).

An East Lombok Village

The rural village community in which I lived in northeast Lombok is traditional and conservative. The villagers are Sasak and Muslim, though there are a few descendants from Balinese families who have embraced Islam and the Sasak language (see also Grace, this volume). The village, Elah, is situated over 400 metres above sea level on the slopes of Mt. Rinjani (see Figure 7.1, above). It is typical in structure to other mountain villages around. There is one main road which passes through the village, lined by the cluster of administrative offices, the village mosque, the sports ground, a *warung* (foodstall), a kiosk or two, and housing. Another smaller road turns north to the last village on this side of the mountain. It too is lined with houses and the *Puskesmas Pembantu* or *pustu* (Health Sub-Clinic). The village is divided into four *dasan* (S) (hamlets), two of which are separated from the main village and administrative centre by ricefields and gardens. Those who have been educated speak Indonesian, but women and older people especially do not speak Indonesian well. Education is not a priority. In contrast, religion is of fundamental importance. East Lombok is well known throughout the rest of Indonesia as being *fanatik* (adhering strictly to) about religion. There are two religious *aliran* (ideologies): *waktu telu* and *waktu lima*. *Waktu telu* is the most ancient and traditional; its followers are nominal Muslims with a heterodox combination of beliefs from an animistic and Hindu-Buddhist pantheon, ancestor worship and supernatural forces. In contrast, *waktu lima* is rigidly orthodox, intolerant of other religions, hegemonic, proselytising and modern. The government recognises *waktu lima* rather than *waktu telu*, and supports the largest *waktu lima* organisation on Lombok, Nahdlatul Wathan, in return for votes at election time; village government officials follow this ideology. The *karyawan* (state functionaries) carry out their duty of mobilising mass support for the government and its programs especially at the time of elections. The *floating mass* doctrine prevents any other political activity at village level and hence reinforces the structural significance of religious organisations such as Nahdlatul Wathan at village level.

Village PKK

Information about the operations of PKK in the village in which I lived is difficult to document because of the inert nature of the organisation. I attended two PKK meetings, one in 1991 and the other in 1992, neither of which drew a large number of women, less than thirty from an adult female population of about 1800. The head of PKK is not the village head's wife but a young school teacher from an influential family who holds all three offices of president, secretary and treasurer. The main activity is *arisan*: the credit society and savings scheme. There was no official business discussed at the first meeting and no ongoing projects involving women. At the second meeting, there was a discussion about the impending visit of the sub-district leader of PKK, the wife of the sub-district head. The focus of her visit was on giving the appearance of keeping the PKK books in order rather than demonstrating any activity.

Several women were disappointed and disillusioned with PKK. One member, an immigrant from Flores, confided to me that she had tried several times to introduce new ideas at meetings but there was little enthusiasm. She consistently questioned the legality of one office bearer being in charge of three offices, but this was ignored. Another neighbour, an older woman, told me she used to be involved with PKK but she has given up attending because she does not always agree with the younger women. Sullivan's (1983) findings at the local level reflect similar tendencies: informal politicking, socialising and pecuniary interests, although this inertia does not apply to all villages in the sub-district or at least not to the same degree. Nor does it necessarily apply to other sub-districts. But PKK activities tend to reflect middle class values and attitudes which are far removed from rural village life, and the distance between class interests sustain PKK ideology and practice and rural needs. Hull (1976) believes that if PKK activities serve women's interests at all, it is mostly those of the middle-class who benefit from bureaucratic state policy through their husbands' positions.

In comparison with Balinese women (Warren, 1993), although some Sasak women are active in economic affairs outside the home, their involvement in the local political organisation is negligible, and their participation in village affairs is dependent on factors such as their husbands' approval and sanction. The only example I know is a daughter of the current village head. Some years ago she was appointed as head of section 5 (the environment) in the Village Public Security Council (LKMD). About four years ago she moved from the village to a larger town, and no-one has replaced her.

EMBODYING WOMEN IN DEVELOPMENT

Despite the virtual non-functioning of PKK, section 7 of the Village Public Security Council (LKMD), Health and Family Planning, is operative. In line with the central government's push to provide equity in health and welfare services to all villagers and control population growth by controlling women's fertility, this dimension of development is actively promoted through government servicing and village functionaries who enlist community participation, and validated by the notion of *pemerataan*, social justice and welfare. Besides controlling women's bodies through fertility control programs, there are other issues confronting women's bodies. One of these is women's relationships with their children.

Posyandu

Pos Pelayanan Terpadu or *posyandu* (Integrated Health Post) is a meeting place where villagers with children under five and pregnant women come to receive maternal health care, nutrition, advice, diarrhoea control, family planning advice and supplies, and immunisation. Women with babies (0–1 year) and children under five (*balita*), and pregnant women, are called to *posyandu* once a month by village officials: the hamlet head in the ward in which they live and *posyandu kader* (health volunteers). A *posyandu* session is the primary source of maternal and child health care (including immunisation) for the rural poor.

Structurally, *posyandu* is a village community participation program, part of the Department of Home Affairs at the local level, through the Village Public Security Council (LKMD) via PKK. The *Pusat Kesehatan Masyarakat* or *puskesmas* (Health Clinic) staff who provide technical services at *posyandu* are part of the Department of Health. *Posyandu* implementation is facilitated by these two groups. Community participation is promoted as beneficial for villagers: it allows them to take the initiative in defining their goals, increasing their access to health care, and at the same time facilitates the further encroachment of state intervention, the legitimation of power and discipline.

The organisation of *posyandu* sessions varies significantly within and between villages in both the frequency and quality of execution. The most isolated communities have poor access to all health services including *posyandu*. Transport problems and distance affect service delivery, and where the hamlet head and/or health *kader* are ineffective, sessions are irregular. Women and children are disadvantaged to a greater degree than men; they are less mobile, less knowledgeable and less experienced in going outside the village than men.

Posyandu Clients

These are rural village women with young children, many of whom are poor, their education level is low, and few have graduated from primary school. Their ages range from mid teens to late forties or early fifties. Many of them do not speak Indonesian well; their local language is Sasak. Their families and friends are mainly

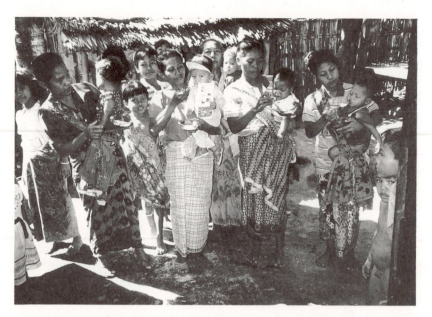

FIGURE 8.1 A group of mothers with their children at *posyandu*, East Lombok. (Photo: C. Hunter).

in the village or nearby. The majority are married to local men of similar background; some as first wives, some second. Among themselves they are noisy, talkative, friendly, argumentative and happy. With outsiders they are shy, reticent and inarticulate to varying degrees, depending on whether they are on their home territory (their own home, ricefield or hamlet) or in a place away from it or out of the village. Only a few of them become *posyandu kader* (health volunteers) but most have incorporated the activities of *posyandu* into their idea of maternal responsibility. PKK is predicated on the assumption that women's primary function is as mothers, but this does not reflect the Sasak village women's experience. On the morning of *posyandu* sessions one feature in particular attests to the opposite. The disorganisation of *posyandu* reflects a bureaucratic assumption that women's time is of no value compared to that of the clinic.

Hamlet heads announce a *posyandu* session over the mosque PA system early on the morning. However health personnel never arrive at the announced time. Mothers arrive slowly. They are in no hurry because they know that the *kader* (health volunteers) are not ready and the nursing staff have not arrived. If they come early and have their babies weighed, they then have to sit around and wait for the immunisations. The women see this as wasting time; they have work to do at home or they are anxious to get to the ricefields.

There are other features which signify women's subordination. One hamlet head is fond of playing loud *dangdut* (popular Indonesian music) throughout the session. In one such session which I witnessed, there were fifty women in the

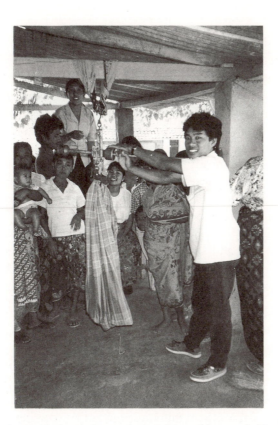

FIGURE 8.2 Mothers with their babies at the weighing table attended by a male *kader*. (Photo: C. Hunter).

houseyard. One mother's child was apparently underweight: the nurse asked all mothers to listen while he explained about nutrition, using the food examples on the back of the health card to illustrate — a lesson that was futile since there was no attempt made to turn down the music. Another instance of staff disorder occurred in regard to immunisation. The nurse arrived and set up the immunisation equipment. He began by breaking the glass vial of the BCG vaccine but then spent time finding the appropriate needle and syringe from a box which contained an assortment of needles and syringes. Each baby was finally inoculated and its immunisation status recorded on the health card.

Theoretically, the head *kader* together with the hamlet head are responsible for several *posyandu* registers. To keep mothers' health cards is additional work which in reality falls to the head *kader*. In the absence of sufficient health *kader* (five is the recommended number), the head *kader* hands a bundle of cards to someone hovering and asks her to find the card for each child whose weight is recorded. This person may have little or no training in the procedure — what he/she knows has been "picked up" by watching others.

The Citizen as Child

Sometimes mothers do not have a health card and there are no new cards available. Immunisation is then recorded by the nurse or health *kader* on a piece of paper, or in the back of an exercise book, to be written in a new health card at a later date. Mothers are not consulted or given any information about this procedure. Health personnel patronise women in this way. Some mothers bring their child's health card with them but the majority are kept by the head *kader*. Mothers would like to keep their child's card, know about their child's weight each month, and have the immunisations explained to them, but this is discouraged in the face of efficiency and security against loss. The nurse turns away babies for immunisation if he thinks they have a fever. One mother of five went three times to *posyandu* for immunisation and was refused each time because the nurse said her baby had a fever (*panas*). The child had not been sick at home before. Such patronising attitudes or *bapak*ism by staff create disillusionment and distrust in mature and experienced mothers.

From the Citizen as Child to the Records which Count

In another instance which illustrates the disorganisation of the *posyandu*, a mother brought an infant of five months for the first triple antigen dose. The mother explained she had not been to *posyandu* before, therefore, her baby had never been immunised. The *kader* could not find a card from a previous occasion. The nurse pondered: had it been lost or could the mother be relied on to know this was her first time at *posyandu*? The nurse was sceptical; the infant should have received one triple antigen before now; he recorded the current immunisation as the second dose on the health card, then immunised the child. Clinic staff set more store in records than mother's knowledge. Women may not know how to read their child's health card, nor know the names of childhood immunisations or which ones their child has had, but they are likely to remember how many times their child has received an injection. Time and again nurses informed me that one had to disregard villagers' knowledge because "they are still ignorant/dumb" (*orang di desa masih bodoh*).

In another example, there was a discussion concerning an infant's age. The weight chart showed that last month the infant's age was recorded as six months. The mother is adamant the baby is only six months old this month. Someone filled in the card incorrectly, a common mistake which many health *kader* and some nurses make. Despite the inadequacy and mistakes in record keeping, the records are what stand. This is part of the rationalising discourse of modernity. The health of the population is controlled and disciplined according to the records, regardless of the manipulation needed to reach government targets.

Village Administrators

Posyandu health *kader* (usually women but sometimes men) are ostensibly voluntary workers. In reality, they are chosen or coerced by the head health *kader* and hamlet head to serve in an administrative capacity for *posyandu* matters (cf. Stephens, Feirman and Wirawan, 1989:17). Ideally, there are two training courses. The first, *akselerasi* (acceleration), is a 4–5 day basic training course in record keeping, baby weighing, use of vitamin A supplements and nutrition. The second, *eskalasi* (escalation), is of 3–4 days and is for management and leadership; usually only the head health *kader* has attended this course.

Young, unmarried women become health *kader* but drop out when they marry. According to Stephens, Feirman and Wirawan (1989:vi), the attrition rate for *kader* exceeds 50%. They may be motivated early on with the promise of training in the *puskesmas* (health clinic) or some monetary incentive. However, motivation wanes because training sessions are irregular and there is no infrastructure for health volunteers to receive a salary. *Kader*, even if they have the training, lack the self esteem or confidence to operate as state functionaries in this modern arena. Some *kader* told me they could not continue this work because their husbands prohibited it. In general, the exception to this is the head health *kader*. For example, Inaq Mas, the head health *kader* in Dasan Gubuk Pare, is an older married woman who has finished childbearing. She is married to the principal of one of the Islamic schools and she does not need to work. Her husband is also the head of the religion section of the Village Public Security Council (LKMD). She became the head *kader* when a representative from the central family planning organisation (BKKBN) asked her to become the family planning volunteer. She says that at the time she did not want the position because she did not feel competent, not having finished primary school, but was persuaded because of her sense of public duty as a consequence of her husband's position.

Despite the authoritarian tactics and obvious involvement of village officials to recruit health *kader*, there is often an assumption by doctors and health clinic staff that health *kader* in the community serve the *puskesmas* (health clinic) rather than the community. In part, this explains the superior attitude of clinic staff to *kader* who are considered to be on the lowest rung of the health bureaucracy. In fact, village women consider them to be most knowledgeable and superior.

Family Planning and Maternal Health

Antenatal services in the village are supplied by the *pustu* or *Puskesmas Pembantu*, *posyandu* and eighteen *belian ranak* (S) (indigenous midwives), three of whom are state trained. *Posyandu* services are supposed to include family planning, antenatal examinations and immunisation services. Often there is a staff member of family planning (BKKBN) present who recruits new acceptors for the pill or injection methods of contraception but not other methods. Tetanus toxoid immunisations are given to pregnant women. However, other maternal health services are often not undertaken. The *pustu* was staffed only by a male paramedic whose antenatal and midwifery services were underutilised because of Islamic constraints on men internally examining other men's wives for IUD contraception and internal pregnancy examinations. Up until 1991 no professional staff midwife lived in the village.

In a survey of 40 women in the village,[5] less than a quarter (20.0%) had tetanus toxoid injections during their pregnancies, and only a quarter (25.0%) had been examined antenatally by health personnel at the *pustu* (health sub-clinic) in the village or at *posyandu*. Almost three quarters of the women (72.7%) had been examined by *belian ranak* (indigenous midwives);[6] others (17.5%) had no antenatal examination of any kind. Of those examined by traditional methods, just over half (54.0%) went to one of the three state trained indigenous midwives. As Grace (this volume) describes, state trained indigenous midwives attend a two to three day course at the health clinic (*puskesmas*) at the subdistrict or district level. They are instructed in confinement hygiene, the observation of danger signs which might arise during pregnancy or childbirth, and neonatal care. They are encouraged to work with professional midwives in areas where they are located. They receive a kit bag containing items such as cottonwool, scissors, thread, soap and mercurochrome, plus a white jacket. A number of men and women stated that the state trained midwives had more expertise than those untrained.

Because of the lack of a professional midwife in the health sub-clinic until May 1991, women and men expected to call on the services of indigenous midwives at the time of confinement. The survey revealed few (8.0%) used a health clinic or village professional midwife, most (92.0%) used indigenous midwives. Almost half (44.5%) of these used state trained indigenous midwives. The main reasons given for not using the professional midwife were not because of cultural resistance but social, economic and distance barriers (see also Grace, this volume).

Although the national health services are still incomplete at the village level the National Family Planning Coordinating Body has been very active. Only 13.8% of the men surveyed[7] reported no use of family planning methods (although none had reached their desired number of children), and 86.1% had wives who were using family planning. None of the men were responsible for contraception themselves, although condoms are easily accessible and vasectomies are also available. Of the wives using contraceptive methods, the most common methods were the injectable depo progestin, the pill, implants, and IUDs[8] (see also Jennaway, this volume).

The slogan of the National Family Planning Coordinating Body, *dua anak cukup* (two children is enough), is prominently displayed on billboards throughout the country and most people are aware of its meaning. The men surveyed were cognisant in the sense that they knew what the government was urging — smaller family size — but it was clear that there was no consensus on this issue. In response to the question "How many children is the right number?" less than half agreed with the government view (see Table 8.1), and almost three quarters were reluctant to say that any fewer than four children was the right number.

The slogan "two children is enough" is an ideology based on an urban middle class notion unlikely to be attractive to poor rural villagers. The two most important aims of Sasak women and men is marriage and the production of children. Women who do not marry are scorned by men and looked down upon by women; women who marry but remain barren are divorced or become co-wives of men and pitied by women. Orthodox Islamic beliefs affect the types of contraception women use.

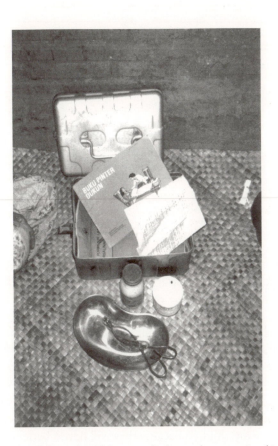

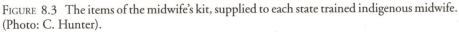

FIGURE 8.3 The items of the midwife's kit, supplied to each state trained indigenous midwife. (Photo: C. Hunter).

However, the government also urges women to control their bodies. They should control their sexual desires and therefore, their reproduction. Consequently, in the government's view, for health purposes their bodies are objects of control, not subjective bodies.

The above slogan is less likely to be followed in Nusa Tenggara Barat (Lombok and Sumbawa), which has the highest infant mortality rates (IMR) in Indonesia. In 1992 these rates showed the smallest decline for all of Indonesia — 145/1000 live births — and the projected rate for the year 2000 was still over 100 (Kasto 1992:18). Because of the cultural significance attached to their domestic and maternal role, and the high infant death rate, women need to have a large number of children to ensure some reach adult age and can provide for their parents in their old age. Women are assiduous in trying to find cures for their sick infants (Finerman, 1984; Nations and Rebhun, 1988; Hunter, in preparation), and are pluralistic in seeking cures (Young, 1981) and choice of medical practitioner. Women in the village who had just lost

TABLE 8.1   The right number of children.

Number of children	"Right" number		Actual number		"Too many"*	
	N	%	N	%	N	%
1	0	0.0	9	25.0	0	0.0
2	16	44.4	8	22.2	2	5.6
3	8	22.2	7	19.4	8	22.2
4	3	8.3	3	8.3	9	25.0
5	2	5.6	1	2.8	4	11.1
6	1	2.8	3	8.3	3	8.3
7	3	8.3	3	8.3	2	5.6
8	0	0.0	0	0.0	3	8.3
9	0	0.0	0	0.0	0	0.0
10	3	8.3	2	5.6	1	2.8
11	0	0.0	0	0.0	2	5.6
12	0	0.0	0	0.0	2	5.6
Total	36	100.0	36	100.0	36	100.0

*"Too many" refers to respondents perceptions of their own family size at time of survey. (Source: Author's field survey, 1992).

infant children display a kind of fatalism but I would argue that this reaction to death is partly explained by a deep grief and partly by Islamic religious belief in pre-destination (cf. Scheper-Hughes, 1992). Young babies who die are considered called by Allah and *masuk surga* (enter heaven immediately) without sin. The younger, modern women in the village express a desire to space their children so that they can have the time and resources to bring them up to be healthy. They say that by doing this they will not need to have as many children because they will have a better chance of survival, and the mothers will have an easier childrearing task.

The government's rationalisation, based on a need for population control, security, surveillance and discipline, places the obligation on individual ethical conduct. The government has consistently promoted population control since the inception of the National Family Planning Coordinating Body in the 1970s (Manderson, 1974; Hull, 1976). For a number of years Indonesia has been pressured by the World Health Organization and other international agencies to control population growth, the concept of which is linked to the capitalist notion of a healthy labour force. Each year in villages throughout the country there are family planning drives to recruit new participants. These drives enlist the assistance of local state functionaries in the village. In 1992 in a campaign of this kind in Lombok, the village and hamlet heads rounded up eligible women from their wards and brought them to the *pustu* (health sub-clinic). On this occasion the head of an outlying ward acted on behalf of his group, bargaining with the health clinic staff about the price of contraception. "The women are poor", he said, "and can only pay a small amount". On the same day, the village head and head of another ward, together with health sub-clinic staff, strongly opposed the wishes of two young women who wanted contraceptive implants.

Reproductive health does not receive the same attention as fertility control. Many women suffer from various side effects of contraception to which they attribute symptoms such as lack of energy, continual bleeding, fatness, thinness, headaches, dizziness, fatigue and hair falling out; this causes anxiety. Many have tried more than one method of contraception to overcome these difficulties. Women have taken their complaints to staff at the health sub-clinic but say they rarely receive satisfactory answers, helpful advice or cures. Seldom are women referred to a doctor in a *puskesmas* (health clinic).

In the above examples sex has become political issue through the disciplining of female bodies in order to regulate population in accordance with the aims of a state intent on nation building. Foucault's (1978:143) notion of "bio-power" (see above) describes the position of the state controlling and regulating the bodies of its population in order to bring about a transformation in society. The progressive nation state requires healthy Indonesian citizens suitable for economic progress, free from pestilence, poverty and overcrowding. The management of health is crucial in this endeavour. Foucault (1978:147) says "at the juncture of the 'body' and the 'population', sex [becomes] a crucial target of a power organized around the management of life rather than the menace of death".

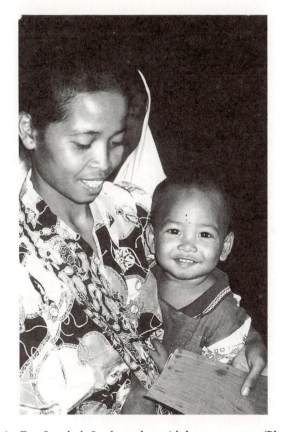

FIGURE 8.4   An East Lombok Sasak mother with her young son. (Photo: C. Hunter).

WOMEN'S OWN AGENCY

Women possess an alternative rationality from that of the government or their menfolk. They have their own particular problems with their bodies' health as well as controlling pregnancy and spacing children. Women sense rightly that they are disempowered. Almost without exception and regardless of topic, in the village in which I lived, if men and women are gathered in the household and questions are asked of women, the men reply. Often women engage in activities such as *posyandu* or family planning at the directive of their husbands. Yet women demonstrate their own agency when, in the absence of men, they discuss issues which affect their daily lives, including issues which directly affect their bodies.

Women's Views on Maternal and Child Health

Women say that *posyandu* sessions are good to check their babies' weights, but they do not like the immunisations because after an injection a baby often has a fever for a couple of days. This makes them anxious and slows down their working ability as more time is spent pacifying (nursing) an unhappy baby.

Mothers comment unfavourably on *posyandu* sessions now, compared with a few years ago. At that time *posyandu* were held at the village head's house. He was very diligent about having nutritious food available. There was always *bubur hijau* (bean porridge), fruit and peanuts for the children. It was more orderly (*tertib*) than it is now.[9] Mothers could comfortably bring their young children and serve them food while attending to a baby in need of weighing and immunising. Porridge is regarded as a sign of a good *posyandu*, of better organisation, a local indicator of order and competence which bureaucrats take seriously. Now, in this village, a *posyandu* session with porridge or any other food is rare. Women attend only because they are told it is good to have their babies weighed regularly and immunised.

When questioned about possible improvements to *posyandu*, several mothers expressed their wish to have sessions earlier in the morning so that they can get on with their domestic chores and start their work day in the ricefields or in other economic activities. In a well-administered health clinic, there is no reason why health personnel could not comply with such a request. The health clinic opens at 7.30 am. *Posyandu* duties are scheduled according to a six monthly timetable and therefore, known well in advance. Allowing for a short delay due to late staff arrivals and problems of transport to the village, sessions could begin at about 9 am. But where there is disorganisation in the health clinic, staff are not prepared and sessions do not begin until 10 or even 11 am.

As already described, the relationship of nurses with village women is marked by dominance and subordination. To a Westerner's eyes the nurse is didactic in his/her message giving, authoritarian, patronising and interrogative in eliciting information, in a tone of voice which is clinical and detached. To many villagers these people are *sombong* (arrogant). Little or no instruction is given about medicines or disease etiologies. Very occasionally, as in the case above, the nurse will give a lesson in nutrition or diarrhoea control. The opportunity for group discussion could be encouraged, but there are few questions asked of mothers as a group and little eliciting of information on health knowledge.

Women's Perceptions of Themselves

The majority of village women spend their entire lives rearing children and working the *bangket* (S) (ricefields), tending the garlic crop and growing vegetables, or engaged in other seasonal activities such as making kapok bedding. While working at these activities women would chat to me about their lives. The word used most often to describe themselves is *bodoh* (ignorant). The meaning is used in two senses: they are not worldly wise in the sense of having hold of the facts about the world; and they have little or no formal education. The perception of them held by health personnel is *masih bodoh* (still ignorant), where the implication is one of "backwardness" or "country bumpkins", a temporary state which will disappear when they get the idea that "progress is good". The women's usage suggests a more enduring situation. When I suggested to the women that their situation may change I was greeted with smiles, laughter, even amusement. Krulfeld (1966) suggests that Sasak demonstrate a fatalistic attitude toward their lack of political control above the local level. I would suggest women partially demonstrate this at the local level; because the means of change are perceived as beyond their immediate reach, change is not aspired to.

Women resist taking on roles which they do not feel competent to carry out. Rural women cannot be expected to volunteer for formal positions outside the home when they have little experience of such outside matters. The persuasion and coercion by village officials exemplifies the situation found in many villages. Inaq Mas has learnt her skills "on the way". She has attended several courses. Her knowledge and competence at the tasks is better than other health *kader*, but not perfect. She possesses some leadership qualities and skills and is looked up to by the other health *kader*, and many of the mothers, as a person who may have answers to their questions and someone they can approach. Her better economic position and her personal and social networks,[10] which extend outside the village, give her an appearance of assurance and competence unsurpassed by most of the others. However, the fact remains that a person like her is expected to take the role, rather than having any choice in the matter. State functionaries require additional personal qualities based on experience.

Masyarakat — The Community

The groups described above are part of the insiders, the *masyarakat*, the village community. Their relationships and interactions are prescribed by status, kin, social and spatial sensibilities. In a conservative mountain village with little migration in or out of the village, social networks, administrative roles, personal networks and relations by marriage and birth are intertwined and closely knit. Women feel they are victims of a system which comes to them from outside their village and over which they have little or no control. It is easy to see why. The Department of Health is a huge bureaucracy with its own agenda and its own momentum. It is a hierarchical system, staff at each level taking orders from those at the level above. In comparison, villagers, especially women, follow their husbands' directives or the strict codes of fundamental Islam. However, both men and women express aspects of resistance in the face of an encroaching state. The cultural context is determined by adherence to *adat* (custom, tradition) and/or *agama* (religion).

At *posyandu*, there is no infrastructure for the villagers to express their concerns or opinions about their children's or their own needs. For example, there is an avenue for women with sick children to receive a letter from the *posyandu* to take the child to the health clinic for free treatment if it is a low income family, but as Grace (this volume) also notes, this is seldom offered to them or used by them. During my research I only witnessed this avenue being used twice. Mothers take their children to the health clinic, but they will pay for the services performed because they do not know the other avenue exists. Despite a notion that *posyandu* is good for checking babies' weight progress and immunisation, mothers and their children are participants in a social situation which they feel is not of their own making and therefore, lacking in purpose. They are participants by virtue of the fact that they are villagers and *posyandu* has been interposed in village life.

The relationship between the health *kader*, village officials and nurses is based on the need to execute an activity — the *posyandu*. The health *kader* have a subordinate role in relation to nurses: record keeping, baby weighing, immunisation of those present. They are receptive to instruction from nurses and look to them or the head health *kader* for guidance in moments of confusion. Sometimes nurses take time to explain a procedure, but more frequently a *posyandu* session is about getting through the activity as quickly as possible, with little or no heed to efficacy or quality of execution. As permanent government employees, the nurses have no job insecurity. Their energies can be directed towards the tasks themselves. All too often, this energy is spent on execution only, on getting rates in registers. The nature of bureaucratic process is such that often the targets become the ends in themselves. The power relations which exist between the government bureaucracy and the village world are based on expediency and pragmatic action, without any underlying understanding of the cultural or historical contexts in which people operate in their daily rhythm of life (see Justice, 1986). The state imperative is *ketertiban* (control), despite the rhetoric of *pembangunan* (development) and *bapak*ism.

Statistics are themselves part of the discourses of the governmentality. In the above examples, sex has become the political issue, through the disciplining of female bodies in order to regulate population (Foucault, 1978:146–7). Sasak culture now not only is regarded as backward, but Sasak villages are found to be "sick" communities; the surveillance of people through government programs and services reveals "problems" such as lack of childhood immunisation and poor weight gain.

In contemporary Indonesia the ideology of the family has woman as the central agent. The order of the five major "duties" promulgated by the PKK tellingly places the Indonesian women's role as "citizen" last, after those of "producer" and "socialiser" of the nation's next generation, "husband's companion", and "household manager" (Hull, 1976:21–2, cited by Warren, 1993:245). The health system is an important component of the processes of vertical integration by which women are incorporated into Indonesian society as "good citizens", but not because maternal health is the priority of the State. Rather, fertility control is a priority, family planning a political tool for population control. I return once more to the quotation by Foucault at the beginning of this chapter. The state remains directly involved in sets of power relations with its population. Women's bodies are politicised, controlled, disciplined and invested according to a state agenda far removed from the contexts and cultures of their historical origins.

ENDNOTES

1. Indonesian words are in italics, while Javanese and Sasak words, also in italics, are followed by the abbreviations (Jv) and (S) respectively.
2. Van Langenberg's approach follows Raymond Williams' (1961, 1983) studies of a lexicon of keywords to understand culture and society.
3. The five principles of *pancasila* are (1) Belief in one supreme God (2) Humanitarianism (3) Indonesian Unity (4) Popular Representation and (5) Social Justice. Since 1985 state law has made it obligatory for all social organizations to adopt *pancasila* as their sole principle, *azas tunggal*.
4. This is maintained through the *floating mass*, the notion that the populace should be free of grass-roots political ties, in order for it to be fully responsive to the directives of the state and the interests of development.
5. The survey was of 40 women of child-bearing age, 10 from each of the four village hamlets, to ascertain their attitudes, beliefs and experience in pregnancy, childbirth and postnatal processes.
6. The discrepancy in the numbers (24 women examined by indigenous midwives and 10 by the health personnel) arises because one woman was examined by both indigenous and modern practitioners.
7. A survey was conducted of 36 men (with the aim of including husbands of the women already surveyed), 10 each from three village wards and 6 from the most isolated ward, about their knowledge of pregnancy, childbirth and postnatal care.
8. There is a discrepancy in numbers here because one man reported for two wives and another had a wife who had used one method for a number of years and then changed to another method.
9. Interestingly they use the term *tertib*, the root word of the New Order value *ketertiban* (orderliness).
10. Inaq Mas has held several positions. Currently she is secretary of the religious organisation, Nahdlatul Wathan, in the village.

REFERENCES

Alexander, J. (1987) *Trade, Traders and Trading in Rural Java.* Singapore: Oxford University Press.
Burchell, G., Gordon, C., Miller, P. (editors) (1991) *The Foucault Effect: Studies in Governmentality: With two lectures by and an interview with Michel Foucault.* Chicago: University of Chicago Press.

Dick, H. (1985) The rise of the middle class and the changing concept of equity in Indonesia: an interpretation. *Indonesia*, **39**, 71–92.

Djajadiningrat-Nieuwenhuis, M. (1987) Ibuism and priyayization: path to power? In *Indonesian Women in Focus, Past and Present Notions*, edited by E. Locher-Scholten and A. Niehof, pp. 43–51. Dordrecht: Foris Publications.

Finerman, R. (1984) A matter of life and death: health care change in an Andean community. *Social Science and Medicine*, **18**(4), 329–334.

Foucault, M. (1977) *Discipline and Punish*, translated by A. Sheridan. Harmondsworth: Penguin.

Foucault, M. (1978) *The History of Sexuality Volume I: An Introduction*, translated by R. Hurley. Harmondsworth: Penguin.

Hull, V. (1979) *A Woman's Place ...: Social Class Variations in Women's Work Patterns in a Javanese Village*. Yogyakarta: Gadjah Mada University. Population Institute Working Papers Series No. 3.

Hull, V. (1976) *Women in Java's Rural Middle Class: Progress or Regress?* Yogyakarta: Gadjah Mada University.

Hunter, C.L. (1995) PhD thesis (in preparation). Newcastle, NSW: University of Newcastle.

Justice, J. (1986) *Policies, Plans and People: Cultural and Health Development in Nepal*. Berkeley: University of California Press.

Kasto, M.A. (1992) Variasi Tingkat Kematian Bayi dan Harapan Hidup di Indonesia menurut Propinsi: Hasil Sensus Penduduk 1990. *Populasi*, **2**(3), 13–23.

Krulfeld, R. (1966) Fatalism in Indonesia: a comparison of socio-religious types on Lombok. *Anthropology Quarterly*, **39**(3), 180–190.

Manderson, L. (1974) *Overpopulation in Java: Problems and Reactions*. Canberra: Department of Demography, Australian National University.

Manderson, L. (1980) Right and responsibility, power and privilege: women's roles in contemporary Indonesia. In *Kartini Centenary: Indonesian Women Then and Now*, edited by A.T. Zain'ddin, K. Lucas, Y. Raharjo, C. Dobbin, L. Manderson, pp. 69–92. Melbourne: Monash University.

Morfitt, M. (1981) Pancasila: the Indonesian state ideology according to the new order government. *Asian Survey*, **21**(8), 838–851.

Nations, M., Rebhun, L. (1988) Angels with wet wings won't fly: maternal sentiment in Brazil and the image of neglect. *Culture, Medicine and Psychiatry*, **12**, 141–200.

Scheper-Hughes, N. (1992) *Death without Weeping*. Berkeley: University of California Press.

Stephens, B., Feirman, H., Wirawan, D. (1989) *Posyandu: Lessons Learned*. Washington: International Science and Technology Institute Inc.

Stoler, A. (1977) Class structure and female autonomy in rural Java. *Signs: Journal of Women's Culture and Society*, **3**(1), 74–89.

Sullivan, N. (1983) Indonesian women in development: state theory and urban kampung practice. In *Women's Work and Women's Roles*, edited by L. Manderson, pp. 147–171. Development Studies Centre Monograph No 32. Canberra: Australian National University.

Sullivan, N. (1994) *Masters and Managers: A Study of Gender Relations in Urban Java*. Women in Asia Publications Series. Sydney: Allen and Unwin for Asian Studies Association of Australia.

Suryakusuma, J. (1991) *The State and Sexuality in the Indonesian New Order*. Paper presented at the Conference on Perspectives on Gender in Indonesia: Women in Society, History and Media. Seattle: University of Washington.

van Langenberg, M. (1986) Analysing Indonesia's new order state: a keywords approach. *Rima*, **20**(2), 1–47.

van Langenberg, M. (1990) The new order state: language, ideology, hegemony. In *State and Civil Society in Indonesia*, edited by A. Budiman, pp. 121–149. Melbourne: Monash University Centre of Southeast Asian Studies.

Warren, C. (1993) *Adat and Dinas*. Kuala Lumpur: Oxford University Press.

Watson, C.W. (1987) *State and Society in Indonesia: Three Papers*, Occasional Paper No. 8. Canterbury: Centre of South-East Asian Studies, University of Kent.

White, B. (1976) Population, involution and employment in rural Java. *Development and Change*, 7, 267–290.

Williams, R. (1961) *Culture and Society 1780–1950*. Harmondsworth: Penguin.

Williams, R. (1983) *Keywords: Vocabulary of Society and Culture*. London: Flamingo.

Young, J.C. (1981) *Medical Choice in a Mexican Village*. New Brunswick NY: Rutgers University Press.

CHAPTER 9

Tso Yueh-Tzu (Sitting the Month) in Contemporary Taiwan

Cordia Chu

Chinese regard the month after birth as the most vulnerable period in a woman's life. It is a period during which she must take proper care of herself or she will suffer long term health consequences such as arthritis, backache, asthma and anaemia. It is the whole family's responsibility to take proper care of her, to provide her with special food, and to relieve her of household duties. Older women such as mothers and mothers-in-law often take it upon themselves to instruct and to assist women in confinement to take proper care, teaching them a set of postpartum behavioural and dietary rules to protect themselves. This observance of proper conduct and confinement during the month after childbirth is termed *tso yueh-tzu*, "sitting the month".

In contemporary Taiwan, the majority of women still observe the traditional form of *tso yueh-tzu* (Chu, 1988). However, due to rapid social change, and particularly decreased support for the new mother and a more hurried lifestyle, *tso yueh-tzu* is harder to observe. In response, beginning in the 1980s, a private postnatal care enterprise emerged, the *tso yueh-tzu chung-hsin*, "Sitting the Month Centre", which combines modern medical facilities similar to those of a hospital or convalescent home, with those of a hotel. Though a modern institution, a closer look at the nature of the services provided reveals that traditional puerperal practices are alive and well. It is indeed old wine in a new bottle, the traditional *tso yueh-tzu* in a modern package. The original "Sitting the Month Centre" (SMC) has grown in popularity, and many such centres have now been established in the major cities in Taiwan.

THE TRADITION OF *TSO YUEH-TZU* AND CHINESE HEALTH BELIEFS

In Chinese culture, women following childbirth are considered to be in a weakened and vulnerable condition, needing to take special care for at least a month to regain their health (Ahern, 1975; Topley, 1976; Pillsbury, 1982). These perceptions and health care measures are to an important extent derived from Chinese medical theories, in particular beliefs about illness causation and prevention. In Taiwan and in most other Chinese communities today, Western and Chinese medicine co-exist, and in dealing with reproductive health problems, women often resort to both, simultaneously or consecutively. For childbirth, Western style hospital delivery has become the norm. However, the Chinese style of postnatal care is preferred.

This paper, based on ethnographic data collected from several field trips between 1982 to 1992, examines *tso yueh-tzu* in contemporary Taiwan. I first explain the traditional concept of *tso yueh-tzu*, to show how puerperal behavioural and dietary rules are derived from Chinese beliefs about health and illness causation. I then describe the observance of *tso yueh-tzu* in rapidly changing Taiwan. Finally, I will describe the nature of the newly emerged postnatal care centres, the SMC, in Taiwan, and analyse how they provide essential services for women to observe *tso yueh-tzu* in a modernised consumer-oriented setting.

BELIEFS ABOUT ILLNESS CAUSATION

Chinese medicine is often classified by researchers in dichotomies such as secular: sacred, classical/professional: magical/religious (Ahern, 1975; Lee, 1980), or classical: popular (Sivin, 1975). The classical or secular tradition refers to medicine based on traditional cosmological theories, of which the primary ones are the balances between the *yin* and the *yang* forces of the universe, the interplay among five elements, and the great interdependence between the Macrocosm and the Microcosm. Sacred or popular medicine, on the other hand, is based on "the belief in supernatural determination of illness and in the application of magical or religious rituals to the treatment of diseases" (Lee, 1980:345–346). Both traditions influence a lay person's health beliefs and behaviour.

The measures a woman takes during the postpartum month to avoid illness are shaped by what she considers causes illness and her vulnerability to it after birth. Explanations of illness causation given by women fall into four categories. The first, most commonly reported, is *shenti neipu ssut'iao*, irregularity or disharmony inside the body, or imbalanced bodily functions. The second most commonly reported is the germ theory (*hsi-chun kan-jan*). Third most common, and mentioned by fewer than one-fifth of informants in a study conducted in 1988 (Chu, 1993), is supernatural causes. These included an offended god, soul loss due to fright (mainly in young children), coming into contact with unclean things or a ghost, becoming possessed by a malevolent spirit, and bad fate due to the wrongdoings of an ancestor. Least commonly reported are magical causes stemming from the universally found principles of homoeopathic and contagious magic. For example, if a pregnant woman watches a puppet show, this may cause the foetus to develop weak or deformed limbs (homeopathic magic, like-cause-like principles); the afterbirth should be buried deeply underground so it is not eaten by an animal, thereby to ensure safety of the child (contagious magic, things which have once been in contact continue ever afterwards to act upon each other) (for details, see Chu, 1993:44–57).

These four causes are not mutually exclusive, and informants sometimes identified more than one cause for the same illness and consequently took more than one type of treatment for the same set of symptoms. It is also common for informants to identify different causes for different stages of a malady, or to change the diagnosis and the purported cause if a particular treatment proves ineffective. I will illustrate this by reporting one informant's explanation of postnatal ill health:

> I went into labour three weeks prematurely and that was because I "let" my husband have relations (sex) with me in the last month of pregnancy and offended away the foetus god. That's why I had a really long and difficult birth this last time and lost a lot of blood and energy. Thus, after the birth, I became very weak, and had little resistance to germs. As a result, I became very ill with fever from an infection immediately after birth, and I was quite ill and weak for a long time.

For treatment, she first took an antibiotic given by a western trained doctor to "kill" the germs. Then, after leaving hospital, she visited a traditional Chinese doctor for a herbal prescription to restore her bodily balance. Meanwhile, she ate a lot of liver, sesame oil chicken, and pork spare rib soup to *pu* (replenish) blood and energy. When she became "clean" (*kan-ching*), no longer bleeding and having completed her month of confinement, she went to a temple to offer incense to the gods to ask for forgiveness as well as for their future protection.[2] She believed that it was only after she had carried out all these proper activities that she had recovered her health (Chu, 1993:45–46).

Postnatal practices primarily derive from the first order of causes, beliefs that illness results from an imbalance in the body. This is clearly the most influential and relevant of the four in shaping a woman's health-seeking behaviour on a day-to-day basis during her reproductive life. In analysing this group of beliefs, I will emphasise diet, because food therapy was the most common form of self-care reported by informants.

ILLNESS RESULTING FROM AN IMBALANCE OF THE BODY

These beliefs are based on the view that when one's bodily functions are in order, one is in good health, but when something upsets or alters this state of balance, one becomes ill. Different health systems may have different terminologies and frameworks to describe this imbalance, but whether it is regarded as an imbalance of internal humours, of *yin* and *yang*, or of the three primary "fluids" wind (*feng*), gall (*t'an*), and mucus (*tan*), it is usually believed that one or more of five factors cause the problem. These are diet, physical activity, environment, climatic changes, and emotions. The common responses by many informants when asked why people became sick were: eating the wrong (e.g. unhygienic or inappropriate) food, or eating too much or too little of a certain kind of food; being subject to too much stress or emotional strain; exposure to environmental pollution; experiencing too sudden changes in weather or extremes in temperature; becoming run down from excessive physical exertion and not having enough rest; and doing too much or too little exercise. The common theme of all these responses is that illness occurs when various external factors cause an imbalance within the body.

People in many cultures believe that a balanced diet is very important to good health. But what is considered a balanced diet varies a great deal between and within different societies. There are also many theories and rules regarding food consumption and avoidance to achieve a balanced diet. However, they generally follow one of two alternatives: theories based on the components of food, and theories based on the "nature" of food. The difference between the two is well explained by Garfield (1979:430):

> At the base of this conflict is a difference in world views expressed by the medical systems. Western medicine reduces physical factors to their smallest parts in order to cause a predicted change through altering one or another component. Oriental medicine approaches the organism as a whole and, through a complex intuitive system of analysis, attempts to reassert a better balance.

The former approach tends to classify food in terms of its components such as vitamins, carbohydrates, protein, fibre, and fat. The latter classifies each item of food as a whole and in terms of its nature such as hot and cold, wet and dry, cleansing and poisonous. Modern Chinese women use a dual system, classifying food both in the Western way according to food components and the Chinese way according to the holistic nature of food based on the *yin-yang* principle. It is useful to analyse these two approaches as manifested in dietary practices.

THE COMPONENT APPROACH TO DIETARY PRACTICES

Dietary practices based on Western nutritional concepts of food components are commonly found in contemporary Taiwan and fit comfortably with Chinese medical emphasis on the importance of diet. Foods are classified by their chemical components such as vitamins, protein, water, carbohydrate, fat, fibre, iron, calcium, salt, sugar, and calories. Informants report the belief that the human body needs a certain amount of each of the above components to maintain balance and ensure normal growth. Eating too much or too little of a certain component will cause an imbalance within the body and hence health problems. Current trends regarding a balanced diet, reported by more highly educated Taiwanese women, is to consume adequate protein, restrict the intake of fat, salt, sugar and carbohydrates, and increase the intake of various vitamins and minerals.

Puerperal dietary practices based on the food component theory, commonly reported by informants, were to increase the intake of spare rib soup (calcium), liver (iron), and fresh fruits and vegetables (vitamin C and fibre). Many who breastfed their babies reported drinking more fluid and boiled milk to replenish fluid lost from making milk, and to produce more nutritious milk for the baby. Among informants, especially those from the middle classes, dietary practices tended to follow principles from both the Western component approach, and the Chinese holistic approach. For example, those who consumed more milk to increase protein and calcium also boiled the milk first to decrease the "coldness" of its nature. In order to understand the

Chinese holistic approach to dietary practices, however, it is necessary first to explain its fundamental principle, the *yin-yang* dichotomy.

The Holistic Approach and the *Yin-yang* Principle

Yin and *yang* are the most fundamental concepts in Chinese thought. The *yin-yang* dichotomy was developed in China as early as the sixth century B.C. (Needham, 1970:342). It is regarded as the basis of the entire universe and everything in creation, also as the root and cause of life and death. The terms *yin* and *yang* first appeared in the Hsi-tz'u appendix to the *I Ching*. *Yin* refers to the northern side of a hill, which is to the rear and the more shadowed side. *Yang* refers to the southern side, which receives more sunlight. The two terms have since developed into a very broad set of meanings and can be related both concretely and abstractly to many aspects of Chinese life. *Yin* and *yang* stand respectively for earth and heaven, moon and sun, water and fire, female and male, cold and hot, private and public, and inside and outside. They are two component parts of the universe which are in constant opposition and at the same time complementary to each other, and together they make up the whole. As long as *yin* and *yang* are balanced, the universe is in order.

The *yin-yang* analogy also applies to the human body. The entire Chinese medical system is based on the assumption that the human body is like a small universe and its structure and functions are governed by the *yin* and *yang* principles as well. In Chinese medical texts, from the classics such as the *Huang Ti Nei Ching* (The Yellow Emperor's Internal Classic) and *Shang-han Lun* (Treatise on Cold Disorders), to modern ones such as the *Chung I Chen Liao* (The Diagnosis and Treatments of Chinese Medicine) from Taiwan (Yang, 1964) and the *Hsin-pien Chung I Hsueh Kai-Yao* (The New Edition of the Study of Chinese Medicine) (Kwang-chou Pu-tui Ho-Ch'in Wei-sheng-po Tsu, 1972) from China, the *yin-yang* principle is always described as the theoretical foundation of Chinese medicine and as a major tool for classifying medical or health phenomena.

The general consensus is that in the human body, the upper part is *yang* and the lower part *yin*; the outside is *yang*, the inside is *yin*; the back is *yang*, and front is *yin*; the *fu* (large intestine, stomach, small intestine, urinary bladder, gall bladder) are *yang* organs, and the *tsang* (lungs, spleen, heart, kidneys, liver) *yin* organs; *ch'i* is *yang*, and blood is *yin* (Yang, 1964:5). If *yin* and *yang* are in balance, one will be in good health; but if the energy is displaced in either direction one becomes ill. If *yin* dominates *yang*, one may feel cold, weak, pale, lacking in spirit and energy; one may break out in a cold sweat or suffer from dizziness. If *yang* is overly strong, one may feel hot or feverish, thirsty, restless, or quick-tempered, and one may suffer from a sore throat or insomnia (Yang, 1964:3–4).

The theory of the relationship between health and *yin-yang* balance is well-known among the general Chinese population. In order to maintain health, the Chinese pay attention to *yin* and *yang* symptoms which occur in their bodies and take measures to counter any imbalance. However, lay people who are not acquainted with the formal philosophical terms from classical literature, often call the symptoms of *yin* over *yang* "cold" and *yang* over *yin* "hot".

This "hot" and "cold" dichotomy also applies to food and herbs classification. Food therapy according to the hot-cold balance principle is widely spread among Chinese communities (Wu, 1979; Topley, 1976; Anderson and Anderson, 1975; Koo, 1976). When Chinese complain that they are too "hot", they often take medicine or food of a "cold" nature in order to balance this condition (see further below). Conversely, when they feel too "cold", they may take in "hot-natured" foods or medicine. There are many other concepts which go hand in hand with the hot and cold dichotomy such as dry and wet, clean and dirty, stimulating and calming, acidic and alkaline, and spicy and plain. Each of these dichotomies is associated with certain bodily reactions, symptoms, or functions.

THE *YIN-YANG* PRINCIPLE AND THE POSTNATAL PERIOD

The *yin-yang* principle is the basis of the Chinese classification of food and self-care behaviour. Therefore, in order to understand Chinese puerperal practices, it is necessary first to explain the relationship between the principles and the nature of the postnatal period.

Female and blood are both identified as *yin*. Menstrual blood, *yueh shui* (monthly water), is associated with the moon and the tides, both *yin* (Li, n.d.:25). Therefore, during her menstrual periods and even more so postpartum, a woman has a very strong *yin* influence flowing in her body. She is believed to be in a state of extreme imbalance toward *yin* and thus in a weakened condition. Being vulnerable, the last thing she should do is to add more *yin* into her body. The most commonly related taboo in avoiding *yin* is to avoid coldness, both in terms of temperature and food-nature, because adding coldness will cause abnormalities in the menstrual cycle.

During the postnatal month, a woman should avoid coming into contact with *leng* (cold in temperature): she should not bathe, swim, wash her hair, feet, or face, or work in cold water, nor should she drink or eat food that is cold in temperature such as ice or refrigerated drinks and fruits. This is based on the theory of *hsueh han tse yin* (cold blood freezes). If a woman comes in contact with coldness or eats things cold in temperature during her postpartum period, her circulation system, especially the blood flow, will be impaired and she will suffer cramps; her periods may also stop (Tang, 1935:122).

Foods that are *liang-hsing* or *han-hsing* (cold in nature), on the other hand, are believed to cause the opposite kind of abnormality in the menstrual cycle and thus should also be avoided by menstruating and particularly puerperal women. This is based on the belief that eating cold-natured food adds to the *yin* essence in the body and thus increases the *yin* flow. For a menstruating woman, this means a very heavy period which will weaken her as a result of losing too much blood. One informant even used the term *hsi-ssu jen* (wash a person to death) to describe the seriousness of such a problem. There are many foods cold in nature that informants said should be avoided during menstruation: bitter melon, fragrant melon, water melon, pears, horseradish, cabbage, mustard green, cucumber, pineapple, seaweed, mung beans, crab, unboiled well water, coconut juice, and sugar cane juice are just a few.

Besides avoiding *yin*-natured food, a woman during confinement needs to be concerned with *pu-shen pu-hsueh* (strengthening her body and replenishing her blood) by eating special foods and taking particular tonics. Based on the *yin-yang* balance principle, postpartum women thus increase their *yang* intake in order to restore bodily balance and regain health. Thus, herbs and food eaten during *tso yueh-tzu* are mainly of a *yang* nature such as meat and warming-natured herbs. Most of them — *tang-kuei*, chicken, *yi-mu ts'ao*, red dates (jujubes), sesame oil chicken, pork liver, pig knuckled stew with red vinegar with "red" sugar, and the special herbal prescription *shen-hua tang* ("birth and dissolve" soup) — are taken to dissolve blood clots, replenish blood and energy, and provide warmth. The herb *tang-kuei (Ligusticum acutilobum)* in particular is well known in Chinese medicine for its effects as a uterine stimulant, in breaking blood clots and stimulating the production of new blood. It is an essential ingredient in most herbal prescriptions for any blood-related illnesses (Koo, 1976:227).

Aside from dietary measures, to recover energy lost during childbirth and to prevent further fatigue, a woman must secure complete rest. During confinement, she should stay in bed most of the time, wear warm and long sleeved clothing, and avoid any physical exertion, including all household duties. Thus, for the entire month, the new mother is relieved of most work duties so she can recuperate.

Other than for health protection, the treatment a woman receives during *tso yueh-tzu* is also a form of reward and recognition for her reproductive contribution. Most informants reported that during the puerperium they received more attention from their family and were pampered and well-treated. Those who had given birth to a son felt especially proud and relieved that they had fulfilled their duty, "giving" their husband's family someone to continue the *hsiang-huo* (incense burning), an heir and descendant to continue the family line and provide for the elderly and the ancestors.

Thus, the puerperium is a time to relax, to enjoy special treatment and attention, and most importantly to recuperate and become healthy. A puerperal woman is expected to look better than usual. She is expected to have gained some weight and thus look more *feng-man* (rounded and full), and to have a better and healthier complexion after all the special and nourishing food she has had. Because she has stayed indoors for a long time away from the sun, her skin often becomes fairer, a sign of beauty in Chinese cultures.

It needs to be mentioned that *tso yueh-tzu* practices are not just for the protection of women. The extreme *yin* nature of the postpartum period also means that puerperal women have to observe many behavioural taboos to protect others. This is because menstrual blood, an extremely *yin* essence, is considered polluting (Ahern, 1975; Chu, 1980). During the puerperium, a woman is regarded as even more polluting than during menstrual periods because of the heavier and longer period of bleeding. There are folk beliefs about specific serious diseases contracted by men from women during the puerperium (Topley, 1970:426). The shame and fear surrounding menstruation carry into the puerperium, and the same behavioural restrictions also apply to this period to prevent women from contaminating others. Puerperal women are not allowed to engage in sexual intercourse, enter a temple, participate in religious or celebrative ceremonies (weddings, funerals, house warmings, etc.), or even to visit other households. However, since the woman has to be confined for a whole month for health reasons anyway, such taboos do not add extra inconvenience. During the puerperium, even though a woman feels embarrassed about her unclean state, the pride and sense of achievement resulting from giving birth and the positive treatment from others usually outweighs any unpleasantness and makes this period a rewarding one.

In short, *tso yueh-tzu* is a traditional set of tightly integrated rules and practices deeply embedded in Chinese culture. The general principles reported by my informants for the puerperium, especially those related to dietary rules, are very similar to those generally held among women in Taiwan, and among Chinese women in Malaysia (Dunn, 1975:311–313), in the United States (Koo, 1976:226–230; Pillsbury, 1982:142–143), and in Hong Kong (Anderson and Anderson, 1975; Topley, 1976); they are also similar to rules I observed growing up in Hong Kong (cf. Hmong women in Symonds, Cambodian women in Townsend and Rice, and Indonesian women in Grace, this volume).

SOCIAL CHANGE AND *TSO YUEH-TZU* IN TAIWAN

Taiwan is noted internationally as an economic miracle because of its rapid transformation from an agriculture society in the 1950s to a strong industrialised economy by the 1980s. Industry as a percentage of GNP rose from 18.0% in 1952 to 46.2% in 1988, and production workers from 20 to 40% of the total labour force from the early 1950s to the 1980s, at which time only 18% were engaged in farming activities (Tien, 1992:35–36). Massive migration from rural to urban areas has also occurred, and opportunities for women to participate in the labour force increased greatly.

Equally notable are the accompanying dramatic and profound social changes and material improvements which made Taiwan in the 1980s a very different place from what it was two or three decades before (Simon and Kau, c.1992:xxi). It has become an affluent, materialistic, fast-paced and consumer-oriented society. In this context, postnatal care centres emerged as an innovative health enterprise.

Between 1978 when I first investigated reproductive beliefs in Taiwan, and 1988 when I concluded follow-up research, I found some differences in *tso yueh-tze* practices, but much remained the same. However, while over 95% of the 300 women surveyed in 1978 observed fully and strictly the traditional *tso yueh-tze*, only two-thirds of those surveyed in 1988 did so.

In a health information needs assessment survey I conducted on behalf of *WOMAN-ABC* (a women's magazine) in 1988 among 200 randomly selected readers (153 returned the questionnaire), data on puerperium practices were also collected.

The majority (87%) reported that they rested a lot; 69% refrained from sex for at least a month; 68% avoided wind (e.g. stopped using a fan, stayed away from windy places); 58% avoided baths (though they regarded warm showers as permissible); 57% avoided touching cold water; 45% avoided washing their hair; 40% refrained from going out; 36% did not lift heavy objects.

Many food restrictions were reported, the most widely reported was avoidance of cold natured food (43%) and "stimulating" food such as chilly or spicy food (16%). In relation to food intake, 35% mentioned consuming traditional herbs such as *shen hua* soup, a "birth-dissolve" soup (an herb mixture especially for women after birth to replenish their blood and to dissolve blood clots); *si-wu* soup, a soup with "four herbs"; *chung-chiang*, a special replenishing herbal soup; and *shih-chuan ta-pu* (ten complete replenishing herbs). Twenty-seven percent ate more vegetables, 23% consumed more fruit, 19% ate more liver and kidney, and 15% ate more fish. Sesame oil chicken, consumed by 90% of puerperal women surveyed in 1978, on the other hand, had decreased in popularity; only 19% of the 153 respondents reporting consuming this, the rest avoided it because they thought it was too fattening (Chu, 1988:118).

What emerged as an alternative to the traditional *tso yueh-tze* at home was the use of the Sitting the Month Center (SMC), mentioned by three respondents. By 1990 when I revisited Taiwan to conduct research for a cross-cultural study of postnatal depression, there were many different kinds of SMC established in Taipei, ranging from modest to expensive, and from those of a traditional Chinese-style managed by midwives, to those of a modern Western-style run by Western trained obstetricians. Subsequently, I visited and observed the operation of six SMCs and interviewed three women from each centre.

THE EMERGENCE OF SMC

A Sitting the Month Centre was first publicly reported by the *Chung Kuo Shi Pao* (China Times) on 26 November 1982, in an article entitled "Leaving home to take a holiday during *tso yueh-tzu*". According to the article, a marketing survey conducted by the founders of the SMC in major maternity hospitals found that 30% of puerperal women were interested in the concept of a postnatal care centre, and regarded it as both useful and needed in modern society. A new commercial health care business thus emerged to answer the needs of new mothers for postnatal care. The first established was reported to be *Yueh-Tze Tiao Li Chung-Hsin* (Postnatal Month Care Management Centre) run by Mrs Chen Chiang Tsai-yun (56 years old), who had twenty years of nursing experience.[3]

The first SMC began with an intake of four women. Within two years, many similar establishments and commercial SMC chains had sprung up in different districts, varying in cost and in the services provided. Their rapid growth in contemporary Taiwan was due mainly to the changing roles of women as consumers and carers in a rapidly industrialising country, and the desire to observe *tso yueh-tze* in an increasingly fast-pace consumer-oriented society.

As more women became gainfully employed, they also became consumers. The cost for staying a month in the first reported SMC was NT$30,000 (US$1 = NT$40), approximately a month's income of an upper middle-class family in Taiwan at that time. The later establishments varied greatly in their charges. Among the six centres I visited in 1990, charges varied for a single-room, double-room and three to four people shared accommodation, ranging from over NT$1,000 for a single room per day to as little as NT$300 per day for a room shared by four people. The informants I interviewed, one from each class of accommodation, revealed that the cost of staying a month at the SMC was the equivalent of a month of their salary. All except two regarded the cost as reasonable and affordable.

When women were asked why they chose to use the SMC, responses included "I have no one to help me", "much more convenient for everybody concerned", "more comfort and fewer restrictions", "no need to dirty the house", "don't want my mother-in-law around that much", "can truly rest", "affordable", "better care for the baby", "more hygienic and scientific", and "don't know how to prepare the traditional food which the centre can provide". The major reason, however, was the lack of support due largely to the changing roles of women who traditionally provided the care. Many informants reported either that they did not have family nearby to assist them or that they did not want to trouble their relatives, mainly the mother-in-law or the mother. The former were mostly recent migrants from rural areas, the latter tended to be women with mothers-in-law or mothers in the paid work force. One of the informants explained that her mother-in-law was very busy with her own business and had no time or interest in performing the traditional duties of caring for her daughter-in-law during the postpartum month. In some cases, the generation gap appeared to be the reason for not choosing family support. One informant, for example, commented that her mother-in-law "was very conservative and old-fashioned", and that she did not want to be told what to do. Another informant said that she did not get along with her own mother and that her husband's mother was in Mainland China. An obstetrician mentioned that she was very glad to stay at an SMC, because she would have clashed with her mother and her mother-in-law about proper puerperium practices.

Traditionally, apart from her relatives, women could also obtain postnatal care support from a hired servant. Servants decreased in availability as employment opportunities increased in industry. Up to the 1970s, it was common for women from poor families, especially in rural areas, to work as maids in middle-class families. Thus, middle class women were able to rely on maids to help with *tso yueh-tzu* and even those who did not regularly employ a maid could hire someone to perform household duties for the month. Wealthier families in times past could even hire, at greater expense than a regular maid, a *Pei-Yueh* (accompany the month), a nurse-maid specialising in providing the traditional Chinese postpartum care for one month. However, with the increased opportunities for factory work, there are now very few full-time maids available. The *Pei-Yueh*, as an occupational group, has simply disappeared in contemporary Taiwan.

The second common reason why informants chose the SMC was the time and labour saving "convenience factor". As one informant put it, "I could not be bothered with shopping for, let alone cooking all those special foods. Here, you have people cleaning up after you, serving you proper meals in bed, and taking care of the baby in the middle of night when you don't want to get up". Another commented, "I don't want my family to go through so much trouble for me. They are very busy people. This way everybody is happy".

Another important factor was the consumer-oriented service provided by the SMC. In order to compete in the market place, the SMC regarded as important the provision of services to the satisfaction of customers. One informant described this very well: "Here, you are treated very well because you are the boss. Unlike staying in the hospital, where they sometimes treat you as if you are a bother to them. You never get what you want when you want it". A nurse said that many of her colleagues preferred to work at a SMC rather than in a hospital because SMCs have a happy atmosphere, few complications, and most importantly, staff received a higher salary and were given *hung-pao* (red envelope containing money) by every patient whom they served.

OLD WINE IN NEW BOTTLES: THE NATURE OF SERVICES PROVIDED BY SMC IN TAIWAN

SMC often appeared to be a modern approach to postnatal care. This was depicted by the slogan in the brochure of two of the largest SMC chains, "Birthing is not illness, [puerperal women] should have a rich and enjoyable life" and "Nourishment and rest, infant care, beauty improvement, talent and artistic learning [e.g. flower arrangement, painting classes], and fitness — *tso yueh-tzu* is like taking a holiday". Indeed there are many services provided by the SMC which a traditional *tso yueh-tzu* at home would not offer. Features advertised by a large SMC included such services as twenty-four hour medical care by doctors and nurses available for both infant and mother, infant care and health education classes for new mothers, facilities and instructions for postnatal fitness exercise, and even recreational facilities. Although the smaller SMCs did not offer such a variety of services, they still provided the most vital services such as twenty-four hour infant care, five meals per day and laundry.

A closer examination of the nature of SMC reveals that underneath the modernised package, the concept is not new at all. Its very creation is rooted in the traditional notion that women needed special care for a month after childbirth to protect their health. This is reflected very well by the slogans listed side by side with the above mentioned slogan on the brochures: "Sitting the month is a Chinese medical specialty" and "Sitting the month well, trouble-free throughout life".

The advice given to women during *tso yueh-tzu* often combines traditional Chinese and Western modern health beliefs. This is reflected in the following instructions listed in the brochure of the two SMCs mentioned earlier:

- rest completely and avoid physical exertion, otherwise backache will result
- be happy; avoid getting upset, angry, or depressed
- keep warm; be careful not to catch cold
- do not use medicinal herbs inappropriately, there should be a balanced intake of replenishing food and herbs; a low-salt diet is important

The daily routine care follows traditional practices even more closely: complete bed rest and the observance of a low-salt special diet which includes replenishing and warming remedies such as *shen-hua* soup and *tang-kuei*. The menu alters from day to day, and details of the five meals provided by the SMC are displayed on a poster board. Special dietary requirements of individuals (e.g. vegetarian, diabetics) are also written on the poster board to remind catering staff. The following is an example of a standard menu of the five meals provided by one of the SMCs:

- Breakfast: milk, bread and sausage or rice congee boiled in meat
- Mid-morning: sparerib soup
- Lunch: three dishes (two meat and a vegetable) and a soup
- Afternoon: pig knuckle and *tang-kuei* soup
- Dinner: three dishes and a soup

In addition, *Sheng-hua* soup would be served in between meals as a hot drink. Other services include laundry, and provision of sanitary napkins, infant diapers, and milk powder for the baby (often provided by a baby formula company).

There is a range of accommodation and services available in different SMCs. The small and less expensive SMCs (six to ten beds) look like small hospitals with plain furniture, and the atmosphere tends to be more casual, homelike, friendly and welcoming. The larger, more expensive SMCs look like hotels, with tasteful interior design and air-conditioned suites. Their services (at the user's cost) even included a limousine to pick up patrons and deliver them home, facial massage, beauty service, postnatal exercise instruction, a recreational room, and television and videos.

Although it is called "Sitting the Month Center", there is flexibility with regard to the length of stay for women and their infants. Women can choose to stay for the entire month or for only a couple weeks. Indeed, some stay for ten days only. On the other hand, if a woman has to return to work immediately after one month of postnatal leave, she may even leave the baby behind for a few months or until she finds satisfactory infant care.

Tso yueh-tzu is a long established traditional practice of Chinese culture. It aims both to reward and protect the health of women with new-born babies. Puerperal behavioural and dietary rules are derived from the traditional Chinese health beliefs which are deeply integrated into all aspects of Chinese culture. In contemporary Taiwan, most puerperal women still believe in the importance of and thus observe the tradition of *tso yueh-tzu*. While the majority can still rely on their family and social network to provide postnatal care, some need help in order to observe *tso yueh-tzu* properly and the SMC provides a much needed service.

Rapid industrialisation and economic growth in Taiwan have brought about profound social changes in lifestyle and in women's roles as consumers and carers. While there are still strong beliefs by postpartum women about the importance of *tso yueh-tzu* for their health, the time-consuming nature of and the decreased family support for traditional practices means that proper observance of *tso yueh-tzu* is becoming harder to achieve for some women. The Sitting the Month Centre, combining both traditional and modern concepts of postnatal care, is an innovative alternative health service in response to consumer needs in a rapidly changing society.

ENDNOTES

1. Data for this paper came from three different studies: (1) a quantitative and qualitative study of 300 Chinese and 300 Australian women on their reproductive beliefs and practices from 1977–1985 (Chu, 1993); (2) a mailed questionnaire survey among two hundred randomly selected readers of a popular Taiwanese magazine, *Family and Women* on the health status of career women in 1988 (Chu, 1988), and (3) a qualitative study of 30 puerperal women and 30 Australian women on "A Cross-Cultural Analyses of Postnatal Depression and Postnatal Health Care" from 1989–1992 (Chu, unpublished fieldnotes).

2. In Chinese folk religion, one often worships different gods for different purposes, e.g. *Kwang Kung* (a legendary heroic figure in the Three Kingdoms period who is wellknown for his loyal and just character and leadership skills) for good business, *Tu-ti Kung* (local earth gods) for household safety, *Chu-sheng niang-niang* (the birth goddess) for early conception of a son, and *Kuan-yin* for peace, health, safety and general well-being. This informant, however, worships *Tien-hou* (the Empress of Heaven) regularly for all purposes.

3. While the *Yueh-tze tiao li chung-hsi* was reported to be the first commercial enterprise by the *Chinese Times*, it was not necessarily the first to offer fee-paying postnatal care services. There have been postnatal care services provided by others informally, e.g. traditional midwives or small obstetric hospitals occasionally allowing a patient to extend her post-delivery stay because of lack of family support and care.

REFERENCES

Ahern, E.M. (1975) Sacred and secular medicine in a Taiwan village: a study of cosmological disorders. In *Medicine in Chinese Cultures: Comparative Studies of Health Care in Chinese and Other Societies*, edited by A. Kleinman, P. Kunstadter, E.R. Alexander and J.L. Gale, pp. 91–113. Washington DC: US Department of Health, Education and Welfare.

Anderson, E.N., Anderson, M.E. (1975) Folk dietetics in two Chinese communities, and its implications for the study of Chinese medicine. In *Medicine in Chinese Cultures: Comparative Studies of Health Care in Chinese and Other Societies*, edited by A. Kleinman, P. Kunstadter, E.R. Alexander and J.L. Gale, pp. 143–175. Washington DC: US Department of Health, Education and Welfare.

Chu, C. (1980) Menstrual beliefs and practices of Chinese women. *Journal of Folklore Institute*, **XVII**, 1, 38–55.

Chu, C. (1988) Shuan Shen Yeh Te Chi Yueh Fu Lu Men Chien Kang Ma? [Health status of career women in Taiwan — a preliminary survey]. *Chia-Ti Yu Fu Lu [Family and Women]*, **62**, 112–118.

Chu, C. (1993) *Reproductive Beliefs and Practices of Chinese and Australian Women.* Monograph No 5. Taiwan Women's Research Program Publication Series. Taipei: Population Studies Centre, National Taiwan University.

Dunn, F. (1975) Medical care in the Chinese communities of Peninsular Malaysia. In *Medicine in Chinese Cultures: Comparative Studies of Health Care in Chinese and Other Societies*, edited by A. Kleinman, P. Kunstadter, E.R. Alexander and J.L. Gale, pp. 297–326. Washington, DC: US Department of Health, Education and Welfare.

Garfield, R. (1979) The philosophical basis of modern Chinese medicine. *Science and Society*, **XLIII**, 4, 430–446.

Koo, L. (1976) *The Nourishment of Life: The Culture of Health in Traditional Chinese Society.* Unpublished PhD thesis. Berkeley: The University of California.

Kwang-chou Pu-tui Ho-Ch'in Wei-sheng-po Tsu, (1972) *Hsin-pien Chung I Hsueh Kai-Yao [The New Edition of the Study of Chinese Medicine].* Peking: Jen min wei shen chu pan she.

Lee, R. (1980) Perceptions and uses of Chinese medicine among the Chinese in Hong Kong. *Culture, Medicine, and Psychiatry*, **4**, 345–375.

Li, C.C. (n.d.) *Peng Ts'ao Kang Mu [Compendium of Materia Medica] [1368–1644 AD].* Ming Edition. **52**, 20–25.

Needham, J. (1970) Hygiene and preventive medicine in ancient China. In *Clerks and Craftsman in China and the West, Lectures and Addresses on the History of Science and Technology*, edited by J. Needham, pp. 340–378. Cambridge: Cambridge University Press.

Pillsbury, B. (1982) Doing the month: confinement and convalescence of Chinese women after childbirth. In *Anthropology of Human Birth*, edited by M. Kay, pp. 119–146. Philadelphia: F.A.Davis Company.

Simon, D.F., Kau, M.Y.M. (eds) (c.1992) *Taiwan: Beyond the Economic Miracle.* Armonk, New York: M.E. Sharpe.

Sivin, N. (1975) *Classical medicine and popular medicine in traditional China.* Unpublished Mimeograph. Cambridge, Mass.

Tang, C.H. (1935) *Hsueh Chen Lun.* Shanghai: Chien Chin ang Shu Chu.

Tien, H.A. (1992) Transformation of an authoritarian party state: Taiwan's development experience. In *Political Change in Taiwan*, edited by T.J. Cheng and S. Haggard, pp. 33–55. London: Lynne Rienner Publishers.

Topley, M. (1970) Chinese traditional ideas and the treatment of disease: two examples from Hong Kong. *Man*, **5**, 426.

Topley, M. (1976) Chinese traditional etiology and methods of cure in Hong Kong. In *Asian Medical Systems*, edited by C. Leslie, pp. 243–265. Berkeley: University of California Press.

Wu, D.Y.H. (1979) *Traditional concepts of food and medicine in Singapore.* Occasional Paper No 85. Singapore: Institute of Southeast Asian Studies.

Yang, T.I. (1964) *Chung I Chen Liao.* Taipei: Wen Kwan To Shu Kung Sse.

PART III:

THE WORKINGS OF THE BODY:
ISSUES OF SEXUAL HEALTH

CHAPTER 10

White Blood and Falling Wombs: Ethnogynaecology in Northeast Thailand

Andrea Whittaker

Grandmother Phai is fifty years old. She has had five pregnancies and has three surviving children, having miscarried her third pregnancy and fifth pregnancy. Last year she fell over whilst working: "It was like my *mot luuk* (uterus)[1] broke or snapped. It stung and stung and now it *ook horn* (gives out heat)" she said. Now, since the fall, she has *maat khaaw* (vaginal discharge): "If I had a lot of *maat khaaw* it is no good, that would mean I had cancer. When I take "Win" [an analgesic] then it is OK. Last year it was so bad I couldn't work either to plant rice or to harvest".

The previous year, she went to a hospital in Roi Et, the provincial capital, where she was given an internal examination and a *yaa kae akseep* (medicine to correct infection) and was told not to do heavy work. She was also given a *yaa naam* (a liquid medicine). The visit cost approximately 200 baht ($A10). After that she went to a private clinic in Roi Et where the doctor did not need to give an internal examination; instead he just put a stethoscope onto her belly and said it was *mot luuk akseep* (an infected/inflamed uterus). That cost her 95 baht.

This year, she went seven times for the treatment of her *mot luuk akseep* and *mot luuk yorn* (prolapse) at a clinic in Rong Kham and was told that her *mot luuk* is *phadong* (referring to a category of diseases causing itchiness). Each time she goes to this clinic it costs 150 baht for the medicine and 70 baht for extra medicine for her *mot luuk yorn*. She was given an injection of "Kaanoo" (tetracycline), but complains, "I am still hot inside and my vagina is hot". She has also tried a herbal medicine of bark and herbs called *sak mot luuk* (clean the uterus) for 20 baht per bundle, which she then boiled and drank. "I'm not going to take it any more as I am not better". At rice planting time she received a series of four injections from the *mor tahaan* (a former army medic) at a nearby district town for 30 baht, so that she could work.

Medical anthropology is fundamentally concerned with the nexus between the body as a physiological entity and as a social entity in relationship to other bodies/society. Scheper-Hughes and Lock (1987:7) have described three perspectives from which we may explore these relationships which they call the "three bodies". Firstly, there is the individual body, the sense of the embodied self as experienced apart from other bodies. The constituent parts of the individual body/mind/self, and the ways in which the body is experienced in health and sickness, are highly variable cross-culturally.

At this level then, medical anthropology is concerned to describe cross-cultural differences in body imagery, disease etiologies and treatments, and cultural differences in the conception of the self. The second level of analysis is that of the "social body, a natural symbol for thinking about relationships between nature, society and culture" (ibid.:6). At this level the anthropologist is concerned with the symbolic uses of the body as a metaphor of society and social relations. The third level of embodiment considered is that of the body politic, referring to the regulation and control of individual and social bodies (ibid.:8). This level of analysis is involved in elucidating the relations of power between particular social groups, or individuals and groups and the processes of socialisation, regulation and conformity to the social and political order.

Likewise, this chapter aims to explore the many levels of meaning within women's descriptions of their gynaecological health. The first part of the chapter is concerned to describe what Kendall (1987:367–376) terms "ethnogynaecology": the indigenous construction of leucorrhoea, other vaginal discharges, and problems that women experience with their uteri. Yet, as in the story of Grandmother Phai above, an examination of women's construction of illness also allows insight into the relations between micro and macro levels of explanation. She describes her conditions of *mot luuk akseep, maat khaaw* and *mot luuk yorn* in terms of humoral concepts of physiology. Yet apart from a mere description of her symptoms and treatment, her narrative also makes reference to the social costs of her condition and the relationship between her position as a peasant farmer and her illness. She explains her condition in terms of the heavy work she must undertake and is advised by the doctor "not to work too hard", advice which she would find hard to follow.

Isaan women's narratives link their reproductive health with the changing status of Isaan women and their socio-economic status. In doing so they make links between health, culture, political economy and individual experience (Singer, Davison and Gerdes, 1988:374). As in the case above, these links are most apparent in women's descriptions of the connection between poor health and the need to work hard, and the links between reproductive ability and productivity. It is this social aspect of their conditions which is explored in the second part of the paper.

The context of this chapter is the social, economic and political subordination of the body politic of Isaan people within the Thai state. The Northeast is the poorest and least developed region of Thailand, with an average per capita income one seventh that of people living in Bangkok (Sheehan, 1993:32). People of the Northeast express a collective identity based upon distinct language, cultural practices and regional history separate from Central Thai people. However, Central Thai culture is the elite culture of Thailand. The Northeast is portrayed as culturally inferior, ignorant, rural and backward, imagery which both reflects and shapes the relations of power between the body politic of Isaan and members of the dominant group and the assignment of resources (see Whittaker, 1995). The final part of the chapter describes how practices and policies operating within health settings mediate the subordinate economic and ethnic status of villagers and are reflected in the attitudes towards and treatment of Isaan women.

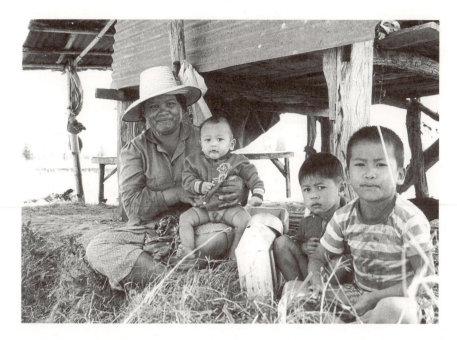

FIGURE 10.1 Grandmother Kaew cares for her grandchildren at harvest time. (Photo: A. Whittaker).

This chapter is based on eighteen months ethnographic research in Northeast Thailand in 1992–1993. Ten months of this time was spent in the remote ethnic Lao community of Baan Srisaket[2] in Roi Et Province which has 740 households and a population of 3,926 people. Research within the village included participant observation, 89 semi-structured and informal interviews with a variety of traditional healers, birth attendants and government health staff, in-depth interviews with 36 women who gave birth within the previous twelve months, and birthing and reproductive health surveys of 67 women. I conducted all interviews myself in the Isaan/Lao language, occasionally with the help of a local research assistant. In addition, two household surveys covering 156 households in the village were completed. These were supplemented by seven focus group discussions on reproductive health with women of various age groups in two other villages, along with hospital and clinic observations concentrating on gynaecological, obstetric and family planning services (see Whittaker, 1995).

BAAN SRISAKET

Baan Srisaket is located in the heartland of Central Isaan, approximately 60 kilometres from the provincial capital of Roi Et. Rice farming is the principal productive activity for the households of Baan Srisaket. The traditional strategy of farmers is to grow enough glutinous (sticky) rice to meet household consumption needs. Additional production is of non-glutinous rice and other cash crops. Rice production is limited to one crop per year due to the often inadequate and unreliable rainfall and infertile soils.

With incorporation into the Thai state, the community has undergone rapid economic and social transformation from a self-contained subsistence economy into a market-dependent capitalist economy. Changes in the mode of production, the introduction of cash crops, fertilisers, pesticides and mechanisation have been paralleled by the introduction of waged labour and an increase in levels of debt and impoverishment. Although owning their land, most farming households have largely lost control over the production process to outside agencies. In 1993, a household survey revealed that 88% of households were in debt to an average of 7525 baht/household (A$376). The average annual income from agricultural sources in 1992 was 14,617 baht/household (A$730). Most households are thus permanently locked into a cycle of debt and rely on labour migration as a strategy to supplement household income.

The villagers of Baan Srisaket are acutely aware of their subordinate position within the Thai state. There is the commonly articulated perception that the state has largely neglected the Northeast, leaving it the least developed and poorest region of the nation and excluding Isaan people from the economic growth and development that has boomed in other regions, particularly the Central Plains. The lived experience of inequality and marginality provides the background for their identification as Isaan people and for their experiences of health and illness.

ETHNOPHYSIOLOGY AND REPRODUCTIVE HEALTH

Within Baan Srisaket the human body is not conceived of as an entity separate from the community, but an embodiment of the relationships of spirits and flesh, *karma* and community. Informants differ on the details of the descriptions of the body according to their expertise or the emphasis they would place on the importance of some elements over others, but the description below draws upon the local beliefs in Baan Srisaket rather than the urban institutionalised forms of traditional Thai medicine.

The human body is said to consist of four *thaat* (elements) derived from Ayurvedic medicine, namely *din* (earth), *naam* (water), *lom* (wind) and *fai* (fire) (see Thailand, Ministry of Public Health, 1986:5 for details; see also chapters by Jirojwong and Chirawatkul, this volume). Disequilibrium of one or more of these elements will result in illness. The body itself is perceived as a cavity supported by bones, covered with skin and with a series of *sen* (channels such as blood vessels, tendons, nerves, muscles) through which circulates the *lu'at* (blood), several kinds of water including *naam khram* (waste water), and several winds such as the *lom beng* (the pushing wind) and *lom chawat* (the pulling wind). Some winds may enter the body and cause illness, particularly after childbirth; some are poisonous (*lom phit*, poison wind).[3] The fiery element of the body is considered a common cause of illness. An excess of *fai* (fire) can cause fevers; a deficiency causes a cold state and weakness. The proportions of heating and cooling properties in the diet may be manipulated to influence the overall balance of these states. Environmental and climatic conditions may also influence the balance of the body.

In addition, a range of other factors are taken into account as important causal factors in disease. Working too hard, drinking too much, thinking too much or being emotionally stressed may all contribute to ill health by either causing humoral imbalance or leaving one vulnerable to the actions of *phii* (spirits). Other physical and supernatural forces may affect the thirty-two *khwan* (souls) which are positioned in various organs of the body. These are likely to flee the body at any time and must be secured back to the body through the *suu khwan* ceremony.[4] The physical body also contains a person's store of *bun* or merit. The Buddhist concept of life as continuous cycles of suffering caused by *karma* underlies beliefs concerning the ultimate aetiologies of disease. While most health problems are believed to arise due to imbalances in the natural, supernatural or social environment, actions from a previous incarnation may have consequences in the present life. Actions to improve one's store of merit are, therefore, in effect health practices to lessen ones' experience of suffering in this life and the next, ensuring physical and spiritual well-being.

Most reproductive illnesses as described in this chapter are understood as due to humoral imbalance. Women are understood to be more vulnerable to bodily humoral imbalance because of the processes of menstruation, childbirth and more recently, the use of contraceptives which disrupt the balance between heat and coolness, wetness and dryness in the body (Irvine, 1982:259; Davis, 1984:66). These humoral imbalances also make women "weak-souled" and hence vulnerable to various spirits and mental disturbance (Irvine, 1982:264–265). Women describe a heavy regular menstrual flow of red blood as indicative of a healthy body. This ensures that the "bad" blood which builds up in a woman's body has been expelled. Such blood may move within the body and cause varied bodily and emotional states: weakness, bad moods, irritability, insanity, skin rashes, headache, "high blood pressure", dizziness, ulcers and paleness (see Chirawatkul, this volume). For this reason there are proscriptions of foods that have "cool" properties that may not be consumed during menstruation or in the postpartum period, as such foods may restrict the expulsion of the blood and cause it to rise dangerously to the head. Irregular menstruation, or variations in the colour or consistency of the blood, are signs of ill health and bodily imbalance.

The state of a woman's gynaecological health is frequently associated with the practice of *yuu gaam/yuu fai*, or the "staying by the fire" after childbirth (see descriptions in Rajadhon, 1961; Pedersen, 1968:136–149; Mougne, 1978; Irvine, 1982; Poulsen, 1983; Jirojwong, and Chirawatkul, this volume). This involves lying close to a constantly burning fire for a period that varies from five to eleven days. Food restrictions are also practised through this time. Staying by the fire cleanses the womb of the accumulated bad blood/lochia and waste fluids that have built up in the body throughout the pregnancy, and "dries" out the womb. If these fluids are not expelled, they will stay within the body and cause weakness, chills and infertility.

Many women complained that their present ill-health, weakness and gynaecological complaints were because they had not been able to stay by the fire for their last birth or because they had not stayed long enough. One woman who had an early stage cervical cancer treated commented "I don't know why I got cancer as I stayed by the fire for all of eight births".

Postpartum rituals of staying by a fire to avoid a "cold state" and consumption of "hot" medicines and foods are associated with the need to restore humoral balance and so ensure long term strength and well-being. "Hot" medicines known as *yaa saatrii* (women's medicines), or *yaa khap lu'at* (medicine to "get rid of the blood"), and manipulation of diet, are the traditional means used to restore the humoral balance of women's bodies (Manderson, 1981a; cf. Townsend and Rice for Cambodian practices, this volume).

WHITE BLOOD: DIRTY WOMBS

I was made aware of the significance of vaginal discharge to women when, upon asking a village Women's Group leader what was the most significant health problem women suffered in her village, I was informed: "*Maat khaaw*. Nearly every woman here suffers from it". *Maat khaaw* refers to leucorrhoea (a normal vaginal secretion) but in Isaan the term is also used to describe a range of abnormal discharges, and implies a state of ill health. Any vaginal discharge other than menstrual blood is read as a sign that the womb is "dirty", not dry and clean (Chirawatkul, 1993:203–205). Medical dictionaries and medical personnel translate this into English as leucorrhoea, but this strict translation is too narrow. An Isaan dictionary gives an explanation which reveals the broader significance of this term. It describes *maat khaaw* as:

> one type of disease that occurs in women. When it occurs it makes the *raduu* [menstruation] spoil. The red colour is white and is called *maat khaaw* disease, *tok khaaw*. It is said that if one boils the bark of the *luum phuuk* tree and the bark from the *muui daeng* [red hardwood] tree and bark from the *muui khaaw* [white hardwood] tree and drinks that, one will be cured (Phinthong, 1989:856, my translation).

Early in my fieldwork, I talked to a 28 year old woman concerned about her infertility. When I asked about menstruation she stated that she did menstruate, but that the colour of the discharge was white to yellow. *Maat khaaw* is understood as equivalent to menstrual blood but white in colour.

Differentiation of vaginal discharges is made by women on the basis of smell, colour, consistency and the volume of discharge:

> If the discharge has a smell it is like *naam khaaw plaa* [water with the stench of fish] and you will be itchy everywhere that the discharge touches and you will get bumps and a rash. Usually *maat khaaw* doesn't smell and it looks like *yaang bakhung* [sap from the papaya], and I get it before and after I menstruate (Aunty Thiaw).

Many women noted that if *maat khaaw* appeared just before or after menstruation it is normal and associated with the cleansing out of the womb. If *maat khaaw* appeared at any other time however, women understand it as a sign of internal problems. Some mentioned that it was a sign of the presence of *chu'arook* (germs) in the womb, associated with the dirtiness of the womb, representing the incorporation of biomedical concepts of disease causation within the indigenous concept of the need for regular cleansing of the womb. Women state that a coloured discharge indicates the presence of a sexually transmitted disease, as does excessive itchiness. Several women, including some nurses, stated that *maat khaaw* is a sign of cervical cancer, and fear of a discharge being a sign of cancer may prevent women from seeking help for symptoms, not wishing to have their fears confirmed.

Experience in health centres in many developing countries suggests that while the incidence of reproductive tract infections (RTIs) and other troublesome conditions is substantial, many women do not seek treatment from the formal health sector for these problems, or else postpone treatment until the condition is acute (Du Toit, 1988:269; Bolton, Kendall, Leontsini and Whitaker, 1989; Wasserheit and Holmes, 1992; Hull, Widyantoro and Fetters, this volume).

INFLAMED WOMBS

Another term used commonly in association with *maat khaaw* is *mot luuk akseep*, an inflamed or infected uterus:

> I have *mot luuk akseep*. I know because I get a lot of *maat khaaw* when I work hard, like when I carry bags of rice. In the past I was never like this. Sometimes the *maat khaaw* has a fishy smell when there is only a small amount, but I have had it for three weeks now. First I went to Rong Kham, to a private clinic and they had a test and gave me medicine to eat and an injection. I didn't get better so I went again and I got more medicine and another injection. Each time cost one hundred and twenty baht [approx.A$6] and ten baht for my transport.
>
> Then I went to a clinic in Roi Et [the provincial capital] and I was told that I had *mot luuk yorn* [prolapse] and then *mot luuk akseep*. I was told not to eat food which is hot or salty and not to work hard and they gave me a *yaa chut* [a packet of unmarked pills to be eaten in combination as a complete treatment and often containing antibiotics]. When my *thorng noi* [lower stomach] started hurting, I stopped taking my contraceptive pills (Aunt Bua).

As is evident in the account above, the term *mot luuk akseep* is understood in indigenous terminology to signify an inflamed/swollen uterus. The same term *akseep* is used to describe arthritic joints. Medical staff use the term *mot luuk akseep* to describe a uterine infection, implying the presence of an aetiological agent requiring treatment, not just the presence of an inflammation. It is also used in Thai medical literature in relation to acute pelvic inflammatory disease. Medical staff usually prescribe antibiotics for women complaining of *mot luuk akseep*. Villagers and untrained healers use the term to mean a swollen and inflamed uterus and associate the condition with the presence of *maat khaaw* discharge and a "hot" state, following the humoral understandings of physiology summarised earlier. Prolapsed uterus is a common gynaecological condition amongst older women in village communities and is frequently associated by women with the presence of *maat khaaw* discharge: "I get something like *maat khaaw* except that it's not the same. It's yellow and white and I have had it for two months with *mak lu'at* [blood colour] in it. Two months ago my uterus collapsed" (Grandmother Thii).

Large numbers of pregnancies and births combined with heavy work have left many older women in Baan Srisaket with prolapses. They are recognised by the local massage doctor who described to me her technique of massaging the womb and then gently pushing it into place again: "A woman nearby was pulling sacks of rice when her uterus came out. She called for me and I got her to lie down with her legs and knees raised. I massaged and compressed her and then gently pushed it back up" (Grandmother Yim). A similar technique is employed by a local midwife to massage a prolapse into its correct position.

The heavy lifting and bending when working in the fields exacerbates the problem and incapacitates women, as Grandmother Bau describes below. Women with painful prolapse speak of manually supporting their pelvis when they walk or harvest rice:

> I get *puat thorng noi* [pain in the lower pelvis] and a pulling down sensation and it pulls to my waist as if I am having a baby and as if my vagina will fall out. I have to hold onto my pelvis when I walk. When it is very bad, I have to stop working hard (Grandmother Bau).

In desperation, Grandmother Seen sought the services of a travelling doctor for help (AW indicates the author speaking, GS indicates Grandmother Seen speaking):

GS: He said he was skilled at pushing up wombs. He said he could do that. He said that if there was anyone who was like that he could push it back for them.

AW: Oh. How did he do it?

GS: He put his hand in and pushed it up into you!

AW: *Oei!*..

GS: Right up into my cunt! [laughter] Really what sort of a doctor! Then Grandfather, he came and saw him enter me.

AW: Yes.

GS: "What sort of a doctor are you!" he said. "Do you have a registration card? ...If you don't leave now you won't leave!" [laughter] "What sort of doctor?" he said. "Do you have your registration card here now?" he said like that. The doctor ran off out of the village there and then. Yeah, he ran off out of this house scared! "I am going to get the policemen to come and get you!" grandfather said."Go! Get out!" he said. [laughter] My husband was angry! [laughter] He didn't even get his money! He had said he wanted five hundred baht!

AW: Oh! That is a lot of money! Five hundred!...

GS: He was so scared he just left from this village! [laughter]

AW: You never saw him again? [laughter]

GS: He was scared we'd catch him. He never came back again.

Another common complaint of women is urinary tract infections, which may be associated with reproductive tract infections. Many women described stinging after micturition and "red" urine, and attributed it to a variety of causes:

> I get red urine and it stings when I work hard and so I buy "Kaanoo" [tetracycline] or drink boiled *nuat maew* ["cat's whiskers", a herb noted for its diuretic properties]. It stings after I pee. One time I thought it was because I was infected with some STD, or because of walking too often, or working too hard, or because of drinking dirty water. I thought that I had a kidney stone, but the doctor told me it was because I had *phae lom* [an allergy]. I stopped drinking rain water (Aunt Dorn).

Incontinence is also a problem for many older women, who may discretely squat to urinate if they cannot reach a latrine. These are problems which are rarely brought to the notice of public health authorities and remain unacknowledged aspects of women's health experiences in many countries.

TREATMENT AND PROPHYLAXIS

There exists a complex indigenous system of gynaecological knowledge and prophylactic and curative practices. A range of treatments are employed by women with these conditions.

Herbal patent formulas sold as *yaa saatrii* (women's medicine) and numerous types of "hot" medicines such as *yaa dong lau* (pickled herbal medicine taken with whiskey), proclaimed to be effective against a range of female conditions, are a common form of treatment and are readily available in village stores. Many women consume large quantities of "hot" medicines in attempts to induce late menstruation and these should be considered as indigenous forms of menstrual regulation.

Folk healers advise women with *mot luuk akseep* to restrict their diet, especially foods such as *tam mak hung* (spicy raw papaya salad), *paa daek* (fermented fish), and pickled foods, bamboo and shrimps. Other foods less commonly cited were quail and *phak khaa* (*Languas galanga*). Pickled and fermented foods appear, like "pickled medicine", to be "hot" food. Metaphorical linkages may also be operating in the banning of strong-smelling, fishy foods so that the discharge will not have such an odour. Seafood and shrimps are said to be dangerous for women with cervical cancer, and are generally recognised as foods that may be *phae* (allergenic) for people causing rashes and itching. It may be for this reason that they are restricted, given that many women complain of vaginal itching when suffering from *maat khaaw* (see also Manderson, 1981a, 1981b, 1986).

Antibiotics are also widely used in self-medication by women suffering from *maat khaaw*. Village health survey data reveals self-medication as the most usual first step in treatment of illness in Baan Srisaket (see also Abosede, 1984; Allen, Jumin and McQuistan, 1989). Women purchase penicillin and a number of different brand names of tetracycline for the symptomatic treatment of discharge, and may consume these in combination with other treatments. These medicines are widely available, sold by the tablet in village stores and pharmacies. A survey of medicines available for sale in six small general stores in Baan Srisaket in November 1992 revealed a total of 76 different brand-name medicines available, as well as numerous different patent medicines. Of these, there were seven different brand-name forms of tetracycline for sale by the tablet, as well as sulphonamides and seven addictive combination analgesics which combine aspirin, paracetamol and caffeine. Brand-names such as "Kaanoo" (500 mg tetracycline) and "Hero" (250 mgs tetracycline) were commonly cited as medicines purchased for *maat khaaw*. The "Kaanoo" packet specifically states that it is for *mot luuk akseep*, wounds, pox or abscesses, pus and any infections. On the front of the packet there is a male and female symbol, suggestive that it is useful for STDs as well. *Yaa chut*, small packets of a mixture of unmarked drugs sold as universal remedies for a variety of complaints, are freely available at local district towns and also are dispensed by the local injection doctors. They often contain potentially harmful and potent medicines. Shopkeepers of Baan Srisaket were unsure of the use of many of the drugs they sold, and some drugs were poorly labelled as to their contents, indications for use, contra-indications and expiry dates.

The widespread use of self-administered antibiotics for *maat khaaw* and *mot luuk akseep* may mask a range of serious reproductive tract infections, including STDs, and may promote the development of resistant strains.

CONTRACEPTIVE TECHNOLOGIES

New contraceptive technologies have been accepted into women's views of their bodies and they present with a range of symptoms and problems they associate with them. As Riley and Sermsri (1974) suggest, clients of family planning services bring to any service or technology a range of pre-existing understandings. The side effects described for modern contraceptives highlight lay perceptions of how these methods work in the context of popular health culture:

> In the past we didn't have the pill and so I had seven children and then after that I went and used an IUD. It was painful and I got a lot of *maat khaaw* and I smelled so strongly that I couldn't get close to other people. I got the doctor to take it out and I had another child right after it was taken out. After that child I took the pill and I got a dry throat and I didn't feel well so I stopped and then I had another child and after that child I made the decision to have a tubal ligation. That was three years ago. Since [I've had] the tubal ligation, I get really tired and can't sleep and have vision problems (Aunt Uay).

Stories of side effects and swapping contraceptives in an attempt to find one suitable to their body and lives are commonly discussed among women. Table 10.1 lists the most common side effects mentioned by village women in interviews and focus groups.

TABLE 10.1   List of common side effects attributed to contraceptives.

Contraception	Common Complaints
PILL	dry throat, tiredness, lack of appetite, skin problems, thinness, dizziness, obesity, abdominal pain, lower back pain
IUD	abdominal pain, heavy discharge, inability to work hard
INJECTABLE	headaches, thinness, weakness, amenorrhoea, dizziness and confusion, coldness, obesity, eye problems, blotchy skin
TUBAL LIGATION	lower abdominal pain, weakness, discharge, forgetfulness, waist and back pain, leg pain, change in consistency of menstruation, amenorrhoea
NORPLANT	weak tired arm, inability to work hard, implant moves through body

Images of gynaecological well-being and problems with contraceptives may have an impact upon family planning programs (Scott, 1978:85). While women may experience side effects that are not considered serious medical conditions, the experiences and side effects attributed to different contraceptives are important because they contribute to discontinuation of contraceptives and switching to less effective methods (Stephen and Chamratrithirong, n.d.:2; see also Suvipakit, n.d.; Charoenchai and Thongkrajai, 1985).

Many of the side effects described by women are culturally specific, referring to humoral concepts of wetness and dryness, heat and cold. But they also reflect understandings of the links between fertility, regular menstruation and vitality. A fertile body is a strong, active, productive body. Modern methods of contraception are understood to disrupt the bodily balance leading to a range of complaints, the most common of which is a loss of vitality and an inability to work hard. In this way, women make explicit links between reproduction and production.

Despite the controversy surrounding the use of Depo Provera in some countries,[5] women in Baan Srisaket appreciate the convenience of injectable contraceptives as there "is no need to remember to take a pill every day". In addition, injections are valued highly in the local culture (Reeler, 1990). Yet injectable contraceptives are frequently associated with side effects (see also Stephen and Chamratrithirong, n.d.). Injections of Depo Provera are said to "make the womb *hiaw* (dry) so you are infertile". Injectables are associated with tired arms, amenorrhoea, thinness, weakness and chills, as the "bad" blood which is normally expelled through menstruation has been absorbed by the body causing a cold state: "After I had the injections [Depo Provera] I never menstruated, I was thin and cold and I had to take warm water baths, whereas in the past I could always use only cold water [to bathe]" (Aunt Naam). The effect of the injectable is likened to menopause. Post-menopausal women also complain of weakness and inability to work hard as a consequence of their lack of menstruation, the build-up of bad blood and infertility (Chirawatkul, 1993). Contraceptives which disrupt the menstrual cycle of women or cause amenorrhoea, such as Depo Provera injections or the contraceptive pill, are disliked because "bad blood" accumulates in the body causing ill health and weakness. Similarly, Norplant,[6] introduced into a nearby district during the time of my fieldwork, was said to cause sore tired arms, amenorrhoea and irregular menstruation, tiredness, weakness and dizziness, and fears were expressed that the small rods inserted in the arms could move through the body. At the local district hospital, 488 women had Norplant inserted in April 1992 and over one hundred women had them removed less than twelve months later. Staff of the district hospital did not acknowledge the cultural understandings of the clients, nor try to address their fears (see also Stayapan, Kanchanasinith and Varakamin, 1983 on Norplant; Charoenchai and Thongkrajai, 1985:89–90 on reasons for methods switching; cf. Jennaway, and Grace, this volume with respect to Balinese and Sasak women in Indonesia).

Women complain of chronic tiredness and weakness, an inability to sleep, vision disturbances and abdominal pain after a tubal ligation. Women's discourses relating to tubal ligations reveal a perceived disruption of the traditional ordering and balancing of the female body caused by the new technologies. Many women say that now women have more problems with their health and are not capable of as much hard work because *bor dai yuu fai lang het man* (they did not stay on the fire after they had a tubal ligation). Women do not stay by the fire after a ligation as the practice is associated with the continued fertility of the women, no longer necessary when a ligation has been performed. Women also say that doctors tell them that staying by the fire after a tubal ligation makes the wound *akseep* (inflamed or infected). Women who do not stay by the fire because they have tubal ligations are encouraged by their mothers and aunts to place a hot water bottle or heated stone on their belly, and all took some form of hot medicinal tonic or *kaeng liang* (a hot soup containing white pepper and usually fish and sometimes banana flowers) (see also Van Esterik, 1988).

THE DISEASE OF NO MONEY: THE SOCIAL BODY AND BODY POLITIC

Is anyone in the house sick?

Yes, I have *rook bor mii ngen* [the disease of no money] (Aunt Jon).

Descriptions of health and illness and therapy seeking are embedded within the economic, political and social conditions in the Northeast. The narratives of village women directly express the relation between their health and their marginal economic position in Thai society:

I went to see the Doctor and got some medicine and the Doctor said to me "Don't work too hard!" But I have to! I don't have the money to get medicine often so that's why the problem's never gone (Grandmother Noi).

I don't go to see the doctor if it's not serious. Everyone waits until they can't stand, or wait until they have finished harvesting (Aunt Ngaam).

Like the majority of rural people living in the Northeast, Isaan women are systematically disadvantaged economically and socially. Women's accounts of their illness and health-seeking behaviour reveal the linkages between gender, class and health in Isaan communities. Women relate their health to the demands of physical labour in domestic chores, in the fields and in the factories of Bangkok, and to the added burdens of reproduction and family planning, all of which combine to make it difficult to maintain good health. Grandmother Noi's statement above clearly links the need to work hard with the continuation of her chronic ill-health. Village women must work because they are poor, yet the forms of work they must undertake because of their poverty are understood as detrimental to their health.

> The trouble with going to see the Doctor is money. I just try to carry on even though feeling pain. Women have responsibility for the other people in the family, my husband and children, and so I will be the last one in the family to go to see the doctor (Aunt Khiaw).
>
> My husband said to me not to go [to see the doctor] because my problem would never get better and if I go we wouldn't have the money to buy something else. Women are the ones who have to save and spend money but not for ourselves (Aunt Lua).

As Aunt Khiaw and Aunt Lua state, the difficulties borne by women in their roles as wives and mothers also affect their access to health care. As primary caregivers within the family, responsible for maintaining household health and treating illnesses, a woman may attend to the needs of others in the household above herself (Browner, 1989). To do so is consistent with the nurturing roles expected of women and the Buddhist view of life as suffering. With the changes in women's productive and reproductive roles that have resulted from the capitalist transformation of the village economy, women combine indispensable economic activities with their domestic workload.

The narratives of women regarding their reproductive health are thus invested with complex meanings referring to a woman's potency as a fertile woman, mother and sexual being, but also as a productive member of society. The discourses of a healthy Isaan woman's body described throughout this chapter is of one capable of labouring in the fields and producing healthy children. The body itself becomes the carrier of meanings associated with the woman's position within the society. An infertile body, whether the result of menopause, contraceptives or surgery, makes a woman less capable of production. At the same time, excessive work/production, forced upon women due to poverty and the increasing demands of the capitalist economy, likewise causes fundamental imbalances in the female body which may become evident in vaginal discharges or prolapses.

THE FORMAL HEALTH SECTOR: ETHNIC AND CLASS SPECIFIC BODIES

Northeastern women's subordinate social status in wider Thai society has direct consequences for their experience of public health care, both in terms of their access to and familiarity with health services and the ways in which health professionals regard them. Few women of Baan Srisaket admitted to ever having had a pap smear or internal examination, except for the young women who had contact with government health services for antenatal care. However, those who had experienced internal examinations spoke of the shame and embarrassment they felt at internal examinations and exposure of the genitals to another person, especially to a male doctor (see also Wangsuphachart, Thomas, Koetsawang and Riotton, 1987:362). In the gynaecology outpatients' section at a major hospital in Khon Kaen, I observed older village women crying and struggling at attempts by staff to take pap smears, weeping with indignation and fear. Some nurses place a cloth over patients' eyes before the examination, despite some patients' requests to the contrary, their explanation being that otherwise the woman would be too embarrassed if she could see the doctor doing the internal examination. Few older women in Baan Srisaket admitted to having had an internal examination, and those who did, had gone for treatment for a specific acute problem and often went with friends for support.

Consultations at the village health centre are very public affairs, easily overheard by anyone waiting or visiting. Few women would wish to discuss intimate symptoms in such a setting. Similarly, in gynaecology and antenatal outpatients' departments and family planning departments at hospitals and public health centres, a number of people may hear intimate details of consultations with doctors and may inadvertently see examinations between hastily drawn curtains. With little priority placed upon privacy, going to see a doctor about intimate matters is an encounter filled with shame and embarrassment. While undertaking observations at a Public Health Clinic in Khon Kaen, I came across a group of five women from the same district as that of my village fieldsite. Although there is a local district hospital in their town, they had hired a pickup truck and travelled 120 kilometres to a clinic, "where no one will know that we have come for internal examinations". Privacy is clearly an important concern of village women, yet I often heard from government health staff that privacy is not a concept prioritised by villagers who live in situations where everything is known by others. Village women rarely fully undress; even bathing is performed while covered with a cloth *phaasin* tied above the breasts, and birthing at home is monitored by the midwife with only the minimal necessary glances under the *phaasin* of the woman in labour. The notion that village women do not need privacy for vaginal examination is a patronising excuse for the indifference of the health staff to the feelings of their patients and permits "cultural relativity" to be used as an excuse for poor quality of care (see Mensch, 1993). In seeking care for gynaecological conditions, women are forced to participate in a process where hitherto secret parts of their bodies are displayed, objectified, explored and medicalised. In this encounter, power and agency is situated in the nurses and doctors. Their failure to provide a private environment completes the depersonalisation of the patient.

Women are critical of the services they receive when seeking care from the public health services and the private registered medical practitioners which constitute the formal health sector in Thailand. The social and economic subordination of Isaan villagers in Thailand is commonly enunciated in public discourse in imagery of villagers as rural, ignorant, traditional, uneducated and impoverished. In larger hospitals staff are often of elite Central Thai or Chinese Thai backgrounds (Cohen, 1989:164–165; Maxwell, 1975:484–485) who tend to look down upon Lao-speaking village women wearing cotton *phaasin* skirts, clearly marking their class and ethnicity. Attitudes of professional health providers are informed by discourses which represent Northeastern villagers as dirty, ignorant and naive and unconcerned about their health: "Very few women come for pap smears. Villagers are not interested in their own health. They only come if they are bleeding or there is something terrible" (Nurse Lii at the local district hospital).

Within a provincial hospital jokes circulate among staff of the "real stories" of Isaan women clients seeing gynaecologists:

> An Isaan village woman was told that she should wash herself before coming to see a gynaecologist, so the next time she did...she washed her hands.
>
> An Isaan village woman was told by a nurse to go to the bathroom and clean up before seeing the doctor. One hour later they realised that she hadn't returned. So they went to the toilets and there she was, cleaning the toilets.

When discussing gynaecological problems of village women at a provincial hospital I was told by one group of interns that: "the reason they [village women] get problems is because they are not clean and their hygiene is poor. This is because they have low education".

Such stories are frequently repeated by the urban middle class and in official discourses about village health. Discourses of development and good health and hygiene frequently disparage the traditional beliefs, practices and knowledge that villagers have about their bodies and health (Cohen, 1989:165). A "Manual for the Commune Council Committee", prepared by the Ministry of the Interior, presents an analysis of problems of underdevelopment that continues to be used:

> The social problem comes from the rural dwellers' lack of education and training. They lack motivation and knowledge to improve their production. They rarely seek knowledge; they are not interested in learning from the mass media, from discussions with experts, or from a study by themselves. More than that, they do not realise the importance of health and sanitation. They will not see a doctor until they have already developed a serious health problem. They do not keep their villages clean and tidy...Most of them are passive (Ministry of the Interior, 1976, cited in Vaddhanaphuti, 1984:308).

A report of "personal and household hygiene" in Isaan in a 1981 study conducted by staff from the Ministry of Public Health and Mahidol University portrays a more lugubrious image:

> The villagers also have...beliefs in black magics [sic] and supernatural beings, for example the belief in the influence in *Devada* or God over the weather conditions or of the spirit over the illness [sic]...Because of a lack of water, especially in summer, the villagers in the two communities take a bath once every day and only the younger members of the households use soap...Another common practice among the villagers is to walk barefooted and not cleaning

them when entering the house. This causes the house to be dirty as well as a health hazard. On the ground underneath the house the villagers keep buffaloes, ducks and hens and their wastes are cleaned only two or three times a year, making the place dirty, filthy and full of parasites (Rauyajin, Predaswat, Plia Bangchang, Dendoung, Upawokin, *et al.*, 1981:12, 16–17).

Descriptions of Isaan villagers as dirty are articulations of their marginal status in the eyes of the elite, sustaining a contrast between Lao villagers as ignorant, uneducated, poor, traditional, dark-skinned and dirty, and the Central Thai elite as educated, wealthy, modern, light-skinned, and clean. Attributions of dirtiness also carry with them assertions of worthlessness, pollution and immorality. In health institutions, such descriptions of impurity are mapped onto the medical parlance of hygiene, germs and disease. Thus ill health is linked in the statement by the interns at the hospital to villagers' poor hygiene and lack of cleanliness, with the implication that ignorance is to blame and that villagers are thereby responsible for their ill health. Health and disease thus become coupled with class and ethnicity. Isaan village women's bodies mediate these discourses in their interactions with health staff and institutions and in their experiences of health and illness.

ENDNOTES

1. The transcription system used throughout this chapter for the Isaan dialect is based upon the Thai Royal transcription system with some modifications by P. Jackson (pers. comm., February 1993). Under this system, long vowels are represented by double letters. Tones are not represented in this system. Thai authors' names within the reference list are listed in alphabetical order according to their last names, not first names.
2. All names of villages, districts and informants in this paper are pseudonyms.
3. It should be noted that there is some debate as to the use of the term *lom* which may mean illness rather than "wind" (Bamber, 1993:430–1). Thus the term *lom phit*, which has been described in the literature as an illness produced by the disruption of the wind element in women's bodies after birth (e.g. Hanks, 1963), may use the term *lom* as meaning illness rather than the wind element.
4. *Suu khwan* ceremonies require the skills of a *mor khwan* (a soul specialist) in which the lost soul is called and fastened to the body through the binding of the wrist with white cotton thread. These ceremonies are performed at any rite of passage such as pregnancy, birth, travel, before ordination and for people with prolonged illness.
5. The injectable contraceptive known as Depo Provera (Depo Medroxyprogesterone Acetate) has not been approved by the Food and Drug Administration in the United States due to reports of higher incidence of breast cancer in beagles and evidence of congenital malformations among infants if accidentally exposed to the drug early in pregnancy (Stephen and Chamratrithirong, n.d.). However, after a review, the United States Agency for International Development (USAID) recommended that Depo Provera should be made available to other countries that request it. The international controversy over the use of injectables has centred around the questions of long-term cancer risks of DMPA, and the ethics of its use in developing countries. A review by Archer (1985) for Save the Children Fund concluded that any long-term cancer risks are outweighed by the

hazards of uncontrolled fertility for women in developing countries and noted that such risks also exist for other hormonal contraceptives. With correct counselling and use, the study concluded that injectable contraceptives provided highly effective, simple to use, and were an undetectable contraception (Archer, 1985:17–18).

6. Norplant is a new contraceptive method that consists of five small tubes containing laevonorgestrel which are inserted beneath the skin of the upper arm and offer contraceptive protection for five years (Sivin, Soledad, Holma, Alvarez-Sanchez and Robertson, 1980).

REFERENCES

Abosede, O.A. (1984) Self medication: an important aspect of primary health care. *Social Science and Medicine*, **19**(7), 699–703.

Allen, S.J., Jumin, L.M.J., McQuistan, D.N. (1989) *Promoting Herbal Medicines in Primary Health Care: A Study in Two Villages in Northeast Thailand.* Unpublished MTH dissertation. Brisbane: Tropical Health Program, The University of Queensland.

Archer, E. (1985) *Injectable Contraceptives. The Role of Long-Acting Progestagens in Contraception in Developing Countries.* London: Save The Children Fund.

Bamber, S. (1993) Diseases of antiquity and the pre-modern period in Southeast Asia. In *The Cambridge World History of Human Diseases*, edited by K.F. Kipple, pp. 430–431. Cambridge: Cambridge University Press.

Bolton, P., Kendall, C., Leontsini, E., Whitaker, C. (1989) *Health Technologies and the Women of the Developing World.* Unpublished Paper. Baltimore, MD.: The John Hopkins School of Public Health.

Browner, C.H. (1989) Women, household and health in Latin America. *Social Science and Medicine*, **28**(5), 461–473.

Charoenchai, A., Thongkrajai, E. (1985) *Reasons for Family Planning Method Switching in Northeastern Thailand: An Experimental Study of a Motivational Strategy.* Khon Kaen: Khon Kaen University.

Chirawatkul, S. (1993) *'Sud Lyad, Sud Luuk', The Social Construction of Menopause in Northeastern Thailand.* Unpublished PhD thesis. Brisbane: Tropical Health Program, The University of Queensland.

Cohen, P.T. (1989) The politics of primary health care in Thailand, with special reference to non-government organizations. In *The Political Economy of Primary Health Care in Southeast Asia*, edited by P.T. Cohen and J. Purcal, pp.159–176. Bangkok: ASEAN Training Centre for Primary Health Care Development.

Davis, R. (1984) *Muang Metaphysics. A Study of Northern Thai Myth and Ritual.* Bangkok: Pandora Press.

Du Toit, J.P. (1988) A cost-effective but safe protocol for the staging of invasive cervical carcinoma in a third world country. *The International Journal of Gynecology and Obstetrics*, **26**, 261–264.

Hanks, J.R. (1963) *Maternity and Its Rituals in Bang Chan.* Ithaca, New York: Cornell Thailand Project, Cornell University.

Irvine, W. (1982) *The Thai-Yuan "Madman" and the "Modernising, Developing Thai Nation" as Bounded Entities Under Threat: A Study in the Replication of a Single Image.*

Unpublished PhD thesis. London: School of Oriental and African Studies, University of London.

Kendall, L. (1987) Cold wombs in balmy Honolulu: ethnomedicine among Korean immigrants. *Social Science and Medicine,* **25**(4), 367–376.

Manderson, L. (1981a) Roasting, smoking and dieting in response to birth: Malay confinement in cross-cultural perspective. *Social Science and Medicine,* **15B**, 509–520.

Manderson, L. (1981b) Traditional food classifications and humoral medical theory in Peninsula Malaysia. *Ecolology of Food and Nutrition,* **11**, 81–93.

Manderson, L. (1986) Food classification and restriction in Peninsular Malaysia: nature, culture, hot and cold? In *Shared Wealth and Symbol. Food, Culture, and Society in Oceania and Southeast Asia,* edited by L. Manderson, pp. 127–143. Cambridge: Cambridge University Press.

Maxwell, N.E. (1975) Modernization and mobility into the patrimonial medical elite in Thailand. *American Journal of Sociology,* **81**(3), 465–90.

Mensch, B. (1993) Quality of care: a neglected dimension. In *The Health of Women. A Global Perspective,* edited by M. Koblinsky, J. Timyan, and J. Gay, pp. 235–253. Boulder: Westview Press.

Mougne, C. (1978) An ethnography of reproduction. Changing patterns of fertility in a Northern Thai village. In *Nature and Man in South East Asia,* edited by P.A. Stott, pp. 68–106. London: SOAS, University of London.

Pedersen, L. R. (1968) Aspects of women's life in rural Thailand. *Folk,* **10**, 136-149.

Phinthong, P. (1989) *Isan-Thai-English Dictionary,* 1st edn. Ubolratchathani, Thailand: Siritham Press.

Poulsen, A. (1983) *Pregnancy and Childbirth — Its Customs and Rites in a North-eastern Thai Village.* Copenhagen: Danish International Development Agency.

Rajadhon, Phya Anuman (1961) Customs connected with birth and the rearing of children. In *Life and Ritual in Old Siam. Three Studies of Thai Life and Customs,* edited by W.J. Gedney, pp. 121–203. New Haven, Conn.: HRAF Press.

Rauyajin, O., Predaswat, P., Plia Bangchang, S., Dendoung, S., Upawokin, P. *et al.* (1981) *Psychosocial Aspects of Rural Health Services in the Northeast Region of Thailand. Research Report Series No. 1, The Anthropological Study of Psychosocial Aspects of Health Workers (Midwives).* Bangkok: Medical Social Science Program, Mahidol University.

Riley, J.N., Sermsri, S. (1974) *The Variegated Thai Medical System as a Context for Birth Control Services.* Bangkok: Institute for Population and Social Research, Mahidol University.

Reeler, A.V. (1990) Injections: a fatal attraction. *Social Science and Medicine,* **31**(10), 1119–1125.

Scheper-Hughes, N., Lock, M. (1987) The mindful body: a prolegomenon to future work in medical anthropology. *Medical Anthropology Quarterly,* **1**(1), 6–41.

Scott, C. S. (1978) The theoretical significance of a sense of well-being for the delivery of gynaecological health care. In *The Anthropology of Health,* edited by E.E. Bauwens, pp. 79-87. St Louis: The C.V. Mosby Company.

Sheehan, B. (1993) *Thailand An Introduction to Thailand, Its People, Trade and Business Activity.* Melbourne: The AustraliaThailand Business Council.

Singer, M., Davison, L., Gerdes, G. (1988) Culture, critical theory, and reproductive illness behavior in Haiti. *Medical Anthropology Quarterly,* **2**(4), 370–385.

Sivin, I., Soledad, D., Holma, P., Alvarez-Sanchez, F., Robertson, D.N. (1983) A four-year clinical study of Norplant implants. *Studies in Family Planning,* **14**(6/7), 184–191.

Stayapan, S., Kanchanasinith, K., Varakamin, S. (1983) Perceptions and acceptability of Norplant implants in Thailand. *Studies in Family Planning*, **14**(6/7), 170–176.

Stephen, E.H., Chamratrithirong, A. (n.d.) *Side Effects of Contraceptive Methods in Thailand*. Bangkok: Institute for Population and Social Research, Mahidol University.

Suvipakit, S. (n.d.) *A Study of the Acceptability of the Routes of Administration of Fertility Regulating Methods in Thailand*. Bangkok: Institute for Population and Social Research, Mahidol University.

Thailand, Ministry of Public Health (1986) *Proceedings of the National Seminar on the Development of Thai Traditional Medicine*. Bangkok: Ministry of Public Health.

Vaddhanaphuti, C. (1984) *Cultural and Ideological Reproduction in Rural Northern Thai Society*. Unpublished PhD thesis. Stanford: Stanford University.

Van Esterik, P. (1988) To strengthen and refresh: herbal therapy in SouthEast Asia. *Social Science and Medicine*, **27**(8), 761–768.

Wangsuphachart, V., Thomas, D.B., Koetsawang, A., Riotton, G. (1987) Risk factors for invasive cervical cancer and reduction of risk by "pap" smears in Thai women. *International Journal of Epidemiology*, **16**(3), 362–366.

Wasserheit, J.N., Holmes, K.K. (1992) Reproductive tract infections: challenges for international health policy, programs, and research. In *Reproductive Tract Infections. Global Impact and Priorities for Women's Reproductive Health*, edited by A. Germain, K.K. Holmes, P. Piot, J. Wasserheit, pp. 7–33. New York: Plenum Press.

Whittaker, A.M. (1995) *Isaan Women: Ethnicity, Gender and Health in Northeast Thailand*. Unpublished PhD thesis. Brisbane: Tropical Health Program, The University of Queensland.

CHAPTER 11

"No Problem": Reproductive Tract Infections in Indonesia

Valerie Hull, Ninuk Widyantoro and Tamara Fetters

> If we go to the doctor we always ask "Doctor, is this [vaginal discharge] serious or not?" The doctor always answers "No problem". We are not satisfied but what can we do — we only have limited time because other patients are already lined up outside (Ibu H., Indonesia).

Reproductive tract infections (RTIs) in women result from a range of causes. They include all the sexually transmitted diseases such as gonorrhoea, chlamydia, trichomoniasis, syphilis, chancroid, genital herpes, genital warts, and the human immunodeficiency virus (HIV). Conditions such as candidiasis or bacterial vaginosis, caused by an overgrowth of organisms normally present in the reproductive tract, are common RTIs. RTIs of both the lower and upper reproductive tract, including pelvic inflammatory disease, can also result from infections introduced during unsafe childbirth, abortion, IUD insertion, or other intravaginal procedures by health providers; and they can be caused by the insertion of preparations or objects for increasing sexual pleasure, or for self-treatment to alleviate discharge or other symptoms (Wasserheit, 1990).

Women suffering from RTIs may experience vaginal discharge which is copious or malodorous, vaginal itching or burning, vaginal dryness, and discomfort during intercourse. Many women experiencing RTIs, however, will not have symptoms, even though the infections are present and in some cases transmissible to sexual partners.

RTIs are treatable and preventable. However, if left untreated, the possible sequelae of RTI include increased risk of HIV transmission, ectopic pregnancy, cervical cancer, foetal wastage, low birth weight, neonatal pneumonia, infant blindness or mental retardation, infertility and even death of woman and infant. Lower reproductive tract infections can be precursors for much more dangerous infections of the upper reproductive tract (Germain, Holmes, Piot and Wasserheit, 1992). Case management involves treatment with antibiotics/sulfa drugs as well as partner treatment in the case of sexually-transmitted infections.

Although RTIs are thought to be widespread, their neglect by health systems and policy makers (Wasserheit, 1990; Aitken and Reichenbach, 1994; Rice and Manderson, this volume) has resulted in their being labelled a "silent tragedy" (Fathalla, 1994). While the burden of RTIs can be significant for men, women and children alike, their impact on women demands special attention for several reasons: these infections have more serious health and social consequences in women than in men; earlier detection and treatment is more difficult in women than in men; women are more likely than men to acquire RTIs both physiologically and because of lack of female-controlled preventive methods; and women are less likely than men to obtain treatment because they are asymptomatic, accept their symptoms as normal, or fear social stigma.

Dixon-Mueller and Wasserheit (1991:1) portray a major reason for the persistence of this "silent tragedy": an entire "culture of silence" which forces women to feel guilt and shame about their sexuality and sex organs, deterring them from seeking timely help:

> Women have internalized the ethic of nobility in suffering such that pain and discomforts emanating from their reproductive and sexual roles are accepted as the very essence of womanhood...Social stigma and hence the culture of silence [are] attached to sexual and reproductive problems, the geneses of which are invariably perceived to be women.

REPRODUCTIVE HEALTH AND RTIs IN INDONESIA

The Policy Setting: Programs and Priorities

Relatively low priority is accorded to public health by the Indonesian government, reflected in both the very low government health spending and in the regressive pattern of allocation which favours richer provinces and especially cities and hospital-level facilities (Griffin, 1992). Government priorities in reproductive health focus on family planning, largely based on a wider demographic/socioeconomic rather than health rationale. More recently there has been attention to Safe Motherhood, particularly in response to widely-publicised regional and international comparisons showing Indonesia's high maternal mortality rate. HIV/AIDs is receiving very recent concern and this has the potential to increase awareness of sexually-transmitted diseases, both because the latter are risk factors in HIV transmission, and because some of the same issues about sex education and related policies apply to both issues. Because of the causes and sequelae of RTIs, their prevention and treatment should in fact be integrated into other public health efforts, including Safe Motherhood, family planning, HIV/AIDs and also child survival programs. In Indonesia there is a network of family planning and health service delivery mechanisms at the community level to which appropriate RTI prevention and treatment services could be added.

Overall, however, efforts in reproductive health in Indonesia remain segregated into vertical programs which are heavily bureaucratised. Although programs involve community workers, all decisions and priorities are determined by the government. There is an absence of grassroots non-government organisations concerned with women's health in Indonesia, so there is no countervailing model to balance the top-down, authoritarian approach of government campaigns. Most importantly, little information exists about women's own health experiences and priorities. Programs to assist in areas such as abortion, adolescent reproductive health and wider sexual health are hampered by politico-religious sensitivities.

The Social Setting: Women and Health in Indonesia

Despite increasing medicalisation of reproductive health processes, women in Indonesia remain the principal guardians of their own and their families' health. As in most societies, women provide health education and treatment in the informal health sector through self-treatment and as traditional midwives, as well as in the formal health sector, where they form the vast majority of paramedical personnel (Hull, 1979).

The position of women more generally in Indonesia varies by ethnic group, religion and especially by social class, but overall Indonesian women have a degree of autonomy both in the domestic and extrahousehold spheres, which has deep roots in traditional economies, where women have played a major role in agriculture and trade in many parts of the archipelago. Within the household, women control family finances; men contribute to child-minding and other household tasks necessitated by women's extrahousehold activities. This description of traditional folk society contrasts with the noble class of indigenous and colonial-period Java, where women were bound to the home, in parentally-arranged, often polygynous marriages, and where income-earning activities were considered inappropriate. It is this elite Javanese cultural ideal which has pervaded Indonesian politics and bureaucracy (Cooley, 1992); however it conflicts with the reality of the lower class women, and the world view of a new generation of women exposed to education and other modernising trends (Raharjo and Hull, 1982). The role of Islam, in particular the recent resurgence of fundamentalist movements, adds further complexity to the blend of tradition and change which affects the lives of women in contemporary Indonesia. The admixture is particularly apparent in the capital city: among the women of Jakarta are university students combining Muslim headdress and blue jeans; women in Javanese *kain* (skirt) and *kebaya* (blouse) carrying heavy baskets of goods for sale; and Western-suited office workers with Gucci accessories. Neither is it unusual to read in the local press, almost daily, calls for more feminist awareness, juxtaposed with laments about the negative influence of globalisation and Western norms on the "traditional Eastern values", in which women's place is in the home.

RTIs in Indonesia

The published anthropological and sociological literature on RTIs and even women's health more broadly in Indonesia is limited; moreover, intensive approaches based on long-term community studies tend to be contributed by foreign researchers (including, for example, various chapters in this volume). The minimal information we have on RTIs is from clinical and epidemiological studies, and until recently, these have focused on STD clinic clients or "core transmitter groups", primarily sex workers. One of the largest study samples which has gone beyond this focus comes from a network of six private maternal and child health clinics in Jakarta managed by the Kusuma Buana Foundation. Of 6,666 women who received pap smears and related clinical examinations from 1987–1994, nearly half had RTIs and 29% had STDs (in this study candidiasis was classified as a sexually-transmitted disease) (Lubis, 1994). Research based on 695 women seeking menstrual regulation in Bali found that 53% of these women had at least one kind of RTI (Susanti and Hull, n.d.). Another recent Balinese study noted that many IUD users experience symptoms of RTI which are generally dismissed or undetected by health providers (Kandera and Surya, 1993).

Indirect evidence for an appreciable prevalence of RTIs in Indonesia derives from evidence of risk factors associated with these infections. There are significant mobile populations of both young men and women; a sharply increasing age at marriage without concomitant increased access to contraception and sex education for adolescents; and widespread prostitution in both urban and rural areas with virtually no condom use. A high percentage of births are attended by untrained personnel without sterile procedures. Statistics on abortions are lacking, but its illegal status means that a high proportion are performed by traditional practitioners under unsafe conditions. There are over five million IUD users in Indonesia, and insertion is often done without proper screening. Self-administered preparations for enhancing sexual pleasure and for genital hygiene are common, and also have the potential to increase the risk of RTI. Finally, there is virtually no effective information and education about RTIs; there is limited access to reproductive health services; and the health system is characterised by inadequate training and quality of care, leading to the potential for inaccurate or missed diagnosis and inappropriate or inadequate treatment.

THE CURRENT STUDY: RTIs IN JAKARTA

Background to the Study

Despite the global consensus for a new emphasis on reproductive health which emerged at the 1994 International Conference on Population and Development, there remains great uncertainty about just what aspects of reproductive health should receive priority — and an overriding ambivalence, shared by developing country policy makers and the donor community alike, about proposals to combine reproductive health programs, including RTI prevention and treatment programs, with family planning services. Governments are reluctant to address the problem of RTIs, in particular because of perceived community sensitivity, their presumed concentration in limited subgroups, and also because they are thought to be expensive and difficult to treat. For effective programs to be developed it is necessary to increase awareness of the problem, to collect baseline data, and to explore the main issues which are relevant to a particular country context. The need to begin this process in Indonesia was the motivation for current research on which this chapter is based.[1]

Specific Study Objectives and Approach

The main priority of the current research was to examine Indonesian women's perceptions and experiences of RTIs, but also to give attention to the views of health providers. Perceptions of the problem of RTIs and reproductive health in the wider "sociopolitical culture" — government and non-government agencies, the donor community and researchers — are also analysed.

The research team involved Indonesian experts with a background in health and health-related areas, and expatriates with extensive and intensive experience in Indonesian community studies.[2] This background was essential; in fact, although the results reported here are taken from focus groups and in-depth interviews conducted over a very short time period, they draw on the team's collective knowledge of the issues and policies necessary to form an understanding of the research problem. All members of the research team were women.

The RTI research involved focus group discussions (FGDs) with women and midwives, and in-depth interviews with physicians. The data collection was carried out in July and August of 1994 in a mixed socioeconomic area of the capital city of Jakarta, and on the island of Lombok in eastern Indonesia. Three FGDs were conducted at each site; one each for midwives and two each for women of contrasting socioeconomic backgrounds. In-depth interviews with four health centre doctors and four obstetrician-gynaecologists were also conducted. This chapter concentrates on the urban Jakarta group, with reference to Lombok women only for points of comparison.

The area of Jakarta selected for research was a neighbourhood of high-density small dwellings connected by what are called *gang tikus* (rat trails, or narrow alleyways). Clusters of households, many of them renting only one or two rooms of a larger house, share wells with attached latrines and washing facilities which are always bustling with users. Families in this urban village or *kelurahan* come from a range of ethnic backgrounds, with about half originally from Jakarta, another 20–25% from Central and East Java (homeland of the ethnic Javanese), 10% from neighbouring West Java (Sundanese), and the rest from a variety of other areas, especially Sumatra. The vast majority are Muslim, though in Indonesia adherents of Islam can range from very strict fundamentalists to what are called "statistical Muslims", those who report themselves as Muslim but who follow a variety of animistic and other belief systems.

In both research sites, women of reproductive age were chosen from lower class and middle class neighbourhoods near the community health centre. Women in the lower-class group tended to have primary school education (nine out of the twelve women); among the middle-class group four had primary education, six had secondary education, and two had attended university. The Jakarta women who participated in the focus groups had on average two to three children; all but one were current family planning users, with the IUD as the predominant method. Midwives participating in FGDs, who were also from the same area, were older and of higher social status than most of the other women.

The closed group discussions were held in a local home or in the health centre during non-clinic hours. Each FGD was led by a facilitator who was a trained counsellor; a medical doctor acted as the focus group recorder.[3] Discussion groups were followed with a question and answer and referral session led by the doctor. General information, including experience of RTIs and characteristics of individual participants, was self-recorded in a questionnaire distributed after the FGD.

WHAT WOMEN SAID

In introducing the subject of RTIs with women, we used both a literal Indonesian translation of the term "Reproductive Tract Infections" as well as the example of *keputihan* (literally, whitish substance) — a well-known common term for vaginal discharge (cf. Whittaker, this volume). The concept of infections of the reproductive tract, as anticipated, turned out to be too broad and abstract for women to relate to their experience. On the other hand, the term *keputihan* is used to describe all forms of vaginal discharge, including non-pathological mucus discharges. In our classification we used a simple breakdown of *keputihan* by colour (white, yellow, green, clear), and characteristics such as itchiness or odour.[4] It was felt that we needed a neutral and familiar term such as *keputihan* to open discussion, rather than give the impression that we were only interested in STDs (known commonly as *penyakit kotor*, "dirty diseases") or severe infections of the upper reproductive tract. It was hoped that women would discuss their own typology of *keputihan* and other symptoms, and how they themselves perceive "normal" signs as opposed to symptoms of illness.[5]

While marital sexual behaviour might be a taboo subject in formal meetings and in mixed sex groups, we found groups of women to be very open — oftentimes raucously so — in describing their problems.[6] Although the questioning always began by neutral enquiries about the situation among women in general, participants quickly brought the discussion around to their own personal experiences and concerns. In response to a direct question on whether RTIs and related sensitive issues could be discussed frankly, respondents in Jakarta summed up at the same time their willingness to be open about these matters, and their sense of community: "As long as it's among women we're not embarrassed; we are all friends".[7]

Experience of RTIs

Most of the women in our focus groups (71% from the self-administered question-naire of respondents distributed after the FGD) complained of having experienced whitish discharge or *keputihan* at some time. Many of these women had also experienced the more specific symptoms of vaginal itching, excessive wetness or malodorous discharge. Inflammation of the vagina or urethra after intercourse was also commonly reported. Bleeding after coitus was experienced by a few women, but lower abdominal pain and fever, symptoms of pelvic inflammatory disease, were reported only twice.

When asked whether virgins/young girls also experience *keputihan*, women discussed their daughters' experiences: they indicated that they took note of signs of discharge when they washed underwear, and some had discussed it with their daughters. This was generally not considered a cause for alarm or medical treatment, though further research would need to determine whether that is due to the nature of the discharge itself, or the assumption that young unmarried girls do not experience infections.

Perceived Causes of RTIs

Women in our study believed (and in some cases were told by health providers) that stress, "too many thoughts" (*banyak pikiran*), and fatigue were the most common causes of their discharge. Lack of hygiene was mentioned by women from Jakarta, though in fact it would have been easier for these women to maintain good levels of hygiene compared to their lower class Lombok counterparts, who usually bathed in unclean rivers, sometimes lacked water for washing after elimination, and used old cloth rather than purchased sanitary products during menstruation.[8]

Women did not feel that there was any relation between the use of particular family planning methods and symptoms of RTIs. Some women reported that certain foods could cause *keputihan*. "Fishy" foods such as salted dried fish or salted eggs were mentioned; as well as some fruits such as pineapple and green bananas; and cucumbers. These are all foods frequently proscribed during pregnancy and lactation as well.

Self Treatment

Most women indicated that they were reluctant to seek help from health providers for *keputihan*. Some felt that their discharge was normal or would clear up on its own; most women did not come to providers with complaints of discharge unless symptoms were very persistent. Even then women were most likely to ask a clinician about their symptoms within the context of a prenatal or family planning examination, rather than a separate visit for the RTI complaint only. Women did not perceive any long-term or even serious short-term health impacts of RTI symptoms, though they did complain about the feeling of embarrassment caused by discharge. Women also were concerned when the symptoms led to the disruption of sexual relations as a result of local discomfort, pain, and also vaginal wetness, which is perceived as undesirable for sexual intercourse. These effects of RTIs need to be pursued further, as important keys to women's perceptions of how they define acceptable vaginal discharge as opposed to discharge which requires action.

Women usually discussed their symptoms with friends and family members before consulting medical providers. *Daun sirih* (betel leaf) was the most popular therapy recommended by these women and their peers. Women either drank the boiled *sirih* or used *sirih* to wash and soak their external genital area; some women did both (*diobati luar dalam* or "simultaneous external and internal medication"). One woman reported using *daun sirih* "as an antibiotic". Many women also believe that *sirih* can increase sexual pleasure[9] by having an astringent effect on the vaginal walls. This leads to its use not only to "dry out" the vagina when experiencing vaginal discharge, but as a regular prophylactic measure. One woman reported, to the amused laughter of other participants, that her husband bought *daun sirih* every morning to boil up for her to drink.

Tongkat Madura (Madura stick) or *tongkat putih* (white stick), a kind of preparation made from alum and herbs, is also used for its astringent effect although some of the women said that it caused the vagina to become very dry and tear during intercourse.[10] In addition, particularly in Jakarta and among better-off Lombok women, commercial products such as packaged vaginal douches and the Avon product "Whim" were used to clean the genitals, particularly after sex. Other traditional herbs mentioned for treating the symptoms of *keputihan* include the skin of *delima putih* (white pomegranate), *temu ireng, temu kunci, temu lawak* (all variations of wild ginger), turmeric, and white pepper, though these tended to be reported more in Lombok than Jakarta. They are either prepared by women themselves, or purchased from stores or from traditional herb-sellers who travel daily through the neighbourhood carrying a variety of herbal mixtures on their backs. The widespread knowledge and use of traditional remedies specifically for women's reproductive health serves as an indicator of the prevalence of vaginal discharge.

Modern Medical Treatment

Many of the women complained that treatment by clinical health providers did not alleviate their RTI symptoms. When *keputihan* was detected by health providers it was usually after examination for family planning (generally IUD insertion), pap-smear tests or antenatal care. Unfortunately, according to women in our focus groups, many of the health providers seemed to give only a limited amount of attention to *keputihan*, and provided virtually no information to the women. One woman said that when she asked the doctor whether she might have *keputihan*, the doctor responded, *Masak perempuan tidak tahu keputihan* (roughly translated, "What woman doesn't?").

According to women's reports, diagnosis was generally made by a brief discussion of symptoms and then women were given a prescription to treat either an infection or fungus. Ampicillin (antibiotic), Antalgin (analgesic) and Chlortrimeton (antihistamine) were some of the drugs mentioned by women while others said that they were given "vaginal suppositories". Women also followed a common practice of purchasing the medications without consulting health providers if the condition returned, or if a particular medication worked for a friend or neighbour. Even prescription drugs are readily available over the counter.[11] The women who sought biomedical care said they hoped that midwives and doctors would give them clear and detailed information about the cause, prevention and treatment of their vaginal discharge but many were disappointed. Ibu H. in Jakarta said, "If we go to the doctor we always ask, 'Doctor, is this serious or not?', The doctor always answers, 'No problem'. We are not satisfied but what can we do, we only have limited time because other patients are already lined up outside".

Partner Communication

When asked whether they discussed *keputihan* with their partners, most of the women in Jakarta[12] said that they had discussed their symptoms with their husbands. Some said, "Of course we tell them, we even show it to them". Lower income women claimed to be embarrassed, but they provided many examples of discussing symptoms with their husbands, including frank discussions of husbands' preference for friction (a dry vagina) during intercourse. In general, women felt that they would not be able to deny their husband's requests for intercourse if they had not informed them of the reason, i.e., *keputihan*. Generally partners respected the need for refraining from intercourse on the wife's request, a finding which confirmed other studies conducted by the research team members. Husbands did not always follow this pattern, however, as Ibu S. from Jakarta related: "My husband wanted to have intercourse but I said 'no' but he forced me. Later he felt itching [of the genitals]. I said, 'You deserve it' ".

Sexual Practices, STDs and AIDS

Discussion of extramarital sex occurred in the context of questions related to possible periods of marital sexual abstinence, which could lead in turn to a partner's seeking sex outside marriage. According to the women, however, marital sexual abstinence during pregnancy or breastfeeding, a feature of traditional rural Javanese society, was not practised in Jakarta. Some women indicated that midwives had recommended that they continue sexual intercourse through late pregnancy in order to facilitate the birth process (*membuka pintu/jalan*, "open the door/way"). Women said that they do not have intercourse during menstruation because it is forbidden for Muslims and because they feel uncomfortable, however there were several reports of variations on the "taboo" and some felt that intercourse in the latter part of the bleeding period was permissible. One woman said that when she told her husband that sex during menstruation was forbidden by religion, he said "but I hear as long as the husband wants it, it's okay".

Although most of the women had heard of AIDS, gonorrhoea, syphilis and cervical cancer, they had little detailed knowledge of the symptoms and the causes of these conditions. Information about those diseases derived from mass media or from their friends and neighbours. Women gave examples of friends and neighbours, often those who had since moved away, who had what appeared to be serious STDs and purportedly high risk behaviour — i.e. either husband or wife were described as *nakal* (naughty). The tendency to ascribe these characteristics to people who had reportedly moved away may have been a less threatening way of discussing these patterns without admitting current "deviant behaviour" in the community or in a partner.

In discussing the issue of partner notification of a sexually transmissible disease in general, however, women in Jakarta were quite forthcoming. They all said it was best for the health provider to tell the woman the truth about the disease, and leave it to her to inform her husband. They felt that if the husband were informed by the provider it would be too embarrassing.

THE CULTURE OF HEALTH PROVIDERS: MIDWIVES

Much has been written about the need for health providers to understand popular beliefs about health and illness — but another important area for research is the belief system and subculture of the health providers themselves, and the provider-client interaction. Midwives in particular are key personnel in maternal and child health in Indonesia.

Discussions with midwives had a good deal in common with women in the focus groups because in fact they shared a similar worldview and experiences with the women they served. The midwives, who worked both in public and private practice, estimated that about 10% of their clients consulted them specifically for various types of *keputihan*. Other clients did not directly seek care for *keputihan* but midwives discovered the symptoms through examinations during family planning check-ups or prenatal care. Initially midwives said they saw no relation between contraceptive methods and RTI symptoms; however, during discussion it emerged that they perceived relatively higher prevalence among IUD users. Of course, IUD users are the women most likely to undergo an internal examination by a midwife. Midwives did not perceive serious long-term or even short-term health conditions linked to RTIs in general, although more concern was expressed about STDs. In Jakarta, the midwives felt that women would never discuss or share private problems such as vaginal discharge or similar symptoms with their own friends but would directly seek professional help. Discussions with women indicated that this was not the case; this perhaps was an example of an idealised response on the part of the midwives.

Diagnosis and Treatment of RTIs

In general, midwives diagnosed infections of the reproductive tract by identifying the characteristics of the reported symptoms. Pelvic examinations were done only during IUD routine examinations and prenatal care. For treatment, midwives recommended Ampicillin, Talsutin, Nystatin, or Metronidazole, though they pointed out that they could dispense prescriptions only through a physician — a regulation which is openly acknowledged as frequently ignored. Along with medication, the Jakarta midwives also suggested clients use antiseptic solution (such as Betadine), vaginal douches or "PK solution" for washing their genital areas. Sometimes the use of *sirih* leaves was also recommended by midwives. One midwife in Jakarta recommended that a couple use Canesten (antifungal) cream inside the vagina and on the shaft of the penis.

Some midwives reported that their knowledge of case management came from assisting gynaecologists in private practice. From our discussions, however, it seemed that midwives had difficulties diagnosing RTI from the symptoms presented. If their initial treatment was not successful, they would refer the clients to doctors or recommended pap smears. The Indonesian health system has recently begun a campaign promoting pap smears, and midwives seemed to ascribe very broad powers to this diagnostic tool. Midwives knew about the use of traditional herbs and food restrictions, and had the same perceptions as the women about stress and fatigue as important causes of *keputihan*. In midwifery school, reproductive tract infections were not discussed as a single topic in the curriculum, although *keputihan* was included as a symptom of STDs. As the discussions continued, midwives expressed their need and desire to learn more about the causes, prevention and management of RTIs: "There has never been any formal training about this topic but if there was a seminar we would attend and we could ask the doctor about these cases". As would be expected, none of the midwives in these FGDs had ever taught RTIs or *keputihan* as a health education topic in the community, though they had given talks on pap smears, family planning, and related subjects.

Sexually-Transmitted RTIs

When midwives discovered symptoms of sexually-transmitted RTIs in their clients, most admitted having difficulties discussing the client's sexual activity and the transmission of the diseases. One Jakarta midwife commented that "Here it is difficult to explain these situations [STDs] because we are afraid of offending someone. For example, if the husband is a good person and we imply to his wife that she got an STD from him, this could cause trouble". Another midwife tells of a case: "There was a woman here once, her husband was the driver of a night bus. In my heart I was suspicious but to explain that maybe her husband...[voice trails off]...Difficult". Only one of the midwives had ever called a husband in for treatment. A few had sent medicine with the wives for their husbands to take but provided no further explanation or follow-up with the men.

A DIFFERENT SUBCULTURE: DOCTORS AND SPECIALISTS

A very different approach to the issue of RTIs was apparent in the interviews with doctors and obstetrician-gynaecologists,[13] who were clearly mainly concerned with basic technical issues of case management.

The two doctors interviewed in Jakarta had, respectively, 13 and 20 years' experience. Although many women, especially IUD users, presented with *keputihan* (an estimated 10–30% of their clients), they had not given serious attention to the need for prevention education or standard treatment. Most cases were diagnosed as candidiasis, and they felt that other types of RTIs were relatively rare. The obstetrician-gynaecologists felt that most of the health centre doctors had enough skill to manage the clinical treatment of the most common reproductive tract infections, although they recognised that women were ashamed to be examined by male doctors. Further, regarding training and emphasis on RTIs, one doctor said, "We've never conducted training or seminars about these infections either for midwives or for the population, because it hasn't been 'programmed' from above [meaning the upper levels of the health system]".

Some Diagnostic Issues

In general, diagnoses were made by asking about the client's symptoms. The providers interviewed did not use the WHO recommended syndromic diagnosis (simple tests) like vaginal PH, leucocyte esterase, swab and KOH odour tests which could be used in the clinic setting. Laboratory tests were recommended by the doctors, however, if they found a very complex range of symptoms or profuse *keputihan*. Although the health centres had laboratory facilities, the doctors in Jakarta and Lombok alike felt that they were inadequate for detecting STDs and RTIs due to lack of skilled laboratory technicians (they can only perform basic tests on urine and blood samples). Even among the specialists, tests like the vaginal PH and KOH odour test are not used due to the time they take or lack of information about these tests. On the other hand, the obstetrician-gynaecologists felt that they were gaining more experience in detecting the symptoms without being dependent on laboratory or simple tests.

Treatment

Health centre doctors recommended similar treatments to those advocated by midwives (antibiotics and/or anti-fungal agents). Pap smears and referrals to specialists were also recommended when the clients returned with the same complaints: "If Ampicillin does not work, we either increase the dose or change medication; if that doesn't work, we refer them to a specialist". Three out of the four specialists interviewed indicated that they often took the approach of using a "bomb" (one of the broad-spectrum antibiotics) rather than trying to identify the causal agent of the symptoms, or dealing with partner notification and treatment.

Sexually-Transmitted RTIs

When dealing with STDs there were only a few reported cases where the partner was specifically invited to be counselled and treated. One doctor gave medication for the husband to the wife. A specialist told us: "A husband once called me, telling me truthfully that he had an STD and asked me to give medication to his wife when she came to my clinic for prenatal care. [He said] 'Please doctor, don't tell my wife that I've called' ". Another obstetrician-gynaecologist based his decisions on the appearance and attitude of the clients:

> If she appears to be a 'naughty' [*nakal*] woman, I will tell her directly about the sexually transmitted disease, but if she appears to be a 'good' [*baik-baik*] woman, I will give her a referral letter for her husband to consult a specialist. If she questions why I will not see him, I explain that I am a doctor for women's problems.

The specialists in fact complained that counselling and giving advice of this nature were not really their function. They were not trained to provide advice of a sensitive nature such as this and felt it to be a "burden". One Jakarta specialist said "It really is the job of a psychologist to inform a patient that she has a sexually transmitted disease".

DISCUSSION

RTIs: Is There Really "No problem"? "No problem" for Whom?

The perception of whether RTIs represent a health problem for women in Indonesia will likely be determined less by epidemiological evidence and cost-benefit analyses, than by prevailing political and religious sensitivities, as well as underlying attitudes toward women and women's problems in general within the health system and larger policy-making context.

Within the health system, part of the challenge for women's health is exemplified by an exchange between one of the women in the study from the lower-income group with her doctor. When she questioned her doctor's dismissal of her symptoms, the response was: "So you want to disagree, you want to see if you're smarter than I am? I'm a doctor and if I say 'No problem' then I know better than you".

Reproductive tract infections in particular are problematic because of their association with sex and immorality. This is manifest in current debate surrounding HIV/AIDS interventions, but was also illustrated by one of the doctors in our study who commented that he based his approach on an assessment of whether his client appeared to be a "naughty" or "good" woman. More fundamentally, and despite the rhetoric on primary health care, commitment to public health in Indonesia is low, and the approach to health programs remains one of largely vertical programs implemented in a top-down manner by a largely male-dominated bureaucracy. What does this mean for women's health problems in particular? A recent quote from a high-level official is illustrative. Although the example refers to bleeding disturbances rather than RTIs, it conveys the difference between problems as perceived by health program managers as opposed to women.

> Women always had bleeding disturbances, and they tolerated them without complaint. Now if the family planning program tells them that menstrual disturbances and bleeding are possible side effects of contraceptive methods which should be reported as health problems, this is a backward step. What were not health problems before have now become health problems.[14]

In fact, some research in Indonesia (WHO Task Force, 1981; Hanhart, 1993) has shown that women did, even prior to influence by the family planning program, perceive bleeding disturbances as a problem — in terms of their health, the interference it caused with religious obligations, and the interruption it made to sexual relations. It is nevertheless possible that women did not consult health providers for bleeding problems because of the sensitivity of discussing menstruation with a male provider, and because of the community norm of tolerating discomforts, and a corresponding low level of expectation that the modern health system could or would help them. In this sense, a real problem for women — be it bleeding irregularities, vaginal discharge, or other problems — may well translate into "no problem" for the health system or the policy maker because it is never acknowledged by the system.

It is possible that survey research or superficially-conducted qualitative research could find that there is "no problem" with regard to a number of women's health issues, including reproductive tract infections. The challenge is not to define problems where there are none, but to ensure that genuine problems for women are not neglected, either due to women's unwillingness or inability to report them, or researchers' inability to objectively document their existence.

Information is Power

The results of our research indicate that women address the problem of RTIs using what knowledge they possess, but operate in a context of limited information, social stigma, and inadequate professional care. Further studies of RTI in Indonesia should develop simple culturally appropriate tools for health education and training materials concerning the causes, symptoms, prevention and treatment of RTIs. Simply, women must learn what risk behaviours are and how to protect themselves.

There will be resistance to such an approach, based on perceptions that factual information on sexual matters is too sensitive to be promoted; that uneducated women in particular cannot absorb information effectively; and that programs can be "successful" by using authoritarian approaches rather than promoting knowledge. It is true that women often cannot understand even the limited information disseminated by government programs, but it is unfortunate that it is the women, rather than the materials and approach used, who are judged inadequate by program managers. Research has shown that educational material prepared with the active involvement of clients, regardless of education level, has the potential to be highly effective (Hull, 1992).

Women themselves expressed a desire for information. The focus group discussions included a specific question which asked whether they would prefer to get information about their complaint when they consulted health providers, or whether they felt just getting treated was the main thing. Women responded that they wanted information; at the same time they were also aware of the constraints of the service system ("we only have limited time because other patients are already lined up outside").

This study has turned up some specific issues which may be of use in devising interventions in Indonesia, but they will need to be developed and tested involving Indonesian women (and men) themselves. Some possible guiding questions for developing educational materials are set out below.

What Can We Tell Women so They Can Recognize When They Should Ignore, Self-treat, or Consult a Professional Provider for Symptoms such as Vaginal Discharge?

We need to have a better idea about what women know now. During the course of this research, not only the women in the focus groups, but also research team members, their colleagues, friends and family members exhibited great curiosity about discharge[4] and when it is or is not normal. There is only limited knowledge about normal cycling and discharge associated with non-pathological causes, so there is a risk that an overly simplified health education message may cause unnecessary alarm or even shame and fear in women experiencing such discharge. Information may need to "go back to basics" of physiology, as well as incorporating information on abnormal symptoms. Health education messages need also to address the commonly-perceived causes of RTIs among women and midwives now: stress, "too many thoughts", fatigue, and eating certain foods.

If it is true, as indicated by the current research and previous research of our study team members (Widyantoro, 1995), that vaginal wetness is thought to interfere with sexual pleasure, this also has health implications. The use of alum and other astringent material, particularly in excessive amounts, may cause tissue injury. The dangers of "dry sex" are now receiving great attention in other countries in the context of HIV transmission. Women also need to know that a high proportion of RTIs may be asymptomatic in women, and that certain medical procedures can put them at risk. They also need to be able to recognise symptoms in sexual partners.

What do Women Need to Know so that They Can Help Prevent RTIs?

Although there will be some formidable challenges in devising appropriate material on basic hygiene and physiological information, the whole area of sexual transmission of RTIs — including the use of barrier methods, negotiating power in sexual relationships, and related issues — will have to confront the same sensitivities and hypocrisy currently faced by Indonesia's proposed HIV/AIDS programs. Because HIV is a better-funded, higher-profile area, however, it may provide important lessons for RTI education and other interventions. Beyond hygiene and knowledge of sexual transmission of disease, women need information to become better educated consumers of health care procedures that can cause infection (see below).

Quality of Care Issues: Implications for Indonesian Health Service Providers

Health service providers admitted to serious limitations in their training and knowledge of proper case management of RTIs, and also in the principles and techniques of counselling and partner notification. Women complained that doctors did not give them information about the infections. Providers also said that laboratory staff lacked the training necessary to make reliable diagnoses. Obviously the system is not furnishing the necessary services even at a limited case management level.

The quality of health services more broadly is an important topic of discussion and intervention in Indonesia (National Family Planning Coordinating Board and The Population Council, 1993). Improvements in the *technical quality of services*, while difficult to achieve, are consistent with the aims of government and the influential professional associations in Indonesia. The broader concept of *quality of care*, however, which focuses on client needs and satisfaction, is a much longer-term goal (Bruce, 1990; Jain, 1992; Huezo and Diaz, 1993). Quality of care involving a client perspective goes to the very heart of class and power relations, individual versus collective rights and responsibilities, and especially for RTIs, gender relations. It can be argued, however, that without a basic respect for clients — without quality of *care* — there is only limited incentive for health providers to improve quality of technical competence.

Interviews with providers, particularly doctors, indicated that they do not see their role as giving information or counselling, and, echoing the perception of the woman about "patients already lined up outside", they feel that they do not have the time to provide this service even if it were appropriate. Women generally expressed a preference for the perceived technical competence of doctors, but found other aspects of the provider-client interaction, especially information exchange, severely lacking.

The need for quality of care in women's health may imply greater emphasis on the role of the midwife, who is generally closer to and more empathetic with women, and in the best position to provide the kind of information required. As providers of regular health education talks, they are also in a good position to help women understand prevention measures. As we have discussed, midwives need to be provided with the necessary information and technical skills in order to better fulfil this role.

Quality of Care Issues: Implications for Consumer Education

Improving the quality of health services will be more effective if health consumers themselves, and particularly women as caretakers of family as well as individual health, are given direct knowledge about quality of care and the motivation to ask questions and make demands of the health system. An ultimate aim would be for women to understand and demand a level of quality of health care services which does not put them at risk of iatrogenic infections, which provides them with information, and treats them with respect. Women need to know the kinds of unsterile procedures during childbirth or abortion which can put them in danger. Women obtaining IUDs need to expect and demand adequate screening, examination and sterile procedures.

The strong class and gender hierarchies prevailing in Indonesia do not provide a supportive environment for client or consumer education, but gradually changes are being seen in provider-client relations as a result of increasing education levels and other modernising influences. Almost daily there are letters to the newspaper complaining about unfair or low quality treatment of both private and government services, including health care, and the private sector is beginning to emphasise and widely advertise the concept of "customer satisfaction". Groups such as the Indonesian Consumers' Institute are becoming active in key areas of health care, including recent activity in women's health.

Involving Men

Our research provided us with some insights into relationships of gender and status which are crucial to developing effective intervention programs. There is a need, however, for more information about men's beliefs concerning RTIs in both males and females, and their knowledge about modes of transmission in order to develop materials for RTI transmission and prevention. The power/gender dynamics in Indonesia between midwives and doctors, between providers and clients (especially of different sexes), between men and prostitutes, and between husbands and wives needs to be better addressed in order to develop effective RTI programs. It may be, as our research suggests, that there is already a pattern of husband-wife relations and communication which is better than found in many cultural contexts, and could be encouraged to be further improved.

Research and programs should begin to explore issues such as the risks of extramarital sexual relationships, the transmission of STDs, and the communication of concerns about sexual and reproductive health between partners. Different approaches may need to be developed to provide women with the capacity and negotiating skills to address these issues with men or people of higher social status. Similarly, there will need to be sensitive efforts to encourage empathy and commitment among men and providers in order to support healthy outcomes.

ENDNOTES

1. This research was part of a broader plan to increase awareness and draw attention to the problem of RTIs in Indonesia through presenting results at an International Congress on Perinatal Infection sponsored by PERINASIA (*Perkumpulan Perinatologi Indonesia* — Indonesian Perinatology Association) held in Lombok, Indonesia in early September 1994. The results of this study were presented in conjunction with a literature review carried out by a team of researchers from the University of Indonesia and PERINASIA, which documented available clinical, epidemiological and behavioural studies of RTI in Indonesia (Daili, Masjkuri and Adisasmita, 1994). The current study was designed to explore women's knowledge, attitudes and practices concerning STD/RTIs, as well as to obtain some information on service provision issues as seen by health providers. The qualitative research was conducted by The Centre for Women's Studies at The University of Indonesia in collaboration with The Population Council in Jakarta.

2. The team's research coordinator was Dra Ninuk Widyantoro, a reproductive health counsellor who is currently involved in research in both Jakarta and in eastern Indonesia and who participated in one of the first RTI studies in Indonesia (Susanti and Hull, n.d.). Medical personnel included Dr Reny Bunyamin, a health centre doctor in Lombok; Dr Inne Susanti, an RTI expert from Bali; Dr Cecilia Boediono of Project Concern Indonesia. The project's technical assistance came from Valerie Hull, Senior Associate of The Population Council and Tamara Fetters, intern of The Population Council, both of whom have undertaken extended periods of village-level fieldwork related to women's reproductive health issues in Indonesia.

3. The researchers on the project used methodological training materials produced by the School of Public Health at The University of Indonesia to practice and refine facilitation and focus group techniques. Focus group recordings were transcribed in full and some of the transcript information was organised using the computer program *Ethnograph*, as part of a teaching workshop on the technique.

4. In the WHO's syndromic approach to RTI diagnosis they further categorise vaginal discharge into clumped, profuse and cervical mucous. The question of how these classifications fit into the ethnovocabulary of *keputihan* is left to be answered by further

research. In a country with over 300 ethnic groups, multiple social classes and generations, however, it may be necessary to identify a type of 'model thesaurus' based on the WHO classification, which can then be adapted by local researchers and programs.

5. The original list of focus group guide questions included trying to probe for issues such as where *keputihan* stands relative to other women's health problems; perceived effects, including on sexual relations; on symptoms as a source of shame; and of specific factors limiting consultation of modern practitioners including cost, status factors, and reluctance to consult male providers. These and other subjects were not able to be pursued given time limits for the discussion groups, but would be worth consideration for future research.

6. There were two exceptions to this general experience. In one group, a woman said that "I don't discuss such things because it is not allowed by Islam". It is interesting that in response to this comment, another woman said, "If you say bad things about your husband that is not right, but as long as you are exchanging experience and advice, that is good". The other exception was the area of *nakal* (naughty) behaviour. In this case, there was a tendency for participants to ascribe high-risk behaviours and STDs to friends or neighbours who had reportedly moved away; this was perhaps an acceptable way to discuss this information, but at the same time avoid bringing shame directly to themselves or current community members.

7. The facilitator was highly skilled in creating the kind of atmosphere which enabled women to talk frankly. Although the focus group guide began with general questions about "women around here", responses quickly took the form of personal experience, not only for frequently-reported symptoms such as vaginal and/or urethral irritation post-coitus where women could take comfort in the similarity of experience of others, but also for rare symptoms such as vaginal bleeding on intercourse which only a few women reported. Even very intimate details of their sexual relationship with their husbands were discussed, such as the preference for dry sex ("my husband buys me *daun sirih* every morning"); a woman who said her husband complains that when he eats fish the tip of his penis itches; or the woman who said her second husband was "cold", never saying anything during sex, so that it was like sleeping with a "water buffalo".

8. It remains to be demonstrated, however, that these factors in fact are linked to increased risk of RTIs. One of the most difficult aspects of the RTI problem is the lack of strong research on which to base basic health messages and interventions.

9. Sexual pleasure for the male is generally most emphasised, but heightened sensation for women was also reported.

10. It is clear that more research on traditional remedies needs to be undertaken to determine the active properties as well as to explore the risks of abrasion and subsequent infection associated with the use of these preparations.

11. For a broader discussion of self-medication and the ready availability of pharmaceuticals, see van der Geest and White (1988); for a comparative discussion for Northeast Thailand, see Whittaker (this volume).

12. None of the women in the low income group in Mataram had ever discussed *keputihan* with their husbands; some of them explained that communication between husbands and wives is very rare and that they only discussed *uang belanja* (spending money).

13. In part this was the result of the choice to use in-depth interviews rather than FGDs for this small group; however many of the questions were the same among all groups.

14. Personal communication to one of the authors, 1994.

REFERENCES

Aitken, I., Reichenbach, L. (1994) Reproductive and sexual health services: expanding access and enhancing quality. In *Population Policies Reconsidered: Health, Empowerment, and Rights,* edited by G. Sen, A. Germain and L. Chen, pp. 177–192. Boston: Harvard School of Public Health.

Bruce, J. (1990). Fundamental elements of the quality of care: a simple framework. *Studies in Family Planning,* **21**(2), 61–91.

Cooley, L. (1992) Maintaining rukun for Javanese households and for the state. In *Women and Mediation in Indonesia,* edited by S. Van Bemmelen, M. Djajadiningrat-Nieuwenhuis, E. Locher-Scholten and E. Touwen-Bouwsma, pp. 229–247. Leiden: KITLV Press.

Daili, S., Masjkuri, N., Adisasmita, A. (1994) *Literature Review on Reproductive Tract Infection in Women associated with Sexually Transmitted Diseases in Indonesia.* Jakarta: Indonesian Society for Perinatology and The Population Council.

Dixon-Mueller, R., Wasserheit, J. (1991) *The Culture of Silence: Reproductive Tract Infections Among Women in the Third World.* New York: International Women's Health Coalition.

Fathalla, M. (1994) Fertility control technology: a women-centred approach to research. In *Population Policies Reconsidered: Health, Empowerment, and Rights,* edited by G. Sen, A. Germain and L. Chen, pp. 223–234. Boston: Harvard School of Public Health.

Germain, A., Holmes, K., Piot, P., Wasserheit, J. (1992) *Reproductive Tract Infections: Global Impact and Priorities for Women's Reproductive Health.* New York: Plenum.

Griffin, C. (1992) *Health Care in Asia: A Comparative Study of Cost and Financing.* World Bank Regional and Sectoral Studies. Washington DC: The World Bank.

Hanhart, J. (1993) Women's views on Norplant: a study from Lombok, Indonesia. In *Norplant: Under Her Skin,* edited by B. Mintzes, A. Hardon and J. Hanhart, pp. 27–45. Delft: The Women's Health Action Foundation.

Huezo, C., Diaz, S. (1993) Quality of care in family planning: clients' rights and providers' needs. *Advances in Contraception,* **9**, 129–139.

Hull, V. (1979) Women, doctors and family health care: some lessons from rural Java. *Studies in Family Planning,* Special Issue: Learning About Rural Women, **10**(11/12), 315–325.

Hull, V. (1992) By and for Women: involving Women in the Development of Reproductive Health Care Materials *Quality/Calidad/Qualité,* Series Number Four. **14**(1–2), 23–24.

Jain, A. (1992) *Managing Quality of Care in Population Programs.* West Hartford, Connecticut: Kumarian Press.

Kandera, I. Wayan, Surya, I. Gde Pt. (1993) *Hubungan antara pemakaian IUD dengan infeksi genitalia (PID) pada wanita yang menderita keputihan (fluor albus) di beberapa fasilitas pelayanan KB Kabupaten Badung, Propinsi Bali* (Relation between IUD use and pelvis inflammatory disease among women with fluor albus in several family planning facilities in Badung, Bali). Unpublished paper.

Lubis, F. (1994) Unpublished data from the Yayasan Kusuma Buana MCH Clinics, Jakarta. (Also reported in *The Jakarta Post* 24 December 1994, 5: "Wives remain victims of sexual diseases".)

National Family Planning Coordinating Board and The Population Council (1993) *Operations Research Regional Workshop on Development of the Principles of Quality of Care in Family Planning Programs in Developing Countries.* Jakarta: National Family Planning Coordinating Board and The Population Council.

Rahardjo, Y., Hull, V. (1982) Employment Patterns of Educated Women in Indonesian Cities. In *Women in the Urban and Industrial Workforce: Southeast and East Asia*, edited by G.W. Jones, pp. 101–126. Development Studies Centre Monograph No. 33. Canberra: Australian National University.

Susanti, I. and Hull, T. (n.d.) *Reproductive Tract Infections in Bali: A Clinical Study of Women Attending a Family Planning Clinic for Menstrual Regulation*. Unpublished paper.

van der Geest, S. and White, S.R. (editors) (1988) *The Context of Medicines in Developing Countries*. Dordrecht: Kluwer Academic Publishers.

Wasserheit, J. (1990) Reproductive tract infections. In *Special Challenges in Third World Women's Health*, edited by The International Women's Health Coalition, pp. 1–15. New York: IWHC.

WHO Task Force (1981) A cross-cultural study of menstruation: implications for contraceptive development and use. *Studies in Family Planning*, **12(3)**, 3–16.

Widyantoro, N. (1995) Learning about sexuality through family planning counselling sessions in Indonesia: personal experiences. In *Learning about Sexuality: A Practical Beginning*, edited by S. Zeidenstein and K. Moore. New York: The Population Council and the International Women's Health Coalition.

CHAPTER 12

Blood Beliefs in a Transitional Culture of Northeastern Thailand

Siriporn Chirawatkul

Cultural conceptions of physiology affect people's understanding of bodily processes and behaviour related to the prevention, diagnosis and management of illness, and the maintenance of health (Helman, 1990). Medical anthropological research on illness, disease and treatment has a long history (Paul, 1955), yet surprisingly, there has been relatively little research on the human body as such, or on its substances: Loudon's paper (1977) on matter — as well as Douglas' enduring work (1966) — are important exceptions to this. Much of the other work on matter has focused on blood, specifically menstrual blood. Blood provides the metaphor for social relationships, health and well-being, kinship ties, personality and psychological states in different cultural contexts (Adams, 1955; Snow, 1976; Like and Ellison, 1981; Martin, 1987; Davis, 1988; Chirawatkul, 1993).[1] This chapter describes beliefs of blood held by villagers in northeastern Thailand, and explores the relationship of the beliefs to perceptions of reproductive health and illness and the influence of these beliefs on women's perception of menstruation, lochia, and menopause. In providing an account of northeastern Thai understandings of the nature and function of blood, this chapter allows comparison both with other papers in this volume (e.g. Rice, Whittaker) and beyond.

Information presented in this chapter was obtained from an ethnographic study undertaken in Baan Mali, a village of northeastern Thailand, in 1990–1991. The village is located ten kilometres north of Khon Kaen town, and has a long history of sociocultural development, which has resulted in an ongoing and rapid process of transition and modernisation (see Chirawatkul, 1993 for details). The data presented in this chapter draw on information collected from unstructured interviews with villagers, including twelve traditional healers, four focus group discussions, in-depth interviews with 23 women, and structured interviews conducted with 150 women aged 35–55 to elicit their experiences of health, illness and perceptions of their bodies' products.

Baan Mali

The history of *Isaan* (northeastern Thailand) can be traced back 5,000 years. *Isaan* people share a cultural and linguistic heritage with people from Laos, and present languages are mutually intelligible. Religious belief has been influenced by both Hinduism and Buddhism, and people believe in merit, demerit, and rebirth. Incorporation of the region into the Thai nation state has been relatively recent — from 1894 — initially through official administrative reform, then with the introduction of formal education (Bernard, 1983; Phongphit and Hewison, 1990).

Baan Mali, a village established by six mahout families in 1891, continues to share more aspects of social structure and culture with villages in Laos than with villages in Central Thailand (Keyes, 1967). The population of this village is homogeneous: Lao ethnicity, Buddhist, with an agricultural base. In April 1991, there were 415 households and a population of 1,853 (897 females and 956 males). Village income is mainly based on agricultural products such as rice, mangoes, tamarind, and flowers. Agricultural production and cottage industry product (garlands, bouquets) are the main income sources of the majority of households. Hired labor is needed for planting rice, harvesting, weeding, spraying pesticide, picking flowers, threading flowers, and preparing garlands and bouquets. Villagers who do not have their own land or gardens become labourers and make money from these activities. Both men and women work for wages. Men prefer to work in the paddy fields while more women work in the garden and flower business. Some families gain income from younger members who work in Khon Kaen town as wage labourers, and a few households have a more secure income through salaried household members. The elderly gain additional income from picking flowers and threading flowers.

Before the booming of the flower business, young female out-migration was quite noticeable. Numbers of women went to work in the textile factories in Bangkok (the capital of Thailand) for a period of around 1–3 years. At that time, few men left the village for wage labor because there was much work in the paddy fields. Today, there are factories in the outskirts of Khon Kaen and the jasmine flower businesses provide opportunities for hired labor, so fewer villagers migrate or leave temporarily. However, a number of young women work in the shopping mall in Khon Kaen town as well as making garlands to supplement their income. People who do move away follow their spouses, continue their education in Bangkok, or seek work there or in other larger cities. Even so they retain a strong tie to the village, returning every year to visit and participate in traditional ceremonies such as *songkran* festival (Thai New Year) and *kathin* ceremony (twelfth month ceremony offering robes and necessities to monks).

Baan Mali is a complex community, and not surprisingly, the health system of Baan Mali is divided into three sectors as described by Kleinman (1980). There is a professional sector of medical and paramedical professionals practising biomedicine; a popular sector of non-professional, non-specialist modalities, where ill health is first recognised and defined, and health care activities are initiated; and a folk sector which includes certain individuals specializing in forms of healing which are either sacred or secular, or a mixture of the two. These folk healers share the basic cultural values and world view of the communities in which they live (cf. Golomb, 1985).

A western medical system was introduced to the village in 1970. A health centre which is responsible for Baan Mali is located in a village five kilometres from

Baan Mali, between Baan Mali and Khon Kaen town. Four health workers are based at the centre. They provide routine services for Baan Mali villagers, including 24 hour services (midwifery, treatment for simple illnesses or injuries, and referral services to the provincial hospital for severe illness), weekly services (vaccination, family planning and neonatal care), monthly services (monitoring of child growth and development by weighing at the village occurs every six months), and yearly services (demonstration of cooking supplementary food for children and monitoring of pesticide poisoning through blood examination).

Baan Mali villagers tend to come to the health centre to ask for contraception and for help with minor illnesses and complaints such as headache, stomach ache, muscle-joint-bone pain, vertigo, fever, minor injuries, diarrhoea, constipation, abscesses, poor appetite, rashes and itching, mumps, cough, otitis, and snake or dog bite. However, villagers who are financially well off or have severe illness or emergency health problems prefer to seek private medical care or to go to the provincial hospital in Khon Kaen town. In the popular sector, villagers distinguish between two categories of patients — *pouy youn* (patients who can maintain their daily life) and *pouy non* (patients who can not move):

> Some persons are sick but they can eat and mobilise themselves. However, they can not carry out hard work. If they do so, they are so tired. People may think that they are lazy because their sickness is inside and it is invisible. A person who is regarded as being severely ill is a person who cannot do anything, is in bed all the time, and cannot be mobilised.

Within families, women are expected to nurse the sick and so women have more experience in caring than men. These experiences position them as health consultants to family members, relatives and neighbours.

Sociocultural change in Baan Mali has led to change in the villagers' livelihood, with some equivocal outcomes. Perceived benefits include economic opportunities, social mobility and access to modern health facilities. Women are more active economically, but need more energy to work, to increase money and property to achieve what they regard as "modern" standards. However, "traditional" beliefs about health and illness retain currency and influence villagers' dealings with health providers.

In the folk sector, the term *maw* is used to refer to persons with speciality knowledge and healing skills. People whose work is associated with health and illness are given the prefix *maw* followed by a term indicating their area of special skills. At Baan Mali, all twelve traditional healers are called *maw*. Among them are three *maw tham* (magic healers), two *maw ya sammunphrai* (traditional healers who use herbal medicine), one *maw khwan* (conducts spirit ceremonies), one *maw gnoo* (treats snake bite), two *maw pao* (healers who blow on sick persons to produce recovery), two *maw namman* (healers who use sacred oil) and a *chum* (a spirit medium). Except for one *maw namman* who is 36 years of age, all are over fifty and none are women. Each healer has his own speciality; of the two *maw namman*, one is a specialist in bone fracture and the other in burns. According to their beliefs about health and illness and their treatment modalities, these healers fall into one of the three categories described below.

The Supernatural

Maw tham and *chum* are in this category. They believe that illness is caused by spirits. Villagers who breach social rules, who for example cut down a big tree without permission from the *phii pa* (the spirit of forest), offend the elderly, do not recognise or take care of ancestors, or make trouble with neighbours, will be punished by spirits. Various symptoms can occur in a person who is believed to be punished by a spirit, such as headache, stomach ache, convulsion, and loss of mind.

Astrology

The *maw doo* or the fortune teller is in this category. *Maw doo* believe that human life relates to the zodiac cycle. Illness is regarded as bad luck that cannot be avoided, but it can be cured by sprinkling holy water on the body or performing a special ceremony. The treatment modalities of *maw doo* tend to encourage clients to release emotional tension and are designed to strengthen the souls of patients.

Medical Theories

Healers within this system include *maw ya samunphrai, maw gnoo, maw pao*, and *maw namman*. They have a common belief that the human body is made up of four humors: earth (*din*), liquid (*naam*), air (*lom*) and heat (*fai*). Each humor has a distinctive nature and function in relation to the other. Illness is caused by abnormal humor(s) and humoral imbalance (see Jirojwong, and Whittaker, this volume). Among them the *maw ya samunphrai* or herbalist is the most popular. This folk healer uses herbal medicine in combination with sacred prayers to cure the patient, using "cold" herbs to redress the imbalance if the patient's body is in a state regarded as "hot", "hot" herbs if the body is "cold".

Herbalists believe that a woman's body during menstruation, pregnancy and postpartum is in a state of imbalance. A woman needs "cold" herbs to maintain good health but should avoid "cold" food to prevent the obstruction of flow. However, "hot" herbs may also be given to maintain the balance of the body and encourage the menstrual or lochial flow. These reasons are similar to those of women in northern Thailand (Muecke, 1976), Chinese women (Gould-Martin, 1978; Pillsbury, 1978; Chu, this volume), Malay women (Manderson, 1981a, 1981b, 1986), and women in the American-Mexican West (Kay and Yoder, 1987).

None of the healers in the supernatural and astrology medical systems have clients who have menstrual problems. However, the herbalists (*maw ya samunphrai*) reported that some women came to see them with problems of irregular bleeding, spotting, headache, dizziness or other problems believed to be due to "blood problems". They treated them with different kinds of herbs, both "hot" and "cold", to regain and maintain "good blood".

DESCRIPTION OF THE TERM "BLOOD"

Beliefs about blood influence perceptions of health and illness, and health practice. A number of ethnographies from quite different areas draw attention to the importance placed on the integrity of the body, the finite nature of blood, and its importance in terms of quality as well as quantity (volume). Adams (1955), for example, recounts the resistance experienced by health personnel from Guatemalan villages to their taking blood samples from children for a health survey, because villagers could not understand how doctors who obviously were weakening their children could claim to be improving their health, since blood is regarded as finite, "non-renewable" or "non-regenerative", which when lost through injury or disease, would permanently weaken a person's resistance to disease (see also Foster and Anderson, 1978: 227). Davis' study (1988) of community health in a Newfoundland fishing community similarly notes villagers' belief that good blood is essential for good health and that bad blood is harmful. They described blood in terms of different characteristics such as red, black, high, low, thick, thin, good and bad. Davis (1988:19) concludes that:

> Popular lay beliefs about the nature of blood are related to a wide range of beliefs and behaviours, which may or may not have negative consequences for the delivery of health care services.... Blood complaints are seen as unifying them in local beliefs concerning birth control, hypertension and cervical cancer.

In Baan Mali, illness is explained by villagers and traditional healers as caused by humour imbalance, especially of blood. A traditional healer states that:

> Mainly, illness is caused by insufficient blood. The healthy person has complete blood. A person who has incomplete blood is prone to sickness and low intelligence. It [the body] is easily invaded by bad blood and good blood becomes bad blood, causing more illness.

Villagers in Baan Mali used the term "blood" to describe a wide variety of bodily and emotional states, personality types, and health or illness status, reflecting conceptions of the relationship of blood to biological function, personality, and health. Women's health, especially as related to reproduction, is described in terms of these beliefs. Villagers believe that blood is one of the liquid humors — the others are serum, bile, sputum, sweat, fat, nasal mucous, tears, joint fluid and urine. Good blood and good air are regarded as essential for good health, although normally the human body has good blood and bad blood. Blood and air have their own pathways, but the two are parallel. If the air pathway is obstructed, air cannot flow freely. The combination of air obstruction and bad blood causes health problems.

Good blood is defined by being of high quality and quantity, red and odourless. A person who has good blood will have red face and palms, and these are regarded as symptoms of good health. But everybody has bad blood inside their body also; bad blood is thin, either light red or dark, smelly and poisonous. Villagers could not provide a clear description of good or bad blood, or of how blood turns bad, but maintain that adults have more bad blood than children or, contrarily, than the elderly. Women also have more bad blood than men, and thus women have to menstruate every month to drain out the bad blood. Men, children and the elderly drain out bad blood by sweating, urinating and bleeding from injury. One informant describes differences in the blood of men and women as follows:

> Women have more bad blood than men. Normally, the bad blood will circulate through the heart at least once a day, causing the person to be in a bad mood and unhappy. Women are more temperamental than men and because woman have so much bad blood, it has to drain out — as a result, menstruation. Men release bad blood by elimination and sweating.

Similarly, according to one woman: "A woman who has good blood is healthy. She doesn't need any special cure. Just like me, I have never been to see a doctor because I have good blood".

Bad blood causes a variety of bodily and emotional states: unhealthiness and weakness, bad moods, irritability and insanity. It can also cause skin rashes, ulcers, paleness, headache and dizziness. A person who has thin blood can easily get sick, may be infertile, and may reach menopause prematurely. In these instances, the relationship between blood and bodily state is taken literally. In addition, blood may be used metaphorically to describe personality. A person who has hot blood is hostile and barely able to control her/his temper, while a cold-blooded person is cruel and evil-minded. Both types of personality are undesirable. Here "blood" is not used to connote fluid in the body, but it is used symbolically only as a characteristic of the mind.

The above description provides a general summary, and hence glosses over considerable confusion. There are, however, contradictory beliefs which occur as a consequence of different personal experience. One individual will state that having bad blood is a natural event and that everybody has it, while another will state that irregular menses or childbirth causes bad blood. Heavy menstruation can be good, therefore, as it drains out bad blood and is a sign of healthiness, but it can be bad since it may cause energy loss. Loss of blood during childbirth can be bad because it may leave the blood volume low, but also good as it drains out bad blood. As two women aged over fifty said:

> I am childless and I have never given birth to a child. Therefore I have never lost blood. Now, even though my period is over, my face is still bright and red.
> When I gave birth, the midwife squeezed out all bad blood so there was no residual and I felt great. No dizziness at all.

Having "good blood" is a symbol of being healthy. Being unhealthy or sick is regarded as a result of poisoning from bad blood. Villagers seek "good blood" by taking herbal medicine, Chinese medicine, and western medicine, some taking medicines from one modality only, others taking a variety of drugs either sequentially or concurrently. As there are several herbalists in Baan Mali, it is convenient for women to see a herbalist and to ask for herbal medicine to ensure good blood. Vitamins are regarded as a western medicine that promotes good health and good blood also, and are both inexpensive and available from the local health centre. Chinese medicine is more difficult to acquire, however, and women have to go to the drug store in the town.

BLOOD BELIEFS AND BODY PRODUCTS

The Meaning of Menstruation

Beliefs about bad blood have influenced women's practices relating to menstruation and childbirth. In menstruation, such beliefs influence women's choice of absorbing and disposing of menstrual blood and of self-care:

> Menstrual blood is bad blood and men are disgusted by it.
> Menstrual blood is bad blood. This blood can be poison to the body.
> In one who has good blood, the menstrual blood will be red. One whose menstrual blood is black has bad blood.

According to these statements, meanings of menstruation derive basically from beliefs about blood. Normally blood is regarded as a vital fluid of life. As I have described earlier, characteristics of blood mentioned by women in this study are "good" or "bad" or "thin". Characteristics of blood indicate health status and body state and therefore, menstruation is regarded as an indicator of women's general health and body state. Village women regard menstruation as a bodily mechanism to drain bad blood, and as a natural event in a woman's life. The occurrence of menstruation is a mark of being a reproductive woman. Healthy women have "good" menstruation: that is, a regular period, heavy flow, and red menstrual blood. A woman whose menstruation is irregular with little menstrual blood is regarded as *lu'at jaang* (thin blood), susceptible to infertility and sickness. In line with this belief, women seek ways to ensure good menstruation.

Yet contrarily, menstrual blood is regarded as dirty, bad blood, since it is unwanted blood; retention can cause headache, stomach ache, and fever. It is also regarded as strong enough to counter the power of amulets, since it comes out from the low part (below the waist) of the woman's body. According to one old man:

> I have seen a dead body that did not burn even though it was in the fire for days. People said the man who had died had a strong power amulet so fire could not burn his body. When a person put a woman's skirt that was soiled with menstrual blood onto the pyre, the body burned.

Because of this belief, several women refused to let their husband touch or wash their bloody clothes, because men like to have amulets to enhance their power or to protect them, and a husband is regarded as a person worthy of respect. As a woman said: "I don't let my husband wash skirts soiled with menstrual blood. It is sinful [to do so]".

Since blood is believed to be "hot", a woman's body during menstruation is regarded as being in a "hot state". If she touches a "cold" vegetable such as mint, it will wither. She is not allowed to grow plants because her hot body will make the young plants die. At the same time, menstrual blood can be clotted by "cold" temperature.

During menstrual periods some women keep themselves warm and avoid "cold" foods and beverages because of their belief that their bodies are in a "hot" state. Menstrual flow will be disturbed by penetration of cold temperature, causing menstrual blood that is regarded as bad blood and hot to be reabsorbed. The "heat" and "poison" would enter the ordinary blood stream, and this blood would then either rise to the head causing headache and fever, be retained in the womb causing stomach ache, or cause skin rashes or emotional disturbance. Women who have a fever at the time of menstruation are said to have it because of the heat of menstrual blood. This fever, specifically referred to as *khai tub radeo* (fever during menstruation), is regarded as dangerous and the woman is considered ill.

According to the belief that menstrual blood can cause illness, the obstruction of menstrual flow is considered a danger to women's health. Several women at Baan Mali prefer to let the blood flow freely and use nothing to absorb menstrual blood while at home, letting it flow freely and soil their skirts instead. Today, even though sanitary pads are sold widely and are very easy to find, women prefer to use sanitary pads or napkins only when they have to go outside the home and on certain occasions. They say it is not beneficial to their health, and that every time they use sanitary pads to absorb the blood, they get headaches and stomach aches. Some women are allergic to the pads, and they say that the pad keeps the menstrual blood in contact with genitalia, causing rashes and itching. In contrast, women believe that cloth can absorb menstrual blood without disturbing the flow, and can be cleaned and reused as well. Women also point out that it is costly to use sanitary pads all night and day during menstruation, and if they were to use sanitary pads every day during their period, they would lose forty five baht (US$2) without any return every month.

Heavy flow is regarded as a sign of healthiness or having good blood. During menstruation several women take medicine to ensure this. Some take herbal medicine with alcohol called *ya dong lao* (*ya* is medicine, *dong* is "to remain a long time", and *lao* is alcohol or liquor), some women take Chinese medicine and liquor. According to one woman "drinking *ya dong lao* during menstruation is very good. Menstrual blood flows very heavily. It flows like a tap has been turned on". *Ya dong lao* is available in the village and can be made by women themselves; many make up a quantity to drink whenever they menstruate. However, if the flow is "too heavy", a woman would lose energy. A heavy flow may also be regarded as a sign of a "dangerous womb" or of severe disease such as cancer. In this case a woman might seek medical advice.

Lochia: Dangerous Fluid

In childbirth, blood beliefs inform the practices that are followed to maintain good health, to facilitate recovery after delivery, and to prevent ill health at a later date. The postpartum practices that pertain in Baan Mali are similar to those reported in several other countries and cultures, where the emphasis is on confinement procedures designed to drain or dry the lochia flow. According to Pillsbury (1978), for example, Chinese women believe that postpartum, a woman has a great mass of dirty blood that needs to be drained to restore healthiness, and to this end she must avoid "cold" and observe behavioural and dietary restrictions that augment "heat" (see also Manderson, 1981b; Chu, this volume).

Women believe that the stomach is full of bad blood after giving birth. Lochia is perceived as a dangerous fluid that poisons the womb (cf. Kay and Yoder, 1987). In Baan Mali, "lying by the fire" (*yuu fai* or *yuu gaam*) is practiced traditionally to drain lochia from the postpartum woman's womb. It makes the womb dry and helps the womb revert to its proper position. *Yuu fai* includes resting on a bed near a hot fire that is kept burning constantly for seven to fifteen days (cf. Townsend and Rice, this volume).[2] The heat of the fire dries out the fluid, and if this is not done women will not regain their health, will be susceptible to illness and will be unable to resume hard work (see also Whittaker, this volume). According to Baan Mali women:

> It is good to lie by the fire. It maintains physical strength and health. No muscle-joint-bone pain.
>
> Lying by the fire, drinking hot water and having good medicine encourages bad blood to drain.
>
> I gave birth at the hospital and had a tubal ligation after that. I did not lie by the fire so I am unhealthy. I am prone to have fever and chills, especially in the cool season.

The diet pertaining to the *yuu fai* period is also carefully selected to establish the normal balance between the elements in the human body. Sticky rice, salt, dry fish, hot water, and herbal medicine (normally the heartwood of tamarind tree boiled in water) are common foods and drinks for postpartum women. These foods and drinks are believed to be effective also as drying agents.

Yuu fai is seen as unnecessary in the case of a woman who gives birth at the hospital, because it is believed that the delivery process has drained out all bad blood from the womb, although as one of the quotes above indicates, not all women share this view. Further, regardless of place of birth, beliefs that a postpartum woman should avoid "cold" and keep "hot" remain. Instead of *yuu fai*, a postpartum woman can keep the stomach warm to dry the uterus and help it revert to a "proper location" by placing a thermos or burnt herbs on the abdominal skin for several days (see Muecke, 1976).

Today very few women postpartum practice *yuu fai*, because it is regarded as inconvenient and out-of-date. Over the past decade antenatal, neonatal, and postnatal care has been widely accepted by village women, and their acceptance of maternal and child health services is regarded as one of the successes of the Ministry of Public Health. Pregnant women prefer to give birth in hospital and they are told that *yuu fai* is unnecessary and may cause burns and electrolyte imbalance. Women also believe that western medicine is better than "traditional" medicine in terms of ease of use, absence of taboos, and because it is "up-to-date". Women who give birth at the hospital come back home with vitamins and capsules of antibiotics to prevent perineal infection.

However, women's belief of dangerous fluid inside the womb after giving birth is still strong. Traditionally, it was held that during postpartum, if the womb was not dried, a woman would become weak, be unable to nurse her child, and would not regain energy needed for hard work. In biomedical settings, gynaecologists or midwives also tell women that the lochia should be drained out and that obstruction of lochial flow will cause infection. These statements confirm women's notion that lochia is dangerous. Women do not use sanitary pads to absorb lochia, lest this impair the flow, and they abstain from hard work and sexual intercourse for at least one month to prevent obstacles to lochia flow and to prevent inflammation or infection. Fever and chill are symptoms regarded as caused by residual lochia: bad blood is absorbed and heat in the blood causes fever; its poison causes chill. The poison of lochia can remain in a woman's body for the rest of her life, and whenever her body is weak or the weather is cool, she will become chilled because of the lochia poisoning.

Beliefs of Blood and Menopause

Beliefs in the importance of the drainage of bad blood, and understandings of the significance of the end of menstruation, affect women's desire or lack of desire for menopause. Women who desire menopause believe that at the time of menopause, bad blood is no longer retained in the body so that the bodily mechanism which produces bad blood ceases. Women who do not wish to reach menopause believe that the process of draining bad blood helps them to maintain their youth and be healthy, and they therefore wish to menstruate for as long as possible.

As mentioned earlier, menstruation is regarded by women as an indicator of good health, and its absence is generally seen as negatively influencing women's health. Menopausal women believe that they became weak at the time of menopause and this continues postmenopausally. Some women believe that when a woman becomes old, there is no bad blood so the bodily mechanism of draining bad blood ceases, that is, there is no period. Residual bad blood causes uncomfortable feelings, but after menopause it will be gone. A lucky woman is one who does not have such residual blood, and therefore will feel no difference before and after menopause. Some women also mentioned atrophy of the uterus and ovaries with age, and associate their failure to produce menstrual blood with this. These explanatory models are concerned with natural body mechanisms and natural events in a women's life. Distress that might be experienced during menopause is accepted as a part of this natural process. As some women said:

> We are not talking about menopause; it is a natural event. After menopause nothing changes, whatever you have done, you still do it.
>
> Now I have reached menopause. It [menstrual bleeding] stops. That's all. I don't do anything about it. It is natural. I don't go to see doctor, because I am not sick. It is normal for the old that menstruation become irregular and then it stops. After menopause I felt dizzy and weak. I feel sick, but I don't think it relates to menopause. It is because of my age.

Only dizziness and headache are associated by women with the cessation of menses. Emotional symptoms, in particular, are considered to be a consequence of stressful life events such as family problems and economic constraint, and are not associated with menstrual irregularity (Chirawatkul and Manderson, 1994). Women believe that dizziness, headache and loss of health may occur in peri- and postmenopause. According to one respondent:

> In premenopause, menstrual blood is cleared out monthly. A good clear-out preserves good health. The heavy flow at the final period is mentioned by some women as the last 'clear-out'. Unlucky women whose last clear-out was not 'good enough' would have some residual [bad blood] in the body. Dizziness and headache, therefore, are the result of the retention of bad blood. The residual blood will be drained out later but in different forms such as sweating and urinating. When all the residue is drained out, all distress will go.

Villagers' understandings derive from the observational experiences of body's elimination. Villagers note that sweat, urine, and faeces are unwanted substances that the body has to drain or clear out. If the body fails to clear them out, they cause discomfort. This notion is also applied to menstrual blood and lochia. Women may not perceive the experiences at the time of menopause as "menopausal symptoms" as described by medical personnel. There is evidence as well to suggest that the symptoms of dizziness, irritability and tiredness are not perceived as "symptoms" in terms of illness, but as unstable conditions of air and blood in the body due to age. Those women with such symptoms sought help by asking health personnel for drugs and vitamins to maintain good air and blood, or asking for herbal medicine for the same purpose from the herbalists. Most women consider dizziness and tiredness to be physical conditions of elderly persons, but may associate irritability as an emotional condition of menstrual changes (cf. Rice, this volume).

CONCLUSION

In this chapter, I have shown that popular lay beliefs about the nature of blood are related to perceptions of reproductive health and illness. These perceptions may or may not have a negative consequence for women's health status and health practices. Beliefs that menstrual blood and lochia are bad blood that can poison the body lead women to avoid the obstruction of the flow and to be concerned with cleanliness. Menstruation is regarded as a normal process, a mechanism designed to eliminate waste; menopause is similarly constructed as normal rather than pathological. Premenstrual distress and menopausal symptoms are not regarded as "syndromes" that can or need to be treated, but rather are perceived as non-problematic aspects of reproductive life. This perception takes a woman away from being in a sick role. Traditional practices to maintain "good blood" and health, such as drinking herbal medicine and lying by the fire, may be perceived as out-of-date by the medical personnel or others influenced by biomedical constructions of reproduction. However, such "traditional" practices have cultural meanings for which there is no western medical substitute. For example, in the process of lying by the fire, the husband has to tend to the fire, provide his wife with food and drink, and help his mother or mother-in-law take care of the baby: such rituals provide a structure that supports the new mother and reinforces family identity. It provides psychosocial support to postpartum women which is not provided by biomedical services. Health providers need to understand these beliefs and gain greater awareness of the cultural significance of "traditional" practices to choose the best way to introduce health services and provide appropriate health care.

ENDNOTES

1. In English, blood provides an enduring symbol of kinship ("blood is thicker than water"), health (poor health is "thin blooded", a strong constitution may be "red blooded"), and calculating personality ("in cold blood").
2. According to Manderson (1981b: 519), the confinement and drying period varies cross-culturally and regionally. In northern Thailand, the total confinement runs for some 30 days, but lying by the fire is observed for 15 days (Muecke, 1976). In central Thailand, the period for lying by the fire varies from 3 to 15 days.

REFERENCES

Adams, R.N. (1955) A nutritional research program in Guatemala. In *Health, Culture and Community: Case Studies of Public Health Reactions to Health Programs*, edited by B.D. Paul, pp. 435–458. New York: Russell Sage Foundation.

Bernard, F.E. (1983). *The Peasants of Isaan: Social and Economic Transitions in Northeast Thailand.* Unpublished PhD thesis, University of Wisconsin, Madison.

Chirawatkul, S. (1993) *'Sud Lyad, Sud Luuk': The Social Construction of Menopause in Northeast Thailand.* Unpublished PhD thesis. Brisbane: Tropical Health Program, The University of Queensland.

Chirawatkul, S., Manderson, L. (1994) Perceptions of menopause in Northeast Thailand: contested meaning and practice. *Social Science and Medicine*, **39**(11), 1545–1554.

Davis, D.L. (1988) "Bad blood" and the cultural management of health in a Newfoundland fishing village. In *Women and Health: Cross-Cultural Perspectives*, P. Whelehan and contributors, pp. 5–20. Granby, Massachusetts: Bergin and Garvey Publishers Inc.

Douglas, M. (1966) *Purity and Danger.* London: Routledge and Kegan Paul.

Foster, G.M., Anderson, B.G. (1978) *Medical Anthropology.* New York: John Wiley and Sons.

Golomb, L. (1985) *An Anthropology of curing in Multiethnic Thailand.* Urbana: University of Illinois Press.

Gould-Martin, K. (1978) Hot cold poison and dirt: Chinese folk medical categories. *Social Science and Medicine*, **12**, 39–46.

Helman, C. (1990) *Culture, Health and Illness: An introduction for health professionals.* Bristol: Wright.

Kay, M., Yoder, M. (1987) Hot and cold in women's ethnotherapeutics: the American-Mexican West. *Social Science and Medicine*, **25**, 347–355.

Keyes, C.F. (1967) *Isan: Religion in Northeastern Thailand.* Data Paper 65. Ithaca, NY: Cornell University, Southeast Asian Program.

Kleinman, A. (1980) *Patients and Healers in the Context of Culture.* Berkeley: University of California Press.

Like, R., Ellison, J. (1981) Sleeping blood, tremor and paralysis: a transcultural approach to an unusual conversion reaction. *Culture, Medicine and Psychiatry*, **5**, 49–63.

Loudon, J.B. (1977) On body products. In *The Anthropology of the Body*, edited by J. Blacking, pp. 161–178. London: Academic Press.

Manderson, L. (1981a) Traditional food beliefs and critical life events in Peninsular Malaysia. *Social Science Information*, **20**(6), 947–75.

Manderson, L. (1981b) Roasting, smoking and dieting in response to birth: Malay confinement in cross-cultural perspective. *Social Science and Medicine*, **15B**, 509–520.

Manderson, L. (1986) Nature, culture, hot and cold: food classification and restriction in Peninsular Malaysia. In *Shared Wealth and Symbol: Food, Culture and Society in Oceania and Southeast Asia*, edited by L. Manderson, pp. 127–143. New York: Cambridge University Press.

Martin, E. (1987) *The Woman in the Body*. Boston: Beacon Press.

Muecke, M. (1976) Health care system as socializing agent: childbearing the north Thai and western way. *Social Science and Medicine*, **10**, 377–383.

Paul, B.D. (editor) (1955) *Health, Culture and Community*. New York: Sage.

Phongphit, S., Hewison, K. (1990) *Northeastern Village Life*. Bangkok: Village Foundation.

Pillsbury, B.L.K. (1978) 'Doing the month': confinement and convalescence of Chinese women after birth. *Social Science and Medicine*, **12**, 11–22.

Snow, L.F. (1976) 'High blood' is not high blood pressure. *Urban Health*, **5**, 54–55.

CHAPTER 13

Only When I Have Borne all my Children!: The Menopause in Hmong Women

Pranee Liamputtong Rice

Menopause is a universal event in the lives of all women. Biomedically, menopause is seen as a biological event and prior to the mid seventies it was characterised as an estrogen deficiency disease (Wilson, 1966; Kase, 1974; Weideger, 1977; Kaufert and Gilbert, 1986). Social scientists argue, however, that menopause is a sociocultural event. The physical changes of menopause are only one part of women's life experiences. They are interwoven with the woman's social status, sex role, personal circumstances, life history and stage of health.[1] Rosenberger, for example, points out that:

> while menopause has a biological base, it is an experience that differs according to cultural values. Menopause draws its meanings from more basic concepts within the culture such as the meaning of women's reproductive power, the role of women in the social structure and the relationship of the physical and the psychological (1986:15).

In her paper on "myth and the menopause", Kaufert (1982:144) puts forward a similar argument. She states that:

> like childbirth and menstruation, there are two levels of reality to menopause. One is the actual physical changes that occur in a woman... all women who survive and have intact ovaries pass through the menopause. 'Passage through the menopause' is also an event occurring within a socio-cultural context. It is this — the cultural dimension of the menopause — which forms the second level of its reality.

Kaufert argues that a woman who belongs to a culture that perceives the menopause as symptom-free will not experience menopausal symptoms related to physical changes in mid life such as hot flushes and depression. These women pass through the menopause without difficulty.

In this paper the experience of Hmong women who migrated from the high mountainous areas in Laos and are now living in Australia is used as a paradigm case to analyse the cultural interpretations of menopause. Following the framework of Kaufert, the paper examines two realities: the meaning of menopause, and the experience of changes as perceived by Hmong women.

THE HMONG

The Hmong women who are participants of this study are refugees from Southeast Asia. They have been accepted as immigrants in Australia since 1975, although the majority of them have recently arrived. The Hmong in Australia come from Laos, where they lived in small villages in the high mountainous areas. Embroiled in the fighting between the American forces and the Pathet Laos, the communist group in Laos, the Hmong were forced to move out of their homeland in the mountains and escaped to Thailand. The majority were then accepted to resettle in the USA. In Australia the main concentration of the Hmong is in New South Wales, though there are some Hmong in Tasmania and an increasing number also in Queensland. In Victoria the Hmong live in close knit groups, mainly in highrise public housing in Fitzroy, an inner Melbourne suburb, and in Coolaroo, an outer northeastern suburb.

In general the Hmong are much poorer than other Southeast Asian refugees. The majority are unemployed. Most did not have any form of formal education in Laos because of the war and their geographic position, and because they are recent arrivals, they are still learning English.

The Hmong are animistic and follow ancestral worship. They believe in reincarnation, the rebirth cycle. They are patrilineal and patrilocal, with family names following the clan system. There are nine clans in Melbourne.

The usual Hmong family is large. Most women in this study have about four to six children, and it is likely that they will continue to bear more children. Traditionally, the Hmong put a high value on having many children, particularly boys, since they can help in farming and continue traditional practices such as worshipping ancestral spirits and caring for their parents in old age. Such traditional customs (except for the farming) are still practised, even though they are now living in Australia.

The demographic characteristics of Hmong women in this study are presented in Table 13.1.

THE STUDY

This chapter reports the results of an ethnographic study concerning reproductive health among Southeast Asian women who are now living in Australia. The groups in this study included Hmong, Lao, Vietnamese, Cambodian, and Thai communities.

I conducted ethnographic interviews covering a number of issues concerning reproductive health, including the beliefs and practices related to childbearing, menstruation and menopause, with 23 Hmong women in Melbourne, Victoria. The majority of the women had experienced childbirth while living in Laos or in a refugee camp in Thailand as well as in hospitals in Melbourne. The women were individually interviewed in their own homes. All interviews were conducted in the Hmong language with the assistance of a bi-cultural research assistant, Blia Ly, who is a Hmong native born woman. She has worked for and represented the Hmong community in Melbourne for more than ten years and is well known and accepted by most Hmong here.

TABLE 13.1   Characteristics of Hmong women.

Characteristics	Number	Percentage
Age		
20–30	6	26.09
31–40	8	34.78
41–50	4	17.39
over 51	5	21.74
Marital status		
Married	18	78.26
de facto	1	4.35
Widowed	4	17.39
Number of children		
1–3	4	17.39
4–6	14	60.87
7–9	1	4.35
10 and over	4	17.39
Level of education		
None	17	73.91
Primary	6	26.09
Current activities		
Home duties	16	69.57
Learning English for migrants	7	30.43
Number of years in Australia		
1–3	6	26.09
4–6	13	56.52
7 and over	4	17.39
Number of family members living in the house		
1–3	2	8.70
4–6	8	34.78
7–9	9	39.13
10 and over	4	17.39
Length of stay in refugee camp in Thailand		
1–3 years	4	17.39
4–6 years	2	8.70
7–9 years	5	21.74
10 years and over	12	52.17
Menopausal status		
Premenopausal	14	60.87
Postmenopausal	9	39.13

Informed consent was obtained after the information about the research and the woman's participation was clearly explained to her. Each interview was tape recorded. The length of the interviews varied, depending on the women's responses. In general, each interview took between two and three hours. Most women were interviewed once. There were, however, a number of occasions when I needed to obtain more information. Those women were then visited for a second time. In addition, participant observation was used to allow me to observe and record the Hmong cultural practices and experiences in Australia more fully. I attended a number of Hmong ceremonies and participated in Hmong activities. The interviews and participant observation were conducted between May 1993 and February 1994.

A content analysis approach was used to derive patterns in Hmong women's beliefs and practices. Put simply, recordings of interviews were transcribed for detailed analysis. The transcripts were examined for the women's explanations related to the concept concerned. From these, several themes were derived. In this chapter, I describe those that relate to women's understandings and experience of menopause.

THE MEANING OF MENOPAUSE

In the Hmong language, there is no equivalent word for menopause. The concept of menopause is understood as *tsis coj khaub ncaws lawm*, which literally means "no more menstruation". In general, menopause is associated with *pog laus*: the terminology used for an old lady, an older person or a grandmother, and is seen as a natural part of "growing old".

No More Children, No More Menstruation

Menopause is interpreted as the consequence of transition from fertility to infertility. Hmong women perceive that women reach menopause only when they are no longer fertile; they have borne all of their children. The following conversation illustrates the point:

Pranee: How old is a woman when her menstruation stops completely?

Xee: After you have all of your children... I don't know how old, it depends on the person. Some will have only seven or eight children and then their children will be finished and have no more, but some others will have over ten children before they finish their children, and that is when you have no more menstruation.

Women were quite definite about this: "With Hmong people their children are definitely finished before their menses stop"; and again, "My children have finished, that is why I don't have it any more. After I had the youngest son in 1985, it just stopped". Most Hmong women believe that in a lifetime, a fertile woman may become pregnant up to 13 or 14 times. Women also believe that early menarche indicates early menopause. Hmong people say that if you have your menses when you are about 10 or 12, you will cease menstruation early also. Even if you are not very old it will stop. But if your menarche is delayed until the age of 14 or 15, then you will still have your menses when you are quite old. All postmenopausal women in this study became menopausal relatively young, when they were in their early 40s (mean age is 43 years old).

Women, once married, are expected to bear many children. Having born her first child, a Hmong woman has fulfilled her most important role for the family since she is able to provide continuity for the patrilineage. Most women believe that they must have at least as many children as their mother or mother-in-law (Symonds, 1991). Children, particularly male children, are the asset of the family. Children are necessary for one's well-being, not only in this life but also the afterlife. If a woman does not bear children there will be no one to look after her in old age. More importantly, if she does not have sons, then there will be no one to care for the family altar and feed the ancestors, including her when she dies. This makes having children a vital part of life for Hmong women (see also Symonds, this volume).

Due to this, some women regretted being no longer able to bear children. However, the majority of Hmong women have already borne many children. They thought that menopause was a positive aspect of their life. The following conversation illustrates this:

Pranee: Do you think no more menses is a good thing or a bad thing?
Dia: It is a good thing.
Pranee: In what sense do you say it is a good thing?
Dia: It is good in that I will have no more children... I am getting old and very tired of looking after children and if I don't have any more then it does not matter.

When I prompted the women with the importance of bearing children and if it would worry them once they had no more menstruation, their answers had much in common with the following explanation:

No more menstruation does not bother me. I think that I have no more children and I am happy that I have finished my children, I have done my duty of being a Hmong woman. So when my menstruation stops I am not worried about it.

Menopause, Change of Role and Status

Hmong girls and adolescents do not have equal social or familial status to Hmong boys and men. However, their status changes when they marry and are able to bear a child. The birth of the first child brings prestige to a Hmong woman. After giving birth to her first child a Hmong woman becomes "Par's mother". She is no longer addressed as "my younger daughter" by her parents, nor as "woman of Lee" by others (Symonds, 1991). Women gain respect and status from all when they produce children. The woman's status changes again once she becomes old. Older women are referred to as *cov txwj laus* (respected elders) and are addressed as *pog laus* (grandmother) by all (Symonds, 1991). Since menopause is associated with old age, postmenopausal women are, therefore, respected and have higher status than when they were still young.

Once women reach menopause, their role shifts from childbearing to childrearing; from caring for their own children to looking after their grandchildren. Women said that their life with children did not end with menopause. By the time Hmong women reach menopause, their daughters or daughter-in-laws have already begun to bear children. Older women help in rearing and looking after their older grandchildren while their daughters or daughter-in-laws are engaged in childbearing, nursing and caring for infants, in conducting other domestic activities, or working (in Laos) in the field. "Older women do not bear more children. At that time your children will be older and you can just relax, but if they have some children then you help them with their children".

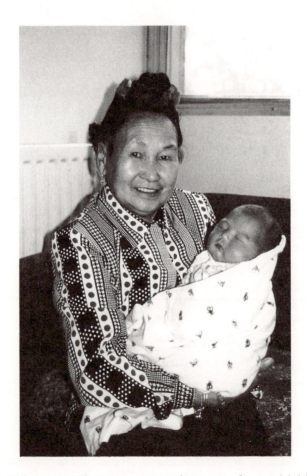

FIGURE 13.1   Older women play an important role in caring for grandchildren. Grandma Va nurses her granddaughter. (Photo: P.L. Rice).

MENOPAUSE AND AGEING

Women associated menopause with ageing. When a woman reaches menopause she is old: "Now I think that I am old and that I will have no more children. I have had many children and that is why it is finished and that is why I don't have any more menses"; "I think that when you are old you run out of that menstruation blood, you have no more of it". The majority of Hmong women did not see ageing as problematic. Since by this time their children would have all grown up, they did not need to be as concerned about the survival and well-being of their children as they were when the children were younger: "I am not too worried about getting old. By that time my children would have all grown up and I don't need to be worried about being poor, if it would be enough food to feed them, or if it would be enough clothes to keep them warm, that sort of thing". The Hmong have a strong belief in the Confucian values of filial piety; traditionally and commonly practised among the Chinese. Adult children have a duty to look after and take good care of their aged parents. Among the Hmong the duty extends to the period after the death of their parents. Male children continue to feed and worship their deceased parents to ensure their reincarnation (Yang, 1992).

However, some Hmong women felt worried about being old. They associated old age with being "near death". To them, this meant that they would not be with their children and grandchildren for much longer: "I am worried that I am getting old and I may not live long any more because when you get old then you will die, that is what I think about"; "I feel sorry that I am getting old and that all that is waiting for me now is death".

UNDERSTANDINGS OF MENSTRUATION

Menstruation, like menopause, is women's business. Hmong women believe that women and menstruation are inextricably linked at a conceptual level. Being a woman means to menstruate. In fact, the term commonly used to mean menstruation by the Hmong is *ua poj niam*, which literally means being a woman. Menstruation is essential for a woman to be able to bear children: "For women, menstruation is a natural part of life and if you don't have it then you will not be able to have children".

During the monthly cycle menstrual blood is retained in the woman's womb. The womb functions as "a dam" and the blood is kept in it to be ready to "make" and "feed" the foetus. If the foetus is not "made" at the end of that month, the blood then turns "bad" and it needs to be expelled. The retaining of the "bad" blood causes ill health in women. Common symptoms include being pale and skinny, having dull eyes, and having no energy. It is also believed to lead to death if the bad blood is retained in the woman's womb for a lengthy period of time.

Despite its importance for conception, menstruation is seen as polluted, shameful and embarrassing, as reflected in the interviews. Very often women made remarks about the embarrassment and shame of menstruation: "I am telling you this, if we talk about your body having that dirty thing, with the Hmong, it is the most embarrassing thing to talk about"; "It is a shameful thing but you have to have it for you to have children. If you say it is a likeable thing, no it is not, I don't like it".

Because of the perceived pollution of menstrual blood, there are a number of prohibitions associated with menstruation. Sexual intercourse during menstruation is avoided. Men do not wish to have intercourse with their menstruating wives due to the "unclean" nature of menstruation. Women are warned not to cross rivers or streams while menstruating, and the clothes worn while menstruating are not washed in rivers or streams as Hmong believe that the spirits of the streams may become angry. The spirits are able to trace a woman through the smell of her menstruation and "strike" her. This causes miscarriage whenever she conceives. Repeated miscarriages in turn cause infertility in the woman, seriously affecting a woman's social status and security (see also Symonds, this volume).

> If you are menstruating and you go into the swamps or river at the moment the spirits wake up you will be struck by them... If the spirits touch you then you are going to miscarry... When you get pregnant they will come and destroy it.
>
> When you have your periods you should not go to wash your clothes in a river or throw the dirty water into the river. If you do this you can be struck by the spirit and this will cause you to be sick. And when you get married it will cause you not to have any children and it is very hard to fix this.

Because menopause meant no more menses, menopause was seen by the women interviewed as a state wherein women were no longer polluted and were clean. Women looked forward to this stage. A postmenopausal woman remarked, "I hated that dirty thing very much so when I became clean, then I was very happy I did not have any more of that, that I did not have to be embarrassed towards other people any more". Very often the women compared themselves, when they reached menopause, as being "clean" like a man — in ways rather reminiscent of Skultans' study of Welsh women (1972). This was particularly so when I asked what they thought about ceasing menstruation. Typical answers were:

> Good, it is the best thing that can happen to you, no more children and you are very clean like the men.
>
> You will just be like a man, if you don't have any of that menstruation, then it is good...it won't be difficult for you ...
>
> For me, my menses became very bad and I hated it so much I got some herbs and took them. After taking the herbs I became very clean like the men.

MENOPAUSE AND HEALTH

Postmenopausal women in the study were asked if there were any physical changes which occurred after the cessation of menstruation. Interestingly, the women could not remember any physical changes after they became menopausal. However, all women could recall that their menstruation became irregular, lighter in particular, in the last year of their reproductive life. "When it nearly stopped it was lighter than usual, it did not come as heavy as usual, and then it stopped...and I have not had it since then"... "It became lighter and lighter and then just stopped. It ran its normal cycle and when it was time it just stopped". No women reported hot flashes, flushes or night sweating, and most said nothing changed physically.

> I have no effect from not having the menses. I still have good appetite but maybe I am old, that is why it is hard for me to have put on weight but my appetite is the same and my health is the same...
> I have not had any bad health since it stopped. I am today the same as I was before, no problems.

Given that older women neither anticipated nor experienced ill health with menopause, a number were surprised to learn that many Australian women experienced some ill health at the time of menopause. They interpreted this as not observing traditional restrictions after childbirth the way Hmong women would do. Hmong women observe particular confinement practices in the first month after giving birth, during which time — at least for the first three days after delivery — the woman must lie near a fire for most of the day (see also Symonds, this volume). They believe that because a woman loses blood in childbirth, her body becomes "cold". The practices to regain body heat lost in childbirth are therefore essential in order to avoid bad health in old age. During the confinement period, a woman must eat only hot rice and chicken soup cooked with several special green herbs. Any cold food such as fresh vegetables and fruits is prohibited. Cold water is particularly dangerous to a new mother (Rice, 1993, 1994). These confinement practices, the Hmong believe, are protective for a woman and hence she will not have any ill health in old age. Therefore, any symptoms of ill health which occur from middle age onward are interpreted as resulting from not following traditional confinement practices during childbearing years.

Women were also asked if they had experienced any emotional change or difficulties during or after menopause. Again women said that they had not experienced any. A common answer was that: "there is nothing, I am very comfortable and very happy...I am happy with my life, my children and my grandchildren. Nothing like that (emotional problems) has happened to me". I also asked women whether their health in general had changed after menopause. Women found it rather amusing that I should ask such a question. Some made remarks like:

> This is a natural part of growing old and when it stops because you are old then there should not be anything wrong with your health.
> When you are old and you just don't have it any more your health will still be the same as before, there is nothing wrong with not having any more menstruation because you are old.

The same question was raised with premenopausal women. Most women believed that the cessation of menstruation would not make them unhealthy. It would, however, have an effect on their "strength": "When you do not menstruate, when you are about forty-five or so, you are old and can't do many things. You won't be as strong as before so you can't do too many things". Women also believed that once menstruation ceased a woman may gradually become blind and this was seen as being associated with old age. "They say that if you don't have that [menstruation] it makes you go blind. I can't thread the needle any more. That is what happens, it is a sign of getting older. When you get older you have no more blood so that you can't see as well as before".

DISCUSSION AND CONCLUSION

This chapter examines the meaning and experience of menopause among Hmong women. Menopause is seen as a natural part of life which any *pog laus* has to experience; it is part of growing old. By the time the women become menopausal they have borne all of their children and their children have grown up. They therefore have done their duty: the duty of motherhood being to ensure the continuity of the family lineage by giving birth to their sons, and to daughters to bring in son-in-laws. Once the women reach this stage they are more respected and they become a "grandmother" to all. As Chirawatkul (this volume) also describes for women in northeastern Thailand, women are pleased that they do not have to deal with the monthly business of menstruation. They no longer feel ashamed about menstruating and do not have to worry about being embarrassed from it. Women are able to feel more relaxed once their menstruation ceases. It is not surprising then that the Hmong women interviewed mostly welcomed menopause. However, some women were ambivalent about menopause, for they saw it as a physical prewarning of entering a "near death" stage; thus they would not have much time left with their children and grandchildren.

In this study Hmong women reported no physical changes apart from irregular menstruation in the last year of their reproductive life. Women did not recall any other physical symptoms that occurred in that year nor after their menstruation had ceased. This positive attitude and experience of menopause can be discussed by examining the nature of menopause within theoretical anthropological frameworks.

Positive Attitudes Toward Menopause

Kaufert (1982:145) writes:

> The menopause marks the end of fertility, and attitudes towards the menopause will be the product of the status of women in society, to the extent that the latter reflects the value attached to their reproductive capacity. To understand what the menopause means in the lives of women in any particular society, the event must be set within the full context of women's role within that society.

Like Kaufert, Brown (1985) demonstrates that in traditional societies the change in a woman's life in middle age appears to be positive. In most pre-industrial societies, a young woman is restricted and her life is "subservience and toil". A number of major changes occur at mid-life. Once she is middle-aged, she has greater authority and is allowed more leisure. They are freed from many restrictions imposed on them when younger, including menstrual restrictions as well as limitations on mobility and lack of personal autonomy. They have authority over younger kin, including the right to make important decisions for them. They are also eligible for special status and this allows them to have more freedom, to no longer be confined to the household. All of these changes improve the status of middle-aged women and it is this improvement that makes the meaning of menopause positive.

Bart's theory (1969) on the influence of status on women's experiences of menopause draws similar conclusions. Bart argues that the increased social status of women with ageing protects them from negative experiences of menopause. This is commonly found in traditional societies where kinship retains its pre-eminent role in social organisation and economic life. According to Bart, there are six cultural characteristics that serve to protect middle aged women. These are "strong ties to family of origin and kin, extended family system, the residence patterns keeping one close to the family of orientation, strong mother-child relationship reciprocal in later life, institutionalised grandmother role, and institutionalised mother-in-law role" (Bart, 1969:14). The Hmong are patrilineal and patrilocal. A woman moves into her husband's home after marriage, but this does not reduce her ties with her natal kin. Extended family networks are maintained and several generations may reside together in one household. The Hmong also have a strong mother-child reciprocal relationship. An aged mother is looked after and taken good care of by her adult children. When her sons are married, daughters-in-law are brought into her house. She then has the duty to teach and train her daughters-in-law to be good wives and mothers. Once she becomes a grandmother, her role changes from bearing her children to rearing grandchildren, and she is respected by all.

Nevertheless, Bart argues that there are three significant cultural traits which improve women's status in midlife: extended menstrual taboos, age valued over youth, and reproductive importance. The relationships between extended menstrual taboos and women's status are also found in studies of menopause among Mayan and Indian women (Beyene, 1986, 1989; du Toit, 1990) . Both Beyene and du Toit found that the majority of the women in their studies did not see menopause as the end of life. Menopause was, in fact, seen as "a very liberating event" that led them to a higher "status". This was due to enforced taboos and rituals associated with menstruation in the women's cultures. Women achieved their "status" when their reproductive role ended, and thus the taboos and restrictions of menstruation were lifted. The Hmong believe in the polluting nature of menstruation and women are perceived as "polluted" or "unclean" when they are still menstruating. This is reflected in a number of taboos associated with menstruation. A Hmong woman becomes "like a man" who has higher status once she reaches menopause. As such, menopause is viewed positively. In addition, the Hmong value age over youth, and women gain status as they are ageing. Once a woman becomes a grandmother her status is much higher than before. These indeed make the meaning of menopause positive for Hmong women.

Barnett's study (1988) in a small Peruvian town found most postmenopausal women were relatively satisfied with their menopausal situation. Barnett argues that their satisfaction was linked to sociocultural factors such as the cultural recognition of adulthood which is only granted to women and men over forty, the end of the daily and direct responsibility of caring for their children, and the satisfaction of fulfilling the role of grandmother. Barnett also suggests that the internal rewards that accompany a woman's sense of accomplishment in her own principal role are equally important and are significant in determining the woman's perceptions of menopause. The present study indicates that at menopause Hmong women believe they have fulfilled their role as a Hmong mother and therefore menopause is seen as a stage to reap the rewards for this. Both Barnett (1988) and Kaufert (1982) note that in traditional societies, older women tend to enjoy great power and prestige. However, this is contingent on their earlier ability to bear and raise children. Women without children — either because they are infertile or their children do not survive — face economic and social deprivation. The menopause ends their hope of becoming pregnant and having children. Women in these situations may perceive menopause as negative and not welcome it. From my data, Hmong women have gained power and prestige by fulfilling social expectations of reproduction: having borne many children and having children survive to carry on their lineage.

The Experiences of Menopause

While menopause is inevitable for all women, physiological and emotional symptoms are not universal (Voda, 1993). Women in some cultures do not experience menopausal symptoms at all; in others they experience different symptoms, or similar symptoms at a different frequency (Kaufert, 1982; Chirawatkul, 1993). Flint (1975), for example, found that very few women of the Rajput caste in the states of Rajasthan and Himachal Pradesh had problems with their menopause other than changes of menstrual cycle. Flint reports that "there were no depressions, dizziness, no incapacitation nor any of the symptoms associated with what we call 'the menopausal syndrome'" (Flint, 1975:162). Similar to Flint, Beyene (1986, 1989) reports the absence of any menopausal symptom in Mayan women. Flint (1975) argues that this absence of symptoms can be explained by the "reward" gained by women when they reach menopause. The "reward" is granted to a woman when she can no longer bear children. At menopause she is allowed to partake of what was "forbidden" during childbearing years. For example, the Rajput women have to live in purdah (veiled and secluded) until their menopause; thereafter they are no longer considered to be polluted. More importantly, their status is much more elevated than before menopause. Flint further argues that most American women suffer severe menopausal symptoms since menopause is a time of "punishment", when children are leaving home and their husbands are suffering various crises of ageing and identity also. American women do not gain status in old age either. The life of Hmong women fits very well with Flint's theory of "reward and punishment", and this may help to explain their absence of symptoms.

Beyene (1989) proposes a "biocultural analysis" to explain the absence and presence of menopausal symptoms. She puts forward three hypotheses for the absence of symptoms. First, this may be due to the women's positive attitudes toward menopause. When childbearing is over, a woman can be free. Second, the low nutritional status of women may lead to early onset of menopause and asymptomatology among Mayan women. Beyene found that Mayan women were already postmenopausal in their mid-forties, while most women in industrial nations are just entering the menopause. Hmong women in this study similarly reach their menopause when they are about mid-forties. Similar to the Mayan women, their nutritional status is low. Their living situations in Laos were relatively poor due to their geographic location, and to the war and its concomitant hardships. Even when they were placed in refugee camps in Thailand and re-settled in Australia, their situation did not improve a great deal. Last, Beyene argues that interference with normal reproductive function through the use of contraceptive drugs and interventions to prevent pregnancy, common among Westernised women, may result in menopausal symptoms. The majority of Hmong women interviewed did not use any western birth control drugs or devices until they came to refugee camps in Thailand or after settlement in Australia. Traditionally, Hmong women keep bearing children until menopause, with little interference with reproductive functions. Beyene's three hypotheses may indeed explain or contribute to the absence of menopausal symptoms among Hmong women in this study.

I have agreed that the Hmong women interviewed in Melbourne continue to perceive menopause as positive and that they experience few so-called menopausal symptoms. However, the longer most Hmong women live here, the greater the process of adaption to living in a western environment. They are faced with many changes and these changes may have consequences for the way in which menopause is perceived and experienced. Because of the availability of western health care and the relative unavailability of traditional herbal medicines and healers in Australia, women seek help from mainstream health services when they experience ill health of any kind. This inevitably puts women in mid life into contact with current medical interpretations of menopause. Roberts (1985) has pointed out that once a woman reaches 40 years of age, doctors tend to bring the menopause into all their discussions of her health; increasingly in industrialised and industrialising countries including Thailand, this has led to discussions of the use of hormone replacement therapy (HRT) too (Chirawatkul, 1993). The question to be asked here is: will this result in Hmong women interpreting menopause as medical event, and in consequence, will they begin to experience menopausal symptoms as many Australian women do? Although evidence from previous studies which have examined women's lives in rapidly changing societies has indicated this may be the case (Datan, Antonovsky and Moaz, 1981; Flint and Samil, 1990; Lock, 1991; Chirawatkul, 1993; Chirawatkul and Manderson, 1994), it remains to be seen what will happen for Hmong women now living in Australia.

ACKNOWLEDGMENTS

An earlier version of this chapter appeared as "Pog laus, tsis coj khaub ncaws lawm: The meaning of menopause in Hmong women" in the *Journal of Reproductive and Infant Psychology*, **13**, 79–92, 1996. Reprinted with permission. I am indebted to the Hmong women who participated in this study and to Blia Ly, my bi-cultural research assistant who assisted me in the interviews and her contributed knowledge about Hmong culture. I should like to thank Rhonda Small and Dr Helen Jonas for their valuable comments in the preparation of this paper.

ENDNOTE

1. See, inter alia, Bart, 1969; Flint, 1975; van Keep and Kellerhals, 1975; Townsend & Carbone, 1980; Lock, 1982; Brown, 1985; Davis, 1986; Beyene, 1986; Barnett, 1988; Kaufert, 1982; Chirawatkul, 1992, 1993; Chirawatkul and Manderson, 1994.

REFERENCES

Barnett, E.A. (1988) *La Edad Critica:* The positive experience of menopause in a small Peruvian town. In *Women and Health: Cross-Cultural Perspectives*, edited by P. Whelan, pp. 40–54. Massachusetts: Bergin & Garvey Publications

Bart, P. (1969) Why women's status changes in middle age. *Sociological Symposium*, **3**, 1–18.

Beyene, Y. (1986) Cultural significance and physiological manifestations of menopause: a biocultural analysis. *Culture, Medicine and Psychiatry*, **10**(1), 47–71.

Beyene, Y. (1989) *From Menarche to Menopause: Reproductive Lives of Peasant Women in Two Cultures,* Albany: State University of New York Press.

Brown, J.K. (1985) Introduction. In *In Her Prime: A New View of Middle-Aged Women*, edited by J.K. Brown, V. Kerns, pp. 1–12. South Hadley, Massachusetts: Bergin and Harvey publishers.

Chirawatkul, S. (1992) *The Social Construction of Menopause in Northeastern Thailand*. Paper presented at the Fourth Tropical Health and Nutrition Conference. Brisbane: The University of Queensland.

Chirawatkul, S. (1993) *'Sud Lyad, Sud Luuk': The Social Construction of Menopause in Northeastern Thailand*. Unpublished PhD thesis. Brisbane: Tropical Health Program, The University of Queensland.

Chirawatkul, S. Manderson, L. (1994) Perceptions of menopause in Northeast Thailand: Contested meaning and practice. *Social Science and Medicine*, **39**(11), 1545–1554.

Davis, D.L. (1986) The meaning of menopause in a Newfoundland fishing village. *Culture, Medicine and Psychiatry*, **10** (1), 73–94.

Datan, N., Antonovsky, A., Moaz, B. (1981) *A Time to Reap: The Middle Age of Women in Five Israeli Subcultures*. Baltimore: Johns Hopkins University Press.

du Toit, B.M. (1990) *Aging and Menopause Among Indian South African Women*. New York: State University of New York Press.

Flint, M. (1975) The menopause: reward or punishment. *Psychosomatic*, **XVI**, 161–163.

Flint, M., Samil, R.S. (1990) Cultural and subcultural meanings of the menopause. *Annals of the New York Academy of Sciences*, **592**, 134–148.

Kase, N. (1974) Estrogens and the menopause. *JAMA*, **227**, 318–319.

Kaufert, P.A. (1982) Myth and the menopause. *Sociology of Health and Illness,*, 4(2), 141–166.

Kaufert, P., Gilbert, P. (1986) Women, menopause and medicalization. *Culture, Medicine and Psychiatry*, **10** (1), 7–21.

Lock, M. (1982) Models and practice in medicine: menopause as syndrome or life transition? *Culture, Medicine and Psychiatry*, **6**, 261–280.

Lock, M. (1991) Contested meanings of the menopause. *The Lancet*, **337**, 1270–1272

Rice, P.L. (1993) *My Forty Days: A Cross-Cultural Resource Book for Health Care Professionals in Birthing Services*. Melbourne: The Vietnamese Antenatal/Postnatal Support Project.

Rice, P.L. (1994) When I had my baby here! In *Asian Mothers, Australian Birth: Pregnancy, Childbirth and Childrearing — The Asian Experiences in an English Speaking Country*, edited by P.L. Rice, pp. 117–132. Melbourne: Ausmed Publications.

Roberts, H. (1985) *The Patient Patients: Women and their Doctors*. London: Pandora Press.

Rosenberger, N. (1986) Menopause as a symbol of anomaly: the case of Japanese women. In *Culture, Society and Menstruation*, edited by V.L. Olesen, N.F. Woods, pp. 15–24. New York: Hemisphere Publications.

Skultans, V. (1972) The significance of menstruation and the menopause. *Man*, **5**, 639–651.

Symonds, P.V. (1991) *Cosmology and the Cycle of Life: Hmong Views of Birth, Death and Gender in a Mountain Village in Northern Thailand*. Unpublished doctoral dissertation. Bardon: Department of Anthropology, Brown University.

Townsend, J.M., Carbone, C.L. (1980) Menopausal syndrome: Illness or social role — a transcultural analysis. *Culture, Medicine and Psychiatry*, **4**(3), 229–248.

van Keep, P., Kellerhals, J. (1975) The aging woman. About the influence of some social and cultural factors on the change in attitude and behaviours that occur after menopause. *Acta Obstetrica Gynecology Scandinavia (Suppl)*, **51**, 19–27.

Voda, A. (1993) Books review. *Signs: Journal of Women in Culture and Society*, Winter: 447–451.

Weideger, P. (1977) *Menstruation and Menopause: The Physical and Psychology, the Myth and the Reality*. Harmondsworth: Penguin Books.

Wilson, P. (1966) *Female Forever*. New York: M. Evans.

Yang, D. (1992) The Hmong: enduring traditions. In *Minority Cultures of Laos: Kammu, Lua', Hmong and Iu-Mien*, edited by J. Lewis, pp. 249–326. Rancho Cordova: Southeast Asia Community Resource Centre.

CHAPTER 14

"Vectors" and "Protectors": Women and HIV/AIDS in the Lao People's Democratic Republic

Angela Savage

The threat of the Acquired Immune Deficiency Syndrome (AIDS) to women in Southeast Asia is largely the result of neglect. Women's risks of infection with the Human Immunodeficiency Virus (HIV) entered the institutional and public consciousness at a relatively late stage in the pandemic (Panos, 1990) and there is an ongoing resistance to seeing AIDS and other sexually transmissible diseases (STDs) as reproductive health issues. On the other hand, the "window of opportunity" (Petersen, 1992:44) for introducing large-scale prevention programs before a critical mass of people were infected with HIV has effectively been lost with an estimated 2.5 million Asians believed to be HIV-positive (WHO, 1994). While the reasons for this neglect are beyond the scope of this chapter, the results must be set against the global context in which the AIDS threat is constructed and responses developed.[1]

The main purpose of the study on which this chapter is based was to generate discussion among Lao and expatriate agencies to develop effective, gender-sensitive AIDS prevention activities at the grass-roots level. At the same time, without substantial changes to the economic and social status of women in developing countries in general, these activities cannot "prevent" the pandemic so much as attenuate its damaging effects.

The greatest risks to women in the Lao People's Democratic Republic for HIV infection are poverty and gender relations. In this chapter I explore AIDS stereotypes to demonstrate how gender relations impact on wider structural factors, in turn to influence perceptions of the AIDS threat and the shaping of the epidemiological profile itself. Women's increased susceptibility to HIV infection is examined and then compared with the diversity of women's perceptions of their own risk. Finally, the implications for the design and implementation of intervention strategies are discussed.

This chapter is based on over two years of fieldwork, initially as a participant-observer, more recently as an AIDS prevention worker, in the two largest cities in the Lao PDR: Vientiane, the capital (population 180,000), and Savannakhet, 640 km south of Vientiane along the Mekong River (population 45,000). It focuses on younger, urban-dwelling, ethnic Lao people[2] whose risk status is influenced by their position at the forefront of the changes presently taking place in the Lao PDR.

TABLE 14.1   Profile of ARC survey respondents by occupation and gender (1,050 respondents).

Occupation	Male	Female	Total %
1. High school student	91	73	15.6%
2. College student	69	28	8.5%
3. University student	56	28	8.0%
4. Farmer	9	3	1.1%
5. Construction/factory worker	100	6	10.1%
6. Business/office worker	85	62	14.0%
7. Merchant	32	61	8.9%
8. Teacher	33	43	7.2%
9. Hotel/restaurant/bar worker	35	84	11.4%
10. Health worker	3	3	0.6%
11. Unemployed	64	37	9.6%
12. Police	9	2	1.0%
13. Soldier	13	2	1.4%
14. Hairdresser	1	–	0.1%
15. *Samlor* driver, transport worker	20	1	2.0%
16. Media worker	–	2	0.2%
17. Housewife	–	1	0.1%

Fieldwork data were tested against the results of a survey of 1,050 young people aged 15–30, in April–May 1994, conducted on behalf of the Australian Red Cross (ARC) to support the Lao Red Cross (LRC) AIDS prevention program and designed to obtain both quantitative and qualitative data. In each city, teams made up of ten local researchers were used in an effort to create a relaxed atmosphere for the interviews. Two Australian women and Lao language students resident at Dong Dok University in Vientiane were deployed to ask 150 respondents direct questions about sexual and drug use behaviour and were used as "outsiders" to ask the more confrontational questions because they could not be identified by respondents as representing the Lao authorities.[3]

A demographic profile of respondents, believed to be a fairly representative sample of the 15–30 year population in the two cities, is shown in Table 14.1.

COUNTRY PROFILE: THE LAO PDR

The Lao People's Democratic Republic is a predominantly mountainous, land-locked country in the centre of the Southeast Asian peninsula, sharing large borders with Thailand and Vietnam to the west and east respectively, and smaller border areas with Burma and China to the north, and Cambodia to the south. The estimated population in 1991 was 4.2 million, comprised of anywhere between 38 and 68 different ethnic groups, depending on the system of classification used. The ethnic

Lao or Lao Loum constitute a 51% majority. The Lao PDR is the most sparsely populated country in Southeast Asia, with the ethnic Lao population concentrated along the Mekong River and the lower valleys of its tributaries. More than 80% of the population rely on agriculture, the majority being subsistence farmers. Average life expectancy is 49 years. In 1990, the infant mortality rate was estimated at 109 per 1,000 live births, and the under five mortality rate at 159. The annual population growth rate is around 2.9% (UNICEF, 1992).

While only 15% of the population lives in urban areas, economic liberalisation and increased commercial activity are attracting more people to the cities. In the ARC survey, 48.8% of the 550 people interviewed in Vientiane had been born in another of the Lao PDR's 17 provinces, most migrating to the capital for education or work. A similar though less marked trend is evident in Savannakhet, the largest urban centre in the south.

One of the poorest nations in Asia, Laos' destiny has always depended on its more powerful neighbours. From its Golden Age origins as the Kingdom of Lane Xang (One Million Elephants), Laos became part of the French colonial empire in Indochina in the late nineteenth century. During the Vietnam conflict, Laos was the site of a brutal "secret war" orchestrated by the Central Intelligence Agency of the United States. A protracted independence struggle finally resulted in the victory of pro-Hanoi Pathet Lao forces and the declaration of a socialist republic in 1975. An ensuing Cold War stand-off led to a period of isolation from which the country has only recently emerged.

The Lao People's Revolutionary Party (LPRP) inherited an economy bankrupted by the former Royalist government's reliance on US aid, exacerbated by the outward migration of the country's educated elite, an economic embargo put in place by Thailand, and a series of natural disasters in the late 1970s. In 1986 the Lao government launched its version of glasnost, the New Economic Mechanism (NEM), under the auspices of the World Bank and International Monetary Fund. Heralded as a "market-driven path to socialism", the NEM aims to generate revenue and attract foreign investment through economic liberalisation, privatisation and structural adjustment in an effort to address Laos' crippling US$1.2 billion foreign debt (UNDP, 1993b:11–25). A subsequent influx of foreign money led to a boom in sectors such as transport, infrastructure, trade, tourism and communications. Negative consequences include widening class gaps; growing unemployment, particularly among the youth; increased rural to urban migration; and a steady rise in what the Lao press refers to as "social ills", among them crime, prostitution, and illicit drug use.

HIV/AIDS EPIDEMIOLOGICAL SITUATION

While the majority of present cases of HIV/AIDS worldwide are in sub-Saharan Africa, the HIV epidemic is believed to be spreading fastest in Asia, with AIDS cases rising from 30,000 to 250,000 since June 1993 (*Bangkok Post*, 1994a; *Nation*, 1994). Of the countries most affected in the Asia region, an estimated 1.5% of the population in Thailand are HIV-positive, with intravenous drug users (IVDUs) and low-charge prostitutes showing the highest rates of infection among detected cases. Similar patterns have been observed in India, where an estimated one million people are HIV-positive. In Burma, anywhere between 150,000–400,000, almost 1% of the population, may be infected (Kahane, 1994; Sakboon, 1994). While reported cases show higher rates of infection among men, the risk of HIV infection for women in Asia is steadily increasing (*Bangkok Post*, 1994b). Seroprevalence surveys have shown HIV infection rates among women attending prenatal clinics of up to 8% in Thailand (*Bangkok Post*, 1994a), 12% in India (Sakboon, 1994), and 1.4% in Burma (Lintner, 1994). Unprotected heterosexual intercourse is believed to be the main route of transmission.

In February 1995, the English-language *Vientiane Times* reported that 55 people in the Lao PDR had been identified as HIV-positive and a further ten were diagnosed with full-blown AIDS, up to the end of December 1994. These figures were derived from 19,220 tests, said to be routinely administered by the National Committee for the Control of AIDS (NCCA) to blood donors, "hospital patients... displaying suspected symptoms", returnees and refugees. All ten AIDS cases were identified in returnees and refugees from Thailand (*Vientiane Times*, 1995:1). The report also noted that two of 250 "bar workers" tested in 1991 were diagnosed HIV-positive. Earlier, the NCCA reported infection rates of 0.7% among "bar workers" and five AIDS deaths (Sakboon, 1994). Of 38 detected cases of HIV in 1993, 19 were among women, 14 among men and five "unknown" (Lao PDR/NCCA, 1994:4).

The following discussion on HIV stereotypes will indicate, however, the impact of social factors not only on perceptions of the AIDS threat in the Lao PDR, but the shaping of the epidemiological profile itself.

THE IMPACT OF STEREOTYPES

De Bruyn (1992:250) notes that the use of the term "risk groups" by the biomedical community to denote categories for epidemiological surveillance has had the effect of reinforcing and expanding negative stereotypes of certain, specifically marginalised groups of people. While she suggests that, since the first decade of the HIV epidemic, the WHO/GPA[4] and others now emphasise "practices" or behaviour rather than "groups" to denote risk, 1994 WHO/GPA reports continue to refer to "population groups considered to be at high risk" (WHO, 1994:1). In the Lao PDR, selective screening practices by the NCCA have been supported by the WHO/GPA under whose auspices the NCCA was established in 1988. At a donor meeting in Vientiane in 1994, pressure was still being brought to bear on AIDS prevention programs and policy statements to dispense with the use of the term "risk groups" (UNDP, 1993a).

De Bruyn's literature review identifies the stereotypes of AIDS as a "homo-sexual disease" and a "prostitutes' disease" as having particularly detrimental effects on women (1992:250). AIDS as a "homosexual disease" is generally not part of the

Lao consciousness and scant attention has been paid by official agencies to HIV risks for men who have sex with men and the female partners of these men. In the ARC survey, although upward of 80% of respondents knew the risk of HIV transmission through unprotected heterosexual intercourse, sharing needles and syringes, and from mother to baby, 57.6% did not know that HIV could be transmitted from man to man during sex.

The first case of HIV infection, detected in 1989, was in a young, asymptomatic Lao woman who, according to an NCCA report, had "probably been infected sexually abroad" (Lao PDR, 1991c:5). Implicit in this assumption is that a "young" (read "single") woman became infected by having sexual relations with a "foreigner", providing the starting point for defining the AIDS threat in the Lao PDR in terms of both illicit sexual behaviour on women's part and as a "foreigners' disease". The Medium Term Plan for the Prevention and Control of AIDS and HIV Infection from which the quotation is extracted was drafted by a WHO consultant, however, thus the assumptions in it are not those of the NCCA alone. HIV stereotypes in the Lao PDR have not evolved in a vacuum, but are connected with wider trends in the global AIDS discourse.

AIDS as a "Prostitutes' Disease"

Summarising information he had gleaned from government radio, a male participant in an AIDS workshop conducted for Lao students of English as a foreign language wrote: "HIV transmission will increase if sexual intercourse with prostitutes increases. Fortunately, the Lao government pays attention to severely punishing prostitutes and this is a way that HIV infection can be prevented". In surveys asking questions about which people are most likely to get STDs such as HIV, 79% (ESF, 1992), 75% (Lao PDR, 1992a:11–12) and 57.1% (in the ARC survey) nominated "prostitutes". This perception has led to the stigmatisation of female commercial sex workers (CSWs) as vectors of HIV infection. In the Lao PDR, where prostitution is illegal and periodic "crack-downs" take place, this has resulted in mandatory HIV testing of "bar workers" — women who may or may not engage in sexual services for commercial purposes.[5] It has also had a negative impact on men's perceptions of their own risk for HIV infection and, subsequently, the risk at which they may place their female partners. A married businessman from Xieng Khouang, for example, suggested he had "no chance" of becoming infected with HIV because "If I play around, it is only with young, pure women, not with prostitutes".

De Bruyn suggests the stereotyping of AIDS as a prostitutes' disease "appears to have a sound epidemiological basis...[g]iven high incidences of HIV infection among some groups of female sex workers" (1992:250), but objects that this leads to stigmatisation rather than intensified prevention education activities. However, the epidemiological record itself may be skewed by selective screening practices which target commercial sex workers (CSWs) and not their clients. In the Lao PDR, two of the NCCA's initial six "target groups" for HIV screening were female "bar workers" and "returnees", the latter comprised mostly of young women forcibly repatriated from Thailand (Insisiengmay, 1992; *Vientiane Times*, 1995). There is no comparable screening of either clients at the "bars", for example, or businessmen, labourers or students returning from abroad.

The sensitivity of prostitution for the Lao government needs to be understood in its historical context. During the "secret war", Vientiane gained a reputation as one of the rest and recreation hotspots for American forces throughout Southeast Asia (Pringle, 1991). According to one expatriate stationed there at the time, "there was a brothel on every street corner". Some expatriates would take pre-emptive doses of antibiotics against sexually transmittable diseases (STDs) before going out for a night on the town. In his account of the CIA's mercenary fliers in covert operations, Air America, Christopher Robbins writes of a "strip" of "exotic bars and specialist brothels" in Vientiane "to keep the most jaded Asia hand entertained" (Robbins, 1988:173). One of the more infamous night-spots, the Rendezvous des Amis, better known for its owner as Madame Lulu's, dealt exclusively in oral sex (Robbins, 1988:174).

A Lao Women's Union (LWU) source describes this as a period when there was an unprecedented tolerance of the "commodification of female sexuality" and the "humiliation of humanity" (National Union of Women, 1989:35) and thus CSW is strongly associated with imperialism. Following the victory of the Pathet Lao in 1975, the brothels were closed down and sex workers and pimps were banished for "re-education" (Pringle, 1991). The vigilance of the state and the uniform poverty of the post-war years appeared to have reduced both supply and demand for commercial sex services (Ngaosyvathn, 1993:55,96). However, the shift to a market economy, widening class gaps and decreasing legitimate employment opportunities for women due to state sector cut-backs, and the attenuated influence of the state as the country "opens up" to the outside world, have contributed to an increase in commercial sexual activity catering to different sectors.

Visible among the new clientele at the top level are Asian and western visitors, notably businessmen from Thailand, for whom escort services can be provided through the major hotels and adjacent nightclubs. In Lao border towns such as Tha Khek opposite Nakon Panom in Thailand, and Savannakhet opposite Mukdahan, women who may not necessarily work in the bars look for cars with foreign number-plates in hotel car-parks, and then enter the adjacent discotheques in search of their owners. At another level are Lao men in the new, burgeoning middle classes who tend to meet women at restaurants, bars and discotheques. Women who work in such venues often do so as a second job and offer sexual favours as the opportunity arises. Some female students sell sexual services through college dormitories, a trend also observed in Thailand (Lyttleton, 1994:142). Additionally, younger, largely illiterate women from the more remote provinces are employed in what are euphemistically known as "beer shops" frequented by poorer workers and male students. The targeting of female commercial sex workers for mandatory testing and the lesser emphasis placed on the role of the male client in sexual exchange indicate, however, that Lao women carry the bulk of the historical baggage surrounding prostitution.

AIDS as a "Foreigners' Disease"

The intersection of gender relations with wider socio-economic factors is also implicated in the construction of AIDS as a "foreigner's disease". The stereotype of AIDS as a "Thai disease" is particular in Southeast Asia. Thailand's AIDS problem has been well-publicised in the Lao PDR as elsewhere and, in the north-west, the Lao PDR shares a land border with Chiang Rai province which records among the highest rates of HIV infection in Thailand. While the risk of AIDS to the Lao PDR is not posed by Thailand's proximity *per se*, human traffic between the two countries is considerable and sexual exchange takes place. The presence of young Lao women in Thai brothels has come to light in reports following police raids (Murdoch, 1991), while some Lao men avail themselves of commercial sex services in Thailand. More significantly, the AIDS situation in Thailand has led to a sub-regional trend where Thai men increasingly procure the sexual services of young women in neighbouring countries where detected rates of HIV infection are lower. Sub-regional intravenous drug use (IVDU) trends and subsequent HIV infection patterns also pose a risk for the Lao PDR (Lintner, 1994).

The targeting of "returnees" from Thailand for screening, however, enhances the notion that HIV is an infection coming into the Lao PDR from Thailand, rather than one with which Lao people can infect one another. This was evident in the build-up to the opening of the Australian-funded Mittaphab Bridge across the Mekong River which links Vientiane and the Thai border town of Nong Khai. People spoke about "AIDS coming across the bridge" and the Committee for Planning and Co-operation (CPC), the central co-ordinating agency for donor activity in the Lao PDR, even mooted the idea of incorporating HIV testing into the customs facilities. "HIV doesn't need a visa", one CPC official told me by means of explanation.

In a letter to the editor of *Vientiane Mai* newspaper in April 1994, amid comments on pollution and increased traffic, the author asked, "When the Mekong Bridge construction is completed, there will be traffic between [Laos and Thailand]; how will the control of AIDS be carried out?" A male interviewee in a snooker hall in Vientiane commented: "Before in Laos, it was free and easy. We did whatever we wanted and didn't think about things coming like AIDS. Now the bridge has opened, many foreigners are coming to Laos, and many may bring the [AIDS] virus with them".

While the perception of AIDS as a "Thai/foreigners' disease" allows Lao people to deny their own risks and responsibilities, these responses represent more than just the stereotype of "blaming others" (Sabatier, 1988). While the Lao PDR remains tightly governed in a single-party system, direct political criticism of the current socio-economic changes is unfeasible. Discourse on AIDS provides an outlet for Lao people to express anxieties, however, as indicated by the central role of the bridge — a concrete sign of the extent of the changes that have taken place to open up the Lao PDR to the outside world. AIDS has become, in part, a metaphor for the potentially negative consequences of that "opening up".

Such anxieties are fuelled by the failure of the expatriate community, from private companies to aid organisations, to take into account the potentially negative effects of their "development" work. While the potential impact of an HIV epidemic on development has been the topic of a national conference in the Lao PDR (Lao Women's Union, 1992), scant attention has been paid to the impact of development on HIV transmission. Projects from road and bridge construction, to logging and mineral exploration, for example, commonly use mobile and/or migrant labour, often importing labourers from countries which have higher rates of HIV infection than the Lao PDR, such as Thailand, Vietnam and southern China. Workers are not encouraged to bring their families, are highly-paid by local standards and are often stationed in remote rural areas characterised by abject poverty. Conditions have been created, albeit inadvertently, for commercial sex work to flourish. Some efforts are being made to encourage companies to take HIV/AIDS issues into account in the design and implementation of their infrastructure projects, to fund workshops, for example, and to supply condoms to their workers. But HIV prevention is generally seen as beyond the scope of such sectors. Even among international aid organisations, proposals to run AIDS workshops for expatriate staff have been rejected on the grounds that the staff "are all highly-educated people who know about AIDS" (read "do not engage in risk behaviour"), despite evidence to the contrary. Western expatriates, predominantly men, are known to engage in unprotected sex with local people, both women and men, and at least one such man was known to be HIV-positive.

Treichler (1989:31) notes that AIDS is "a complex, contradictory, and multilayered discursive construction". This is further illustrated by Lao women's position in the official discourse. Women are seen as "vectors" of HIV infection and "blamed" for its spread, and/or they are increasingly invested with responsibility for the prevention of HIV transmission through the preservation of "cultural standards". Just as stereotypes about AIDS as a "prostitutes' disease" have a negative impact on men's perception of their own risks, the notion that adhering to traditional standards of sexual behaviour will offer protection for women against HIV is equally dangerous as it fails to take into account risks posed by the behaviour of the male partner. As a female teacher from Khammouane said, "I have no chance of becoming infected with HIV because the most important aspect in the Lao tradition is faithfulness to the family".

Guttal (1993:27) points out in her analysis of women's education in the Lao PDR, that "[a]s caretakers of the domestic sphere, the responsibility of preserving and continuing culture through dress, food, language, rules and values is likely to be placed more on women than men". For some women, the caretaker role is a source of self-esteem. A female college student in Vientiane maintained, "Lao women respect Lao culture and keep it beautiful and look after their own honour always". For other women, however, it is an onerous burden. A female high school student in this study said, with visible resentment, "Women are the ones who look after society [and] they are not allowed to forget this".

While such issues are particularly important for ethnic minorities in the Lao PDR, they have become more so for the majority ethnic Lao, and for the Lao government, during the present period of social upheaval. The construction of women as cultural caretakers not only negatively influences individual perceptions of risk but, as the following discussion indicates, it enhances Lao women's risk for HIV infection by shifting attention away from the more significant impact of poverty and gender relations.

LAO WOMEN'S INCREASED RISKS FOR HIV INFECTION

While the risks for HIV infection for Lao women and men cannot be isolated from the poverty of the population as a whole, women's increased susceptibility is significantly affected by gender relations. In their article, "Confronting the HIV epidemic in Asia and the Pacific", Moodie and Aboagye-Kwarteng state:

> For women, the risk of HIV infection is inextricably linked to their socio-economic status in a society. The lower status of women in the home and in society means that women often lack control over their sexual lives and are unable to insist on safe sexual behaviour either in domestic or commercial relationships...[F]or many women the major risk factor of becoming infected with HIV is simply being married (1993:1544).

Gender-related issues both compound wider structural factors and underline risks related to biological or reproductive health factors.

Notions of what constitutes "gender relations" and women's experience of gender as a structuring factor in their lives vary considerably, however, even within the ethnically and socioeconomically homogenous communities of Vientiane and Savannakhet, as the following discussion will demonstrate. On the one hand, traditional gender relations and the status of women have an undeniable impact on some women's perception of both their risk of HIV infection and their ability to protect themselves. On the other hand, to overstate women's passivity is to deny other women's assertions of the power they have both to challenge traditional stereotypes and take action to protect themselves from HIV, in theory if not in practice. The implications of this diversity will be considered in the final section on planning intervention strategies.

Risks Related to Gender Relations

The general consensus in the scant literature on the subject is that Lao women occupy a more favourable position than that of their counterparts in neighbouring countries (UNICEF, 1987; Iinuma, 1992; Ng, 1989), with ethnic Lao women generally enjoying higher status than minority women (Evans, 1990:196). This is believed to be the case in pre- and post-revolutionary Laos. There is no overt son preference and, as Evans (1990:124) observes, a distinguishing feature of the Lao Loum domestic cycle is "preferred matrilocal residence for daughters" who typically inherit the land of their parents. This practice endures, even in urban areas, and provides a basis for economic independence among ethnic Lao women. Combined with the psychological support made possible through proximity to the family home (Ng, 1989:173), women would appear to have a strong basis for asserting control over their sexual lives.

Recent historical developments have, on the one hand, enabled Lao women to make gains in addressing inequities in their social status. On the other hand, they have had limited impact on the more deeply-rooted aspects of gender relations in Lao culture which also serve to limit if not override their "cultural advantages" (Ng, 1989:174). The first steps were taken towards women's emancipation in the Pathet Lao "liberated zones". The Lao Patriotic Women's Association was formed in 1955 as a mass organisation to mobilise women's support for the revolutionary struggle. Since 1975, as the Lao Women's Union, it has promoted women's development and the protection of women's interests. In the post-war period, social policy stemmed from Lenin's dictum that "women constitute half of society; if they are not emancipated, half of society won't be liberated" (Ngaosyvathn, 1993:102). Considerable gains were made by Lao women in access to education, health services and child care, and women were elected to government for the first time (Ng, 1989:174–5).

Lao women had long been marginalised from formal education, both in the Buddhist pagodas and under the elite secular education system created by the French. Despite improvements, however, sons continue to be given preferential access to schooling over daughters who are expected to work in the home. Adult literacy rates are consistently lower among women than men, estimated at 35% and 65% respectively (Insisiengmay, 1992:3). Of the 21 people in the ARC survey who said they could not read or write Lao, 19 were women, including several young women from the more remote provinces working in "beer shops". Lower educational standards marginalise women from legitimate employment, while lack of access to appropriate or intelligible information can result in lower awareness of HIV/AIDS transmission routes and prevention methods.

The traditional division of labour in Lao society further undermines gains made by women in access to child care. With over 80% of the population engaged in agriculture, 60% of farming is done by women (Iinuma, 1992:5) and, on average, women's working day is two hours longer than that of men (National Union of Lao Women, 1989:30). As primary carers in a country with an impoverished health system, an AIDS epidemic would further increase Lao women's workloads. Several people in this study also noted that women's primary responsibilities in the home resulted in increased sexual freedom for men and, by extension, increased risk of exposure to HIV for women through their partners. A female office worker in Savannakhet noted, "if [women] have started a family, they have only their husband. As for men, they like to look for new women all the time. Therefore, it is not equal". An unemployed man from Savannakhet agreed: "Following the theory of Lao people, men are able to leave home more often, but for women it is difficult...[and] this makes for inequality in sexual relationships". Women's lower educational status and their disproportionate workload, combined with stringent conditions for party membership which do not take these conditions into account, contribute to their lack of representation in the higher levels of government (Ng, 1989:175–6). And, as one Lao woman put it, "little will change while policies on women are drawn up by men".

In theory, the Lao legal code provides a strong framework for women to protect themselves from HIV infection. The 1991 Constitution enshrines women's equal rights (Lao PDR, 1991a:9) and Lao women have legal rights to inheritance, property ownership and capital. Under the Family Law Code, men are obliged to take financial responsibility for any children that they father, which can serve to discourage men from engaging in unprotected premarital or extra-marital sex. Women and men are entitled to sue for divorce without the consent of the other partner on grounds including infidelity and the risk of exposure to a life-threatening disease (Lao PDR, 1991b:9). In the ARC survey, 13% of people referred to equal rights under the law as the basis for their belief in the equality between the sexes. As one male merchant from Savannakhet suggested, "These days, men and women can choose their own path of life as well as having choices such as the rights to choose their partner and career". More often, however, women are largely unaware of their legal rights or lack the capacity, due to cultural and structural constraints, to exercise these rights. As one Lao woman maintained, "Men won't accept women having equal rights to men in the matter of sexual relationships". The disproportionate responsibility allocated to women for upholding standards of "proper" sexual or cultural behaviour, for example, impacts on their willingness to sue for divorce which, as a "last resort", might protect them from HIV infection. Lao women are largely "blamed" for the failure of a marriage, even in cases of violence and alcoholism, for "not being a good enough wife". Buddhism plays a key role in this respect in socialising women to be self-effacing (Ng, 1989:175; Ngaosyvathn, 1993:30–40), codifying women as "lower beings" to men (Evans, 1990:132). The Lao wife of a violent and unfaithful husband told me that she had married against her family's advice and must therefore accept her "fate"; when she had approached her family for advice, they told her to "adopt the Buddhist way" and "let everything go in one ear and out the other".

Stigmatisation may also result in loss of financial support. It is significant that while only 6.5% of the total sample of women in the ARC survey had been divorced, 31.8% of female "bar workers" in Savannakhet were divorcees. As observed, the combination of lack of social support and financial dependency dramatically reduces women's power to negotiate safer sex practices in either commercial or non-commercial sexual exchange. A young woman from the remote province of Houaphanh, working in a night club in Vientiane, said "I know how to get it [HIV] and how to protect myself, but I still have sex without condoms. Men say it makes them lose feeling and it isn't enjoyable. Asking a partner to use one can be embarrassing for both parties". Similarly, Lao people frequently refer to inequalities in gender relations which result in increased sexual freedom for men both prior to and after marriage. A male office worker from Bokeo noted, "For most Lao women, when they get married, they must accept sexual activities; men gain knowledge [of sex] much sooner". A female bar worker agreed: "Men have more freedom to sleep around. Women are looked down on by society if they do". The results of the ARC survey suggest that men, if not more sexually active than women, are in a more socially

TABLE 14.2 Number of previous sexual partners of respondents in ARC survey (1,045 respondents).

No. of previous sexual partners	Men	Women	Total
1. Never had sex	33.1%	62.2%	45.1%
2. 0–1	15.6%	25.9%	19.8%
3. 2–4	28.2%	7.7%	19.8%
4. 5–9	12.3%	2.1%	8.1%
5. 10–19	5.8%	0.5%	3.6%
6. More than 20	4.7%	0.9%	3.2%

acceptable position to admit to their sexual experience, as represented by the reported number of previous sexual partners (see Table 14.2).

Almost half the respondents in the ARC survey agreed with this analysis to some degree, though the reasons given for their beliefs varied considerably. Some people, notably men, saw inequities in gender relations as a defining characteristic of Lao culture. As one male shopkeeper in Vientiane said: "Lao society is not like that [where men and women have equal freedom in relationships with the opposite sex]. Lao society is a good, beautiful society and we respect Lao culture". Other people, notably younger women, were critical saying the "culture doesn't progress" because of traditional gender relations. As one female student in Vientiane put it, "Lao traditions don't talk about sexual relationships. This is a problem". Another female university student from Sayaboury commented: "Women aren't allowed to have sex with a man if they're just friends or boyfriends — only when they're married. When they can do all these things, only then will they truly be equal".

In addition to women's primary responsibilities in the home, people also cited women's fear of pregnancy to account for differences in sexual behaviour between men and women. One female office worker in Savannakhet noted that, "[single] women are scared of having children, but men can't have them". Others talked about rape being a key determinant of inequality in relationships between the sexes, with a female college student in Vientiane noting, "women are forced [to have sex]. Men are stronger". In the most severe case, women's choice to protect themselves from HIV infection is destroyed by rape, and most rape occurs between people who know each other. The Lao Penal Code prohibits men from raping "a woman who is not his wife", effectively sanctioning nonconsenting sex within marriage (Lao PDR, 1994:54). This provides no legal protection for Lao women who choose abstinence, a common response to a husband's infidelity, as a means of HIV prevention. Women's capacity to protect themselves from HIV infection through unprotected sexual intercourse will be lower for those who see this situation as "cultural" or "natural", relative to those who seek to actively criticise and challenge it.

Ironically, it is in a climate of relative prosperity that Lao women risk losing many of their gains. Opinions differ as to how this situation has emerged. On the one hand, policies which emphasise gender rights in theory but not gender equality in practice can only have limited impact as they fail to educate men to the same degree as women. As a male translator from Savannakhet maintained, "The customs of Lao people are that women must have independence like all people in Lao society, without question, as well as having equal rights to men. I don't agree with this in many respects as most women must follow the words of men in higher positions".

Indeed, LWU policies have changed since the early 1980s in recognition of this problem. The "Three Goods" slogan, adopted at the 1984 National Congress to encourage women to be "a good citizen, a good wife and a good mother", was altered in 1988 to require women to be "good citizens", "good builders of the family based on the new [socialist] culture", and to develop "good solidarity". The emphasis on building families recognises men's role. As one LWU staff member said, "It's not fair to women. The woman can be a good wife and a good mother, but what if the man is not good?"

On the other hand, the interests of Lao women, like their counterparts in other developing countries, have always been sublimated for the national good. As a senior LWU official told me, "We are Lao citizens first, Lao women second". The Lao government upheld a pro-natalist population policy for over ten years after 1975 in an effort to build a productive labour force, for example, despite the health problems to women caused by frequent pregnancies and alarmingly high infant and maternal mortality rates.

Ng (1989:176–177) suggests the promotion of conservative gender relations is part of the political agenda of the LPRP: "Stressing women's traditional domestic roles as wives and mothers ensures for the party a certain degree of social harmony and stability". She adds that more deeply entrenched concepts of gender identity are equally responsible and that the ideological training of the post-war years has failed to analyse what constitutes sexual equality and women's emancipation.

I would argue, however, that the Lao revolution was ultimately never equipped to address the more deeply-rooted traditions which determine gender relations, contending as it was with the abject poverty of the post-war years. Lao women's struggle for emancipation is inextricably bound up in their material conditions. Lao women essentially know what oppresses them: poverty, and the behaviour of men. They also tend to recognise the ways in which one disempowers them from addressing the other. It does not follow, however, that they passively accept the status quo; as one expatriate worker put it, "They may be downtrodden, but that doesn't necessarily mean they like it!" This is illustrated by women's discussion of AIDS issues. While Ng (1989:179) argues that economic liberalisation may provide opportunities for increasing women's financial independence, it is equally possible that the meaning of the "market-driven path to socialism" for many Lao women is marginalisation from the benefits and vulnerability to the dangers of change. The threat of AIDS in Laos is a case in point.

Risks Related to Biological and Reproductive Health Factors

Risks for HIV transmission through the health sector reflects the poverty of the country as a whole. Infrastructure is poor if not non-existent outside the provincial and district centres. Resources are scarce, staff limited and often inadequately trained, underpaid and unmotivated. In 1993, there were an estimated 1,089 people per doctor in the Lao PDR; medical staff are concentrated in the provincial centres (UNDP, 1993b:3). There is one blood bank in Vientiane at the LRC where the blood supply is screened. Donations number less than 2,000 units per year, however, and other formal and informal blood transfusion services operate. While a recently drafted national blood policy will improve controls, standards are undermined by lack of infrastructure and equipment.

Women's reproductive roles increase their susceptibility to transfusion with unscreened blood. In the Lao PDR, high rates of post-natal haemorrhage occur, due either to the prevalence of malaria-related anaemia or traditional birthing practices, which can lead to retention of the placenta. As many of the ethnic groups in the Lao PDR practice colostrum denial, including the Lao Loum, the new-born is seldom placed directly on the breast which might facilitate delivery of the placenta. Instead, tugging of the umbilical cord occurs, often leading to haemorrhaging (Lao Women's Union, 1992:112–113). In western-style hospitals where the majority of urban women give birth, women in labour literally queue for beds and no sooner than one has delivered her baby, another woman takes her place on the bed. The beds are often little more than wooden benches and may not even be sluiced clean, let alone freshly covered between births. Such conditions increase the risk of exposure to HIV-infected fluids for the mother, baby, and birth attendants, who are predominantly women.

Cultural expectations concerning motherhood play a role in women's exposure to risk. While birth spacing and even birth control are gaining more popularity in urban areas, women's status as wives is still connected to their reproductive ability. As one Lao woman, a student of English, put it, "Lao people feel very strange if the wife doesn't give [her husband] a baby". This student connected the desire to have a baby to Lao couples' reluctance to use condoms and the subsequent risk of exposure to HIV infection.

The risk of HIV exposure is greatly enhanced by the presence of other STDs, which are believed to be more efficiently transmitted from men to women than from women to men (Panos, 1990:13–14). Reliable data on STD rates in the Lao PDR are unavailable as STDs are not notifiable diseases and there is no national control program. People — particularly women — are reluctant to be tested, due to shyness, embarrassment, or fear of public censure.

The one STD clinic in Vientiane, the Centre of Dermatology and Venereology, is advertised solely as a dermatology clinic, partly because of its limited capacity to respond, and partly because people will be deterred from using its services. One respondent in the AIDS survey commented that he had "never seen an STD clinic in Vientiane". Few people use the clinic's screening and treatment services: in 1993, the centre reported only 26 cases of STDs, 22 among men and four among women. Though the director of the centre is a woman, women do not appear to use the service; according to one female office worker from Champassack, "We discuss [STDs] in private — we don't like to discuss them openly".

An informal survey conducted by the non-government organisation (NGO) CARE International found approximately 25% of women seen daily in the Outpatients Department of Mahasot Hospital are diagnosed as having pelvic inflammatory disease (PID), a secondary infection of gonorrhoea or chlamydia which often renders women infertile. Mahasot Hospital in Vientiane reported 434 cases of PID in 1992, while Sethathirath Hospital reported 126 cases of PID in 1993. Detected cases of genital herpes have also been increasing in Vientiane since 1990 (pers. comm.).

Several respondents in the survey referred to STDs as "women's diseases", suggesting that women are also allotted disproportionate "blame" for infection. STDs are largely associated with illicit or commercial sex and Lao women fear social censure in the health sector, even when the most likely source of infection are their husbands (Panos, 1990). The majority self-medicate through pharmacies, which has resulted in drug-resistant strains of STDs throughout Southeast Asia, particularly during and since the Vietnam war. While stigmatisation of STD patients is neither exclusively a Lao nor non-western phenomenon, the association of STDs with that period of Lao history may compound the obstacles for infected women to seeking treatment.

De Bruyn (1992:252) notes that "[c]ertain beliefs relating to health and disease may put both women and men at risk of transmission because preventive measures such as condom use are rejected". In the ARC survey, women were three times as likely as men to suggest that condom use was bad for their health (9.1% of women) — that it "may cause a miscarriage", for example. Condom use was also said to "reduce strength" or render men infertile. These beliefs may stem from indigenous concepts of the body derived from Ayurvedic theory, as explored by Escoffier-Fauveau and Pholsena (1993). Women commonly spoke about conception as the coming together of male and female "seeds". Sperm was seen as "the quintessence of blood" and women suggest frequent intercourse during pregnancy as necessary for the sperm to nourish the foetus (Escoffier-Fauveau and Pholsena, 1993:35–37). Condom use would thus block the release of sperm with "negative" consequences for both the man and woman and, in the case of pregnancy, the foetus.

These opinions may, however, reflect lack of familiarity with the product. One male university student commented, "I don't think there are any disadvantages [to condom use], just that people don't know how to use them". Poor condom quality may also be a factor as a number people in the survey mentioned "inflammation" as a disadvantage of condom use, and a surprising number of questions have been posed in AIDS workshops concerning possible "allergies" to condoms. Non-consenting sex and subsequent lack of lubrication may also be a factor for women experiencing discomfort with condom use.

In this study, factors related to gender were more significant than indigenous concepts of health in determining potential for safer sex practices. In the ARC survey, while just over 70% of men and 62.5% of women said they would use or ask their partner to use condoms, nearly 10% of the men qualified their answers saying "if with a prostitute, not a girlfriend", "if someone we don't know", "in circumstances outside the home", or "have to look at the person first", further reflecting the influence of HIV stereotypes. Men were four times as likely as women to nominate "loss of feeling" as a disadvantage of condom use (16.7% of men).

A higher proportion of women to men said that they "lacked confidence" to negotiate condom use with a partner. Surprisingly, though, a much greater proportion of men than women (23 out of 29 people) said they were afraid to "upset their partners" by raising the issue of condom use. As a male construction worker in Vientiane said, "There are no disadvantages to Lao people — put condoms in your pocket or bag. If your wife sees them [however], it's not a good thing. She'll think that you're being unfaithful". This points to the complexity of gender relations among the ethnic Lao, as everywhere, including industrialised countries. In the Lao case, men's "fear" of their wives' reaction may be connected to the wider repercussions of living in close proximity to the wife's family and the pressure a wife's family can bring to bear on the husband.

Of the 148 people asked direct questions about their sexual behaviour, 90 indicated they were sexually active (60.8%). Of these 90 people, 40 men (69%) and 19 women (55.9%) said they had used condoms in the past; 51 of the men (87.9%) and 29 women (85.3%) said they had had sexual intercourse without using condoms in the past. Women were more likely to have had unprotected sex in the context of marriage, however, with three-quarters of the men being single compared with less than half of the women.

Condom use has the capacity to reduce dramatically the risk of exposure to HIV and other STDs through heterosexual transmission. Current research suggests it is twice as easy for women to contract HIV from men than it is for men to contract HIV from women through unprotected heterosexual intercourse (Panos, 1990:13). While lack of access to affordable, high-quality condoms and lack of knowledge about correct condom use impact on both women and men's ability to protect themselves from HIV infection, risks are enhanced for women through an association of condom use with CSW, men's greater control over condom use, and women's lesser capacity to negotiate condom use due to structural and cultural factors.

IMPLICATIONS FOR INTERVENTION

Overcoming HIV Stereotypes

The results show the negative influence of HIV stereotypes on concepts of risk for HIV infection. People name "prostitutes", "people who play around" and "clients of prostitutes" as people at highest risk, rather than "people who don't use condoms during sex". This results in discrimination or even persecution of people whose behaviour may not be putting other people at risk and, equally importantly, shifts attention away from understanding personal risk through one's own behaviour and that of one's regular partner. It is interesting to note that, in the ARC survey, more people named "people who share needles" than "drug users" as being at risk, indicating a capacity to distinguish between behaviour and identity, which can be expanded.

AIDS education programs should carefully distinguish between "identity" and "behaviour". Instead of talking about "risk groups", AIDS education programs need to talk about "risk behaviour" or "risk situations". It is both more accurate and less discriminatory to talk about behaviour such as "unprotected sex", "sex without condoms" and "sharing needles" as the real risks for HIV infection. The behaviour of both partners needs to be clearly articulated as the basis for understanding personal risk. As Manderson, Lee and Rajanayagam (1996) note in their review of the literature on the use of condoms in heterosexual sex, condom use appears to be significantly influenced by perceptions of personal risk.

Developing Gender-sensitive Programs for Risk Reduction

Trying to understand people's perceptions of gender relations for the design and implementation of AIDS education programs is important partly for practical reasons. The results of this study suggest, for example, that men spend more time out of the home where they are more likely to engage in risk behaviour, than women. Therefore, programs which target men may need to be implemented in public places where men meet, while programs which target women may need to be home-based and/or be directed through community organisations such as LWU.

Information on gender relations also helps program planners to understand risk behaviour and to design appropriate messages which are culturally acceptable. However, as the diversity of the results show, there is no one method or message which will be appropriate for everyone. Whether people believe gender relations are "cultural" or "natural", some take them for granted and passively accept them; some believe they should be maintained; others seek actively to challenge and change them. Gender relations may be politicised, personalised, or seen as an interplay between wider structural and interpersonal factors. It is important, then, that people are equipped to develop appropriate choices about how to protect themselves and their families.

At the grass roots level, both men and women need to assess their risk status on the basis both of their behaviour and, particularly for women, their partners' behaviour. It is evident that many women, notably married women, do see a link between personal risk and the sexual behaviour of their partners. As one Lao woman, an architect, graphically explained in an English language exercise: "Men in Vientiane can go out of the home, maybe go abroad to places such as Thailand. Sometimes they go to brothels and go to bed with another girl. And the man gets drunk, so forgets to use a condom. And some people simply don't want to use condoms. They may then become infected with HIV. After they come home, they don't know if they have HIV infection or not because people infected with HIV may not show any symptoms. So they have sexual intercourse with their wife without using condoms...Because of the traditions, the Lao woman must be monogamous and faithful with her husband; so it is her husband who will infect her with HIV". However, not all of these women feel as if they have the ability to protect themselves from HIV infection.

At the same time as men need to be educated to change the behaviour that places their partners at risk, women need to be empowered by education programs to take action to protect themselves and their children with the widest possible range of alternatives. These options may include monogamy, emphasising the need for both partners to be monogamous in order to avoid HIV infection. Changes to the law to cover rape within marriage could provide legal protection for women who choose abstinence as a means of protection from HIV.

Condom use, both in and outside of marriage or regular relationships, is another option. The results of this study suggest that, with improved supplies, communication and skills training, condom use can become more widespread in the Lao PDR. Manderson, Lee and Rajanayagam (1996) reached the same conclusion, that training in negotiation skills and peer support, in addition to the provision of information, "would appear to be most successful in encouraging condom use...regardless of population, sub-group, gender, or risk category". Increased promotion of condom use for birth spacing may help to overcome negative associations of condom use with only extramarital or illicit sex. While STDs prevention and birth spacing have different objectives, links can be articulated between sexual health and fertility.

While women's capacity to negotiate condom use varies, there are Lao women and men who demonstrate confidence and openness. Nearly 60% of the married women in the ARC survey said they would ask their partner to use a condom, some seeing it as a means of protecting themselves from "unfaithful husbands" and "making sure" of their partners. Similarly, some single women also suggested they would use condoms in marriage to avoid a husband placing them at risk in the future. These people were not asked, however, if they had actually ever used condoms and safer behaviour cannot necessarily be gauged by positive inclinations (Manderson, Lee and Rajanayagam, 1996). One female high school student said simply, "If [a man] doesn't wear one [a condom], I won't have sex with him". Another teenage man expressed a similar sentiment: "Before we are going to have sex, we must know each other. If we don't use a condom, we don't have sex". While these people are in a minority, they represent a great resource for AIDS prevention programs as peer educators and illustrate the scope of what is possible.

Condom use can also be promoted specifically outside marital or regular monogamous relationships, an option called "negotiated safety". Some people in this study felt that they could avoid HIV infection if they or their partner used one every time they had sex outside the relationship. As one young woman in Savannakhet noted, "Have [him] wear one if he has sex with someone else. If it is with me, I don't make [him] use one". While it is difficult to guarantee that a partner will use a condom 100% of the time outside of marriage, this may be a viable option for some people. It can protect the marital or regular partner and enables both parties to enjoy unprotected sex with each other, therefore also helping to minimise the objection that total condom use results in a "loss of feeling" and prevents couples from having children as desired.

The impact of alcohol consumption on sexual behaviour needs to be taken into account, however, in advocating negotiated safety. Alcohol consumption is conspicuous among Lao men to the point of being a ritualised part of male social activity both in and outside the home. Lao women are less likely to drink to excess with the exception of festive occasions which, in rural areas, may constitute little more than the visit of a guest from beyond the local village. Contexts in which CSW is negotiated, from beer shops and bars to discotheques and nightclubs, almost invariably involve alcohol. As one male construction worker from Savannakhet noted, "When going and playing around, I drink and get drunk and can't control myself. I lose my wits and don't think about the diseases which may come afterwards".

Steps must be taken to guard against discrimination of women who have no choice but to leave or divorce a husband whose behaviour puts them and their children at risk. The creation of legitimate employment opportunities for women will help in this respect, as well as providing some alternatives to CSWs.

All these options require strong community support for women, particularly through an organisation like the LWU. Women's participation in program design, implementation and evaluation will be crucial to the success of prevention programs. One of the most valuable resources at the grass roots level are women who feel confident and able to negotiate condom use with their husbands or partners who may be recruited, trained and equipped to become peer educators.

Risk reduction through effective STDs management and improvements to the health care system are long-term activities which require significant funding and additional research. In the short-term, peer education programs can also be used to address issues related to STDs treatment and prevention, while AIDS awareness components can be incorporated into health worker training, including the training of traditional birth attendants.

CONCLUSION

The Lao case study demonstrates the impact of HIV/AIDS on women's reproductive health and the subsequent importance of a gender-sensitive approach in AIDS prevention programs. While the poverty of the country as a whole remains a significant obstacle to the development of effective programs in all sectors, increased community participation, particularly of women, in the research, design, implementation and evaluation of AIDS prevention activities will help to mobilise community resources and strengths in the hope of minimising the damaging effects of the epidemic.

While greater financial commitment is needed on the part of international agencies and NGOs, efforts also need to be made to overcome the ongoing use of terms such as "risk groups" and references to HIV stereotypes in recognition of their negative impact on perceptions of the AIDS threat. STDs and specifically AIDS need to be emphasised as reproductive health issues for women, to encourage integration of prevention components into a wide range of development sectors, thus maximising the use of financial and community resources.

AIDS education programs can be accused of attempting to "change" a society. To some extent this is the case, as effective AIDS programs aim to change behaviours which, as Moodie and Aboagye-Kwarteng (1993:1545) observe, "are expressions of deeply embedded societal norms and values relating to — among other things — sexuality and the status of women". As this study demonstrates, however, the status of women is not homogenous and women's experience of gender as a structuring factor in their lives varies, even when ethnicity, age, class and other variables are taken into account (cf. Manderson, Lee and Rajanayagam, 1996).

For nationalist elements throughout Southeast Asia, particularly in countries such as the Lao PDR, resistance to change is embedded in a history of long and bloody struggles against colonialism and imperialism. The promotion of an homogenous model of female sexuality may be seen in this context as a strategy for unifying and thus strengthening national identity. On another level, vested interests are also served among the ruling elite who are almost invariably older men and for whom diversity and specifically women's challenge to the sexual hegemony represent a threat to the maintenance of power.

These interests are served, to an extent, by the stereotypes embedded in the global AIDS discourse: in the epidemiological category of "(female) commercial sex worker" rather than "(male) client"; in discussions of "risk groups" rather than "risk behaviour"; and in programs which emphasise the provision of health information, failing to take into account the diversity of the population receiving that information and the structural and cultural factors impinging on women's ability in particular to act on that information.

There is a risk that exposing the diversity of women's perceptions of gender relations, even within relatively homogenous communities, will lead to the conclusion that gender is not a significant structural factor; or that the existence of diversity *per se*, calling into question the generalisability of research findings, will subsequently stand in the way of developing effective AIDS prevention strategies. By contrast, recognition of difference within the category "women" contributes to an understanding of the complexity of gender relations and calls us to examine the interplay of gender with other factors, as illustrated by examples in this study. Similarly, recognition of diversity among Asian women in developing countries, all too often characterised as uniformly passive and submissive (Lyttleton, 1994:138), reinforces the importance of women's participation in the design and implementation of AIDS prevention programs. The importance of peer education is also implicated.

The key strategy in effective AIDS prevention programs in developed countries, notably Australia, has been the provision of information, coupled with peer education and skills training. Such an approach recognises the validity of participatory programs and takes into account the diversity among and within what are loosely termed the "communities" that constitute a society (Delahunty, 1994). It makes sense, then, that in extending the gains of these programs to women in developing countries such as the Lao PDR, the diverse impact of structural and cultural as well as interpersonal factors is taken into account to realistically equip and empower people to adopt safer behaviour.

ENDNOTES

1. I would like to acknowledge and thank the following people for their contributions: the Lao women and men who responded to the survey (under condition of anonymity); research assistants Jo Miller and Rachel Dechaineux; survey team members (in Vientiane) Phonesavan, Latsadah, Khampraseud, Phetsamone, Vilaysack, Visouka, Khampone, Khamkhine; (in Savannakhet) Viengsay, Lanthasen, Phongsay, Le, Khankeo, Bounmy, Sengaloune, Pavisinh, Bouthavy, Khamphao; team trainer Dr Sounthone Nanthavong-douangsy; for collaboration on the questionnaire, Bridget Gardner and Somthong Srisudhivong; for training on Epiinfo, Chuanpit Chua Oon; for editorial assistance, Kim Spurway. Thanks also to the Lao Red Cross, Vientiane and Savannakhet; Lao Youth Union, Savannakhet; Lao Women's Union, Vientiane; Alan Crouch, Australian Red Cross; Høkan Björkman, UNDP; Nicholas Russell, International Federation of Red Cross and Red Crescent Societies; Jeanette Redding, Tony Lisle, and Shalmali Guttal. Special thanks to Andrew Nette. While I am grateful to these individuals and institutions, I remain solely responsible for the opinions expressed in this chapter.
2. The classification of the Lao PDR's diverse ethnic groups remains a point of contention. Most popular is the figure of 68 different groups, though the Institute of Ethnography identifies 38 and the 1985 census distinguished 47 different groups (UNICEF, 1992). Self-assessment surveys place the figure closer to 800 (personal communication). Using the ethnographic standard of language as the basis for classifying the major southeast Asian groups, the Lao PDR is made up of TaiKadai, Austroasiatic and SinoTibetan tribes and subtribes (UNICEF, 1992). These groups fit loosely into the official Lao classification system, based on habitat, of Lao Loum (lowland Lao), Lao Theung (midland Lao) and Lao Soung (highland Lao) respectively. For the purposes of this study, "ethnic Lao" refers to people who have self-identified as Lao Loum and/or who are ethnic Lao Tai (Tai speaking).
3. While clear distinctions were drawn between research and health education in an effort to avoid interviewer-prompting, researchers were also trained to provide information at the end of the interview. Each interviewee also received a pamphlet on HIV/AIDS to help address concerns that may have been raised by the interview process.
4. Global Programme on Aids of the World Health Organization.
5. Although reports refer only to the testing of 250 bar workers in 1991, routine, mandatory testing of women working in the bars and discotheques in Vientiane is known to be ongoing (personal communication from bar workers).

REFERENCES

Bangkok Post (1994a) Women on losing end as AIDS hits Asia, 13 April, Bangkok.

Bangkok Post (1994b) 60% rise in AIDS cases, 2 July, Bangkok.

de Bruyn, M. (1992) Women and AIDS in developing countries. *Social Science and Medicine,* **34**(3), 249–262.

Delahunty, Brendan (1994) Strategic focus. *National AIDS Bulletin,* 7(11), 12–13.

Escoffier-Fauveau, C.S., Pholsena, P. (1993) *Women and Reproductive Health in the Lao PDR.* Vientiane: Save the Children Fund UK/United Nations Development Programme.

ESF (1992) Survey of cartoons about AIDS, spreadsheet. Vientiane: Ecoles Sans Frontières.

Evans, G. (1990) *Lao Peasants Under Socialism.* New Haven and London: Yale University Press.

Guttal, S. (1993) *Strategies for the Promotion of Basic Education for Women and Girls,* draft report. Vientiane: World Education.

Iinuma, T. (1992) *Country Gender Analysis for the Lao People's Democratic Republic.* Vientiane: Swedish International Development Authority.

Insisiengmay, S. (1992) The epidemiological situation of HIV/AIDS in the Lao People's Democratic Republic. In *The Implications of HIV/AIDS on Social and Economic Development in the Lao People's Democratic Republic: Strategies for Preventing an Epidemic,* UNDP, pp. 46–48. Vientiane: United Nations Development Programme.

Kahane, T. (1994) AIDS alarm sounds in Burma. *Bangkok Post,* 15 July.

Lao PDR (1991a) *Constitution of the Lao People's Democratic Republic.* Vientiane: Supreme People's Assembly.

Lao PDR (1991b) *Family Law* (in Lao). Vientiane: State Publishing Enterprise.

Lao PDR (1991c) *Medium-Term Plan for the Prevention and Control of AIDS and HIV Infection.* Vientiane: Lao PDR.

Lao PDR (1992a) *National AIDS Programme.* Vientiane: State Publishing Enterprise.

Lao PDR (1992b) *Penal Code* (English translation). Vientiane: State Publishing Enterprise.

Lao PDR (1994) *Annual Report 1993.* Vientiane: National Committee for the Control of AIDS.

Lao Women's Union (1992) Women and AIDS in the Lao PDR. In *The Implications of HIV/AIDS on Social and Economic Development in the Lao People's Democratic Republic: Strategies for Preventing an Epidemic,* UNDP, pp. 109–117. Vientiane: United Nations Development Programme.

Lintner, B. (1994) Plague without borders. *Far Eastern Economic Review,* 21 July.

Lyttleton, C. (1994) Knowledge and meaning: the AIDS education campaign in rural northeast Thailand. *Social Science and Medicine,* **38**(1), 135–146.

Manderson, L., Lee Chang Tye., Rajanayagam K. (1996) Condom use in heterosexual sex: a review of research, 1985–1994. In *Prevention of HIV Infection,* edited by J. Catalan, L. Sherr. Chur: Harwood Academic Press.

Moodie, R., Aboagye-Kwarteng T. (1993) Confronting the HIV epidemic in Asia and the Pacific: developing successful strategies to minimise the spread of HIV infection, *AIDS,* 7, 1543–1551.

Murdoch, L. (1991) Sex slavery. *The Age Saturday Extra,* 14 September.

Nation (1994) WHO report says Aids cases up 60 pc in one year. 3 July.

National Union of Lao Women (1989) *Status of Women: Laos.* Bangkok: UNESCO.

Nette, A., Savage A. (1993) Laos confronts the spectre of AIDS with empty pockets. *National AIDS Bulletin,* 7(5), 30–31.

Ng Shui Meng (1989) Social development in the Lao People's Democratic Republic: problems and prospects. In *Laos: Beyond the Revolution,* edited by J. Zasloff and L. Unger, pp. 159–183. Basingstoke: Macmillan.

Ngaosyvathn, M. (1993) *Lao Women Yesterday and Today.* Vientiane: State Publishing Enterprise.

Panos (1990) *Triple Jeopardy — Women & AIDS.* Budapest, London, Paris, Washington: Panos Institute.

Petersen, G. (1992) The epidemiological situation of HIV/AIDS in Asian and Pacific countries. In *The Implications of HIV/AIDS on Social and Economic Development in* the Lao People's Democratic Republic: Strategies for Preventing an Epidemic, UNDP, pp. 40–45. Vientiane: United Nations Development Programme.

Pringle, J. (1991) Laotian backwater embraces fresh reign of hope. The Australian, 4 April.

Robbins, C. (1988) Air America. London, Moorebank, Henderson: Corgi Books.

Sabatier, R. (1988) Blaming Others: Prejudice, Race and Worldwide AIDS. Washington, London, Paris: Panos Institute.

Sakboon, M. (1994) SE Asia's eyes closed as plague worsens, Nation, 17 June.

Savage, A. (1994) HIV/AIDS and Sex in Vientiane and Savannakhet. Unpublished draft report. Vientiane: Australian Red Cross.

Thaitawat, N. (1993) Laos deals with AIDS at its borders. Bangkok Post, 10 August.

Treichler, P. A. (1989) AIDS and HIV infection in the third world: a first world chronicle. In Remaking History, edited by B. Kruger and P. Mariani, pp. 31–86. Seattle: Bay Press.

UNDP (1993a) HIV/AIDS Donor Meeting, Lao PDR, March. Vientiane: United Nations Development Programme.

UNDP (1993b) Development Cooperation Lao People's Democratic Republic, November. Vientiane: United Nations Development Programme.

UNICEF (1992) Children and Women in the Lao People's Democratic Republic. Vientiane: United Nations Children's Fund.

Vientiane Mai (1994) Letters to the editor, 12 April. Vientiane.

Vientiane Times (1995) National AIDS conference sets focus for 1995 plan, 2(5), 1. Vientiane.

WHO (1994) AIDS Surveillance Report Western Pacific Region, No 2, January. Manila: World Health Organisation.

Notes on Contributors

Josefina Cabigon is a demographer and is Associate Professor of the Population Institute, College of Social Sciences and Philosophy, The University of the Philippines. Her research interests are fertility, mortality, family planning evaluation, nuptiality and demographic research techniques. Her most recent publications are concerned with the effect of fertility patterns on child survival in Southeast Asia (with Chai Bin Park, Andrew Kantner, Marina F. Jose, and Josefa S. Zafra, 1993) and Life Table Estimates for the Philippines (with Wilhelm Flieger, 1994).

Siriporn Chirawatkul is a psychiatric nurse and medical anthropologist and is Associate Professor of Psychiatric Nursing in the Faculty of Nursing, Khon Kaen University, Thailand. Her books (all in Thai) include *Psychiatry for Nurses* (1981), *System Theory and Nursing* (1983), *Mental Health and Mental Illness: Handbook for School Teachers* (1983), *Communication for Quality Nursing Care* (1988, 1991, 1993), and *Menopause* (1994). Her primary research and publications, both in Thai and English, relate to women's health, culture and illness, transcultural nursing, and psychiatric nursing.

Cordia Ming-yeuk Chu is a Senior Lecturer and the Convener of Master Program of Environmental and Community Health, Faculty of Environmental Sciences, Griffith University, Queensland, Australia. She is a medical sociologist and anthropologist, and has been teaching social sciences in public health since 1989. Her research areas are reproductive health, women's health, workplace health promotion, and community development in health. Her books include *Workplace Health Promotion in Queensland* (1992), *Reproductive Health Beliefs and Practices of Australian and Chinese Women* (1993), and *Ecological Public Health: From Vision to Practice* (edited with R. Simpson, 1994).

Tamara Fetters has worked as an anthropologist in Indonesia, an advocate/community service worker for migrant farm workers in California, USA, and as a legislative assistant in the Iowa State Capitol. From 1990–1991 she conducted research on traditional and biomedical health care behaviour of pregnant women in rural Bali, and subsequently also worked as a Community Service Project Leader in Bali. She is presently an MPH candidate in the School of Public Health, UCLA.

Jocelyn Grace has an Honours Degree in Anthropology from the University of Western Australia, and is currently completing a PhD in Humanities at Murdoch University. Her doctoral research on women and health development in rural Indonesia focuses on the delivery and utilisation of primary health care services for women and infants in a village in East Lombok. Since completing fieldwork, Jocelyn has also worked as a short-term consultant on health-related development projects in Indonesia.

Valerie Hull is currently a Senior Associate with the Population Council in Indonesia, providing technical advice to government and non-government groups working on projects to improve the quality of reproductive health care. She is on leave from the Australian Aid Agency (AusAID), where she was Director of Health and Population. As a researcher, she has held positions at Gadjah Mada University in Indonesia and the Australian National University, carrying out studies and publishing on a wide range of reproductive health issues of relevance to national programs and policies.

Cynthia L. Hunter has a Master's Degree in Anthropology from the University of Western Australia, and is currently a PhD candidate in Anthropology and Sociology at the University of Newcastle, New South Wales, Australia. Her chapter is based on fieldwork conducted as part of doctoral research in Lombok 1991–1992. Her research interests include illness and healing in pluralistic medical contexts, maternal and child health, and national health services in rural Indonesian communities.

Megan Jennaway is a graduate of the University of Sydney and is currently a PhD candidate in medical anthropology at the Tropical Health Program, Australian Centre for International and Tropical Health and Nutrition, the University of Queensland. This chapter is based on fieldwork conducted as part of doctoral research in North Bali 1992–1993. Her research interests centre on gender, health, and institutional and ideological controls over women, particularly polygyny.

Sansnee Jirojwong is Senior Lecturer at the Faculty of Health Science, Central Queensland University, Australia. She received a bachelor's degree in nursing and midwifery in Thailand in 1978, and from 1978–1991 lectured at the Faculty of Nursing, Prince of Songkla University, Thailand. During this period she undertook an MPH program in the Philippines, and a second master's degree in Australia. In 1993–94 she accompanied her late husband, Michael Skolnik, to Brunei Darusalem and was an education officer at the College of Nursing. Her research is in the area of psychosocial factors influencing women's health and maternal and child health. She has a doctorate from Melbourne University.

Lenore Manderson is an anthropologist and social historian and is Professor of Tropical Health in the Australian Centre for International and Tropical Health and Nutrition, the University of Queensland. Her books include *Women, Politics and Change* (1980), *Australian Ways* (editor, 1985), *Shared Wealth and Symbol* (editor, 1986), *New Motherhood* (with Mira Crouch, 1993), and *Sickness and the State: Health and Illness in Colonial Malaya, 1870–1940* (1996). Her primary research interests and publications relate to infectious disease in resource-poor communities, and to gender, sexuality and women's health.

Makiko Nakayama is Associate Professor at Naruto (National) University of Education, Japan, teaching courses on women's studies and the family. She received a master's degree from Ochanomizu University in 1990 for a study on how Japanese women who bore their first child in the 1980s view their pregnancy. Her major works include: "Reproductive health and self-determination for Japanese women: technology, information, and choice" in *Proceedings of 1994 Tokyo Symposium on Women: Empowerment of Women* (1994) and "Sekushuariti to jyosei no karada [Sexuality and women's bodies]", in *Enpawamento No Jyosei-gaku [Empowerment of Women's Studies]* (1995).

Pranee Liamputtong Rice is Senior Lecturer at the School of Sociology and Anthropology and Research Fellow at the Centre for Study of Mothers' and Children's Health, La Trobe University, Melbourne, Australia. Pranee was born in a small Malay town in the south of Thailand, and has a master's degree from a Thai university and a doctoral degree from Monash University, Melbourne. Currently she is engaged in a study of pregnancy, childbirth, childrearing and reproductive health among Filipino, Turkish, Vietnamese, Cambodian, Lao, Hmong and Thai women. Pranee has written two books: *My Forty Days: A Cross-Cultural Resource Book for Health Care Professionals in Birthing Services* (1993) and *Asian Mothers, Australian Birth: Pregnancy, Childbirth and Childrearing — The Asian Experience in an English Speaking Country* (editor, 1994).

Angela Savage is an HIV/AIDS peer educator and is a graduate of the University of Melbourne, Australia. She worked as a research assistant at the Key Centre for Women's Health in Melbourne, studying non-English speaking background women's experiences of the Australian health care system, and evaluated HIV/AIDS training of trainers courses. In February 1992 she travelled Laos to collect data for an anthropology doctorate. Within a year however, she was a full-time AIDS prevention worker with the Australian Red Cross; the results of her research have provided the basis for the HIV/AIDS prevention program of the Lao Red Cross. She began work as coordinator of a Red Cross HIV/AIDS Network for the Greater Mekong sub-region in January 1995. She is based in Hanoi with her partner, a journalist.

Patricia V. Symonds was born in Liverpool, England, in 1932, and moved to the United States to study at Brown University, Providence, Rhode Island. Her master's degree was on adolescent pregnancy among the Hmong (entitled *A Flower Full of Honey Ready for the Bee*, 1984). She has since conducted field research in north Thailand regarding HIV/AIDS knowledge, and consequently implemented a grass-roots project for HIV/AIDS education and prevention (1994–95). She teaches at Brown University.

Kimberley Townsend completed her BAH in Philosophy and Psychology in 1989 at Queen's University in Canada. She worked with Cambodian refugees at Site 2 Camp on the Thailand Cambodian border from 1992 to 1993. Her position as Mental

Health Coordinator enabled her to observe different health care practices. She is presently studying in Canada to become a naturopathic physician.

Andrea Whittaker has a PhD in Tropical Health from the University of Queensland, Australia, specialising in medical anthropology. For this she conducted eighteen months ethnographic fieldwork in a rural village, studying women's reproductive health issues and primary health care services. The chapter in this volume is based on part of her thesis. She is currently a researcher in the Discipline of General Practice and the Department of Anthropology and Sociology, University of Newcastle, Australia.

Ninuk Widyantoro is a consulting psychologist with a major interest in women's reproductive health issues. She is founder and consulting psychologist of FENOM-ENA, a psychological consulting bureau in Indonesia. She has been working for many years in clinics and villages, in both urban and rural settings, in Indonesia. Ms Widyantoro has written a number of articles on abortion, contraceptive choice and women's reproductive rights.

Index

305